AIDS Epidemiology: A Quantitative Approach

Monographs in Epidemiology and Biostatistics
edited by Jennifer L. Kelsey, Michael G. Marmot, Paul D. Stolley, Martin P. Vessey

AIDS Epidemiology:
A Quantitative Approach

Ron Brookmeyer
Department of Biostatistics
School of Hygiene and Public Health
Johns Hopkins University

Mitchell H. Gail
Epidemiology and Biostatistics Program
National Cancer Institute

New York   Oxford
OXFORD UNIVERSITY PRESS
1994

Oxford University Press

Oxford   New York   Toronto
Delhi   Bombay   Calcutta   Madras   Karachi
Kuala Lumpur   Singapore   Hong Kong   Tokyo
Nairobi   Dar es Salam   Cape Town
Melbourne   Auckland   Madrid
and associated companies in
Berlin   Ibadan

Library of Congress Cataloging-in-Publication Data
Brookmeyer, Ron.
AIDS epidemiology : a quantitative approach / Ron Brookmeyer
and Mitchell H. Gail.
p. cm.   Includes bibliographical references and index.
ISBN 0-19-507641-9
1. AIDS (Disease) — Epidemiology.   2. Biometry.
3. Epidemiology—Statistical methods.   I. Gail, Mitchell H.   II. Title.
[DNLM: 1. Acquired Immunodeficiency Syndrome—epidemiology.
2. Epidemiologic Methods.   WD 308 B872a 1993]
RA644.A25B75   1994
614.5′993—dc20
DNLM/DLC
for Library of Congress   92-48337

9 8 7 6 5 4 3 2 1

Printed in the United States of America
on acid-free paper

To Robin and Claire (R. B.)

To my wonderful parents (M. G.)

Preface

The purpose of this book is to review the contribution of statistical science to our understanding of the acquired immunodeficiency syndrome (AIDS) and to summarize and interpret the major epidemiological findings. Statistical ideas and approaches have contributed to an understanding of factors that promote transmission of the human immunodeficiency virus (HIV) and of strategies for preventing transmission, to an accurate description of the natural history of disease associated with HIV infection, including the "incubation" distribution of the time from infection to the onset of AIDS, to the design and analysis of therapeutic clinical trials and impending vaccine trials, and to an assessment of the scope and likely course of the HIV epidemic and of the incidence of AIDS. In some cases, non-standard statistical ideas are absolutely crucial to avoid misleading interpretations of data, because standard methods of analysis for chronic disease are not always suitable for studying a rapidly growing epidemic and because non-standard "samples of opportunity" can lead to severely biased results unless the mode of sampling is taken into account.

Two examples illustrate these phenomena. If we plot the crude numbers of incident AIDS cases reported to the Centers for Disease Control (CDC) against calendar time, the most recent counts will be misleadingly small because delays in reporting will reduce recent counts. To avoid misleading interpretations of AIDS incidence data, we must adjust for reporting delays. As a second example, the earliest estimates of the incubation distribution of AIDS were obtained by studying the incubation times of persons who developed AIDS as the result of a contaminated blood transfusion. Because the available cases in such a sample necessarily had relatively short incubation times, a naive analysis of such data would tend to seriously underestimate the usual time it takes to develop AIDS.

In other contexts, statistical thinking has helped define problems and assess the extent and sources of uncertainty associated with given conclusions. For example, the quality and type of information available from a cohort of individuals whose dates of infection are unknown ("prevalent" cohorts) differ from that of a cohort whose dates of seroconversion are known ("incident" cohorts). As another example, estimates of the numbers of persons infected with HIV-1 in the United States are obtained either from seroprevalence surveys in selected populations or by "back-calculation" using AIDS incidence data and information on the incubation distribution. Each of these methods is subject to large random and systematic sources of error, yet the two approaches are based on complementary types of information. In making estimates of the numbers infected, it is essential to consider a variety of sources of information and to report realistic assessments of uncertainty.

It is our hope that this book will introduce epidemiologists to statistical ideas that are helpful in analyzing and interpreting epidemiologic and clinical data on AIDS. Likewise we hope to introduce statisticians to some of the unusual features of epidemiologic and clinical information on AIDS so that they may appreciate the need for specialized statistical methods in this area. Finally, we hope some readers will be interested in the story of data interpretation and discovery in a rapidly evolving scientific context.

Topics Covered

We review the discovery of risk factors and the associated methodologic difficulties of interpreting cohort and case-control data in a rapidly evolving epidemic (Chapter 2). The statistical features of special studies on the uninfected sexual partners of infected persons (partner studies) are also reviewed and discussed (Chapter 2). Chapter 3 describes the results of surveys to estimate trends in HIV seroincidence and seroprevalence. We also discuss the difficulties of interpreting data from non-representative samples and of assessing the extent to which general surveys are biased because persons at high risk of HIV infection refuse to participate. We describe the special statistical approaches used to estimate the incubation distribution and review available results in Chapter 4. Age at infection is the only well documented factor that influences the incubation distribution, but many markers, especially CD4 + T lymphocyte levels, have been used to monitor the progression of HIV illness following infection. Chapter 5 describes statistical issues that arise in interpreting information on cofactors that might influence the incubation distribution and on markers. We discuss the reliability of assays to detect HIV infection and the effectiveness of screening for HIV to protect the blood supply in Chapter 6. Chapter 7 outlines surveillance methods used to monitor AIDS incidence, including methods for delay correction and extrapolation procedures. Back-calculation procedures for estimating the infection curve from AIDS incidence data and for projecting AIDS incidence are presented in Chapter 8. Transmission models are developed to help understand factors that influence the infection curve and to help define and evaluate possible prevention strategies (Chapter 9). Chapter 10 stresses the need to integrate a variety of sources of information in order to understand epidemic trends and applies those ideas to studying trends in underdeveloped countries, to forecasting in small geographic areas, and to projecting pediatric AIDS. Statistical issues in vaccine development and experimental therapeutics are described in Chapter 11.

Readers particularly interested in the natural history of HIV infection in individuals may wish to concentrate on Chapters 1, 2, 4, 5, 6 and 11. Those interested in monitoring and forecasting the epidemic in populations may wish to emphasize Chapters 1, 3, 6, 7, 8, 9 and 10.

Although this book is self-contained, there are a number of excellent general sources for background information. *AIDS: Etiology, Diagnosis, Treatment and Prevention* (edited by DeVita, Hellman and Rosenberg, 1988) and *AIDS Pathogenesis and Treatment* (edited by Levy) provide a comprehensive introduction to biological and medical issues, and *The Epidemiology of AIDS* (edited by Kaslow and Francis, 1989) describes the epidemiology of specific risk groups. The three books, *Confronting AIDS: Directions for Public Health, Health Care and Research* (Institute of Medicine, 1986), *Confronting AIDS: Update 1988* (Institute of Medicine, 1988) and *The Second Decade* (edited by Miller, Turner and Moses, 1990) document progress in scientific understanding and an evolution of thinking on social, legal and ethical problems associated with the AIDS epidemic. Jewell (1990) reviews statistical issues and innovative statistical methods used to cope with AIDS data. The February, 1988 issue of *Science* includes papers on AIDS epidemiology in the United States (Curran, Jaffe, Hardy, et al., 1988), international perspectives (Piot, Plummer, Mhalu, et al., 1988), economic impact (Bloom and Carliner, 1988), prevention (Fineberg, 1988) and other aspects.

Baltimore, Md.   *R. B.*
Rockville, Md.   *M. G.*
January 1993

Acknowledgments

Our work in AIDS epidemiology benefited from the help and ideas of many people. We would especially like to thank our close research collaborators including Drs. Philip Rosenberg, James Goedert, Robert Bigger, and Jiangang Liao. We were stimulated and assisted by discussions with many colleagues including Peter Bacchetti, Raoul Benveniste, William Blattner, Samuel Broder, John Brundage, David Byar, James Curran, Ann Damiano, Klaus Dietz, Tim Dondero, Susan Ellenberg, Robin Fox, Lytt Gardner, Tim Green, Herbert Hethcote, Nicholas Jewell, John Karon, C. C. Law, Ira Longini, James Massey, Mads Melbye, Meade Morgan, Steven Piantadosi, Dale Preston, Thomas Quinn, Michael Simberkoff, Patty Solomon, Wei-Yann Tsai, Sten Vermund, Sue Wilson, and Scott Zeger.

We wish to thank a number of colleagues for helpful comments on various chapters including Klaus Dietz, Dennis Dixon, Roger Dodd, Tim Dondero, Susan Ellenberg, Trena Ezzati, Ralph Folsom, Genoveffa Franchini, Joseph Gastwirth, James Goedert, Herbert Hethcote, Dan Horvitz, Nicholas Jewell, Peter Nara, Wasima Rida, Philip Rosenberg, and Wei-Yann Tsai. We are grateful to all those who gave permission to reprint their published illustrations and graphs, and to Greg Wilson for producing a number of graphs and illustrations. Ron Brookmeyer is grateful to the Department of Mathematical Sciences at Johns Hopkins University for providing office space during the early stages of the preparation of this book.

A very special thank you goes to Patty Hubbard for her excellent and unflagging assistance in preparing and editing the manuscript.

Finally, we thank our wives, Robin Fox and Dorothy Berlin Gail, who encouraged us to begin and to continue.

Contents

5. COFACTORS AND MARKERS, 113

6. SCREENING AND ACCURACY OF TESTS FOR HIV, 147

7. STATISTICAL ISSUES IN SURVEILLANCE OF AIDS INCIDENCE, 170

8. BACK-CALCULATION, 189

AIDS Epidemiology: A Quantitative Approach

1

Introduction

1.1 BRIEF HISTORY

In 1981, five homosexual men were reported to have developed a rare illness, *Pneumocystis carinii* pneumonia (PCP) (Centers for Disease Control (CDC), 1981a). Within a few months, 26 cases of a rare tumor, Kaposi's sarcoma, had been identified among homosexual men (CDC, 1981b), and public health officials soon had evidence that both of these rare diseases were related to an underlying deficiency in the immune system (Gottlieb, Schroff, Schanker, et al., 1981; DeWys, Curran, Henle, and Johnson, 1982), reflected in a reduced number of helper T lymphocytes (CD4+ T lymphocytes). In 1982, the new and frightening "acquired immune deficiency syndrome" (AIDS) was defined as "a disease at least moderately predictive of a defect in cell-mediated immunity occurring in a person with no known cause for diminished resistance to that disease. Such diseases include Kaposi's sarcoma, *Pneumocystis carinii* pneumonia and serious opportunistic infections" (CDC, 1982a). A specific list of AIDS defining conditions was elaborated, and some new AIDS defining conditions were added later in response to additional epidemologic evidence and changes in diagnostic practice resulting from the availability of serologic tests for the AIDS virus.

Remarkable medical progress was made in the decade following the identification of this disease. The World Health Organization began surveillance activities on a global scale. In the United States the CDC established a surveillance system to keep track of AIDS incidence within risk groups defined by mode of exposure. This system described the spread of the epidemic and suggested approaches to prevention. Special epidemiologic studies identified the major modes of transmission, which are sexual contacts among homosexual and bisexual

3

men and in heterosexual populations, introduction of the virus into the blood through contaminated needles or transfusion of contaminated blood or blood products, and perinatal transmission. Such studies suggested an infectious etiology. Major breakthroughs occurred (Barré-Sinoussi, Chermann, Rey, et al., 1983; Popovic, Sarngadharan, Reed and Gallo, 1984) when a virus, now called the human immunodeficiency virus (HIV-1), was isolated from the lymph nodes of patients with AIDS. Isolation of the virus and procedures for growing the virus in a laboratory environment (Popovic, Sarnagadharan, Reed and Gallo, 1984) made it possible to develop serologic tests to detect the virus. These assays, in turn, led to epidemiologic studies that provided strong evidence that HIV-1 was the causative agent of AIDS, that further defined the risks associated with specific modes of behaviors, and that further delineated the extent and growth of HIV-1 infection in the population (Gallo, Salahuddin, Popovic, et al., 1984; Sarngadharan, Popovic, Bruch, et al. 1984). Moreover, serologic assays made it feasible to screen blood donors for infection and so to prevent further spread of disease, and serologic surveys suggested additional approaches to disease prevention. Isolation of HIV-1 also led to detailed biochemical studies of the virus, its components, its life cycle, and the resultant human pathophysiology.

Clinical studies on individual patients characterized the natural history of HIV-1 infection, including a wide array of AIDS-defining and other conditions, and provided information on the distribution of times from infection with HIV-1 to development of an AIDS-defining condition (the AIDS "incubation distribution"). Incubation times turned out to be long and variable, with a median of about 10 years. It was therefore appreciated that the numbers of AIDS cases developing in the first decade of the epidemic represented only a fraction of all those already infected and that trends in AIDS incidence could not be relied upon to measure recent trends in the underlying rates of new infections (the "infection curve").

Information on the viral life cycle and natural history of illness led to rational approaches to combat the virus (Broder, 1988), including the development of zidovudine (AZT). Progress has also been made in delaying and treating the many sequelae of immune deficiency, especially opportunistic infections.

Despite this progress, the AIDS epidemic poses an enormous threat to public health. It has been estimated that more than 5 million people are infected with human immunodeficiency virus worldwide (Chin, Sato, and Mann, 1990). In the United States, 206,392 cases of AIDS and 133,233 AIDS-related deaths were reported to the CDC through December 31, 1991 (CDC, 1992a). Quarterly AIDS incidence in the United States is greatest among homosexual or bisexual men and intravenous drug users, but as the epidemic has progressed, the proportion of incident AIDS cases in other exposure groups, such as people exposed through heterosexual sex, has increased (Figure 1.1).

1.2 HIV VIRUS AND ITS CLINICAL EFFECTS

Until 1970, it was assumed that genetic information was always transcribed from DNA into RNA, but in 1970 it was discovered that certain viruses, called "retroviruses," used RNA to carry their genetic information, and, moreover, employed the enzyme "reverse transcriptase" to transcribe the RNA into DNA in the cells of the infected host (Temin and Mitzutani, 1970; Baltimore, 1970). HIV-1 turns out to be such a retrovirus. After attaching to the host cell wall, HIV-1 releases its RNA together with reverse transcriptase into the cytoplasm of the infected host cell (Figure 1.2). Reverse transcription of the RNA code yields viral DNA, which resides in the cytoplasm in episomal (circular) form or enters the cell nucleus and becomes integrated into host DNA. Integrated viral DNA genes may remain latent, or, in

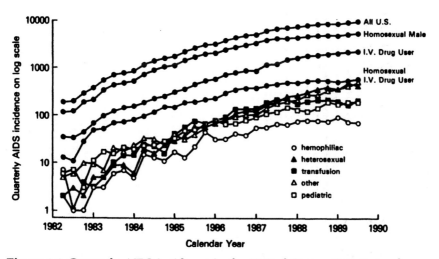

Figure 1.1 Quarterly AIDS incidence in the United States. Counts are shown on a semi-logarithmic scale for eight risk groups and for all cases combined. The incidence data are corrected for reporting delays and are based on information received at the Centers for Disease Control through March 31, 1990. (Source: Gail and Brookmeyer, 1990b.)

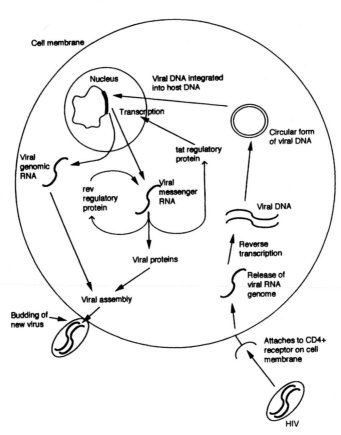

Figure 1.2 Life cycle of HIV-1. (Source: Adapted from figure 2-3 in Shaw, Wong-Staal, and Gallo, 1988 and from figure 3 in Fauci, 1988.)

response to viral and host regulatory proteins, these genes may become activated. When the viral DNA genes are activated, messenger RNA is transcribed. Some of the earliest proteins to be translated from messenger RNA are the regulatory proteins *tat* and *rev*. *Tat* protein promotes the transcription of more messenger RNA. *Rev* protein causes multiple spliced segments of messenger RNA to form singly spliced segments that can be translated into structural proteins, envelope proteins, and reverse transcriptase. These proteins, together with viral genomic RNA transcribed from the integrated viral DNA, are assembled to form new HIV-1 viruses, which leave the infected cell and are available to attack new cells. These phenomena are described in greater detail by Shaw, Wong-Stall and Gallo (1988), Haseltine (1991), and Greene (1991).

Infected humans produce antibody to a variety of antigenic viral

substantial normal variability among individuals and in serial measurements from a single individual. An excellent introduction to the principles of normal and abnormal immune function is found in the textbook on internal medicine edited by J. H. Stein (1990).

The clinical response to infection is complex and progressive (Figure 1.4). Within a few days or weeks of infection, the patient often develops an acute mononucleosis-like syndrome with fever, malaise and lymphadenopathy. Symptoms abate, but an insidious and progressive attack on the immune system begins as HIV-1 bonds to cells with CD4 receptors, for which gp120 has high affinity. In particular, HIV-1 attacks CD4+ T cells, whose name derives from the fact that they contain CD4 receptors. Through incompletely defined mechanisms, HIV-1 kills CD4+ T lymphocytes and progressively destroys the immunocompetence of the host. The CD4+ T lymphocyte levels drop rapidly in the first months following infection to about 800 cells/μl. Thereafter, the decline proceeds at a slower rate of perhaps 80 cells/μl/year.

Within a week or two of infection, p24 antigen appears in the blood, followed in about 6 to 10 weeks by the appearance of host antibodies to envelope proteins and p24 (Figure 1.4). As p24 antibodies appear, p24 antigen disappears. After a period of years, when the CD4+ T lymphocytes have been seriously depleted to roughly 400 cells/mm^3, p24 antibody levels tend to decline, and p24 antigen tends to reappear,

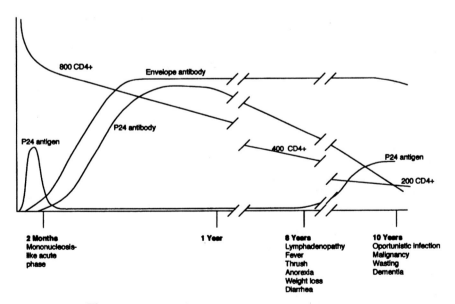

Figure 1.4 Typical clinical course of HIV infection.

often in anticipation of advancing clinical illness. The CDC (1986) has categorized symptoms and signs associated with HIV disease. The term *AIDS-related complex* (ARC) is often used to describe signs and symptoms of HIV infection that do not meet the surveillance definition of AIDS. One definition of ARC is the presence of two or more of the following conditions (but no AIDS-defining condition) in a patient with laboratory evidence of HIV infection: lymphadenopathy, persistent fevers, persistent diarrhea, involuntary weight loss, oral hairy leukoplakia, multidermatomal herpes zoster, oral candidiasis, recurrent Salmonella bacteremia, nocardiasis and tuberculosis. Finally, as CD4 + T lymphocyte levels continue to fall, an AIDS-defining condition appears, such as an opportunistic infection, a malignancy (Kaposi's sarcoma or non-Hodgkin's lymphoma), wasting syndrome, or dementia.

The various risk groups defining mode of exposure to HIV have different distributions of initial AIDS-defining criteria in the United States (Table 1.1). In particular, Kaposi's sarcoma is found mainly among homosexual men (gay men), although this condition has become proportionately less frequent even among gay men than earlier in the epidemic (Lifson, Darrow, Hessol, et al., 1990). Intravenous drug users (IVDUs) tend to have wasting syndrome or dementia as initial AIDS defining conditions more often than gay men. *Pneumocystis carinii* pneumonia (PCP) is common in all risk groups and accounts for about half of all initial AIDs-defining conditions. In Africa, diarrhea and weight loss are common presenting conditions.

The incubation distribution $F(t)$ is the probability that an infected individual develops clinical AIDS within t years of infection. Clearly, $F(t)$ depends on the definition of clinical AIDS, which has been broadened as the epidemic progressed, and on the use of treatments that can delay the onset of opportunistic infections or the progression of HIV infection. We usually think of $F(t)$ as describing the "natural history" of incubation periods, before the surveillance definition of AIDS was broadened in the United States to include wasting syndrome and dementia, and before effective treatments were introduced in 1987. However, models of the incubation distribution that allow for changes in the definition of AIDS and for treatments are discussed in Chapter 8, where these adaptations are needed to obtain projections by "back-calculation" beyond 1987. To estimate $F(t)$ empirically, one usually takes the date of seroconversion as the date of infection, even though seroconversion may follow infection by many months in rare instances. The hazard of developing AIDS within 2 years of infection is very small

Table 1.1 Percentages of Various Initial AIDS-Defining Conditions for Each Risk Group

Risk Group	PCP	Other OIs	Kaposi Sarcoma	Lymphoma	Wasting Syndrome	Dementia	Other
Gay men	51.5	27.3	9.7	2.6	6.0	2.6	0.4
IVDUs	49.6	31.9	1.2	1.3	11.9	3.9	0.2
Gay IVDUs	45.0	31.4	7.5	1.9	9.6	4.2	0.3
Hemophiliacs	45.6	32.8	0.0	0.6	16.1	5.0	0.0
Heterosexuals	50.2	33.4	1.2	2.2	10.1	2.6	0.3
Born in Pattern II countries	39.5	50.0	3.0	0.4	5.3	1.3	0.4
Blood transfusion recipients	46.4	32.7	0.9	3.3	12.4	4.0	0.4
Undetermined	53.3	32.6	3.7	1.3	5.4	3.1	0.7
All risk groups	50.4	29.6	6.5	2.1	8.0	3.0	0.4

Note: Based on cases reported to the CDC in the first half of 1990. The conditions are ordered hierarchically from left to right. For example, a person with PCP and lymphoma is categorized as PCP.

but increases thereafter. By 10 years, approximately half those infected will have developed AIDS.

Infection with HIV-1 is insidious because during the long period of incubation the infected host may be unaware of the infection and can transmit the virus. Infection with HIV-1 is frightening because the illness tends to be progressive and to cause serious illness in a large proportion of those infected. By 5 years nearly all patients have abnormally low CD4 + T lymphocyte levels (Longini, 1990), and by 10 years, about half of those infected have developed AIDS. The median survival following the diagnosis of AIDS depends on the initial AIDS-defining condition but is still only about 2 years, despite progress in treating this illness.

Recently, another AIDS-causing virus, HIV-2, has been identified in West Africa (DeCook and Brun-Vézinet, 1989). Because HIV-2 is not always detected by antibody assays defined for HIV-1, screening procedures are being modified in the United States to detect both viruses. We shall sometimes refer to HIV-1 as HIV.

1.3 MEASURING THE EPIDEMIC

If it were readily estimated, the most useful measure to track the course of the infection in particular risk groups would be the *infection rate curve* $g(s)$, which we sometimes will refer to as the "infection rate" or the "infection curve." The quantity $g(s)$ represents the number of new HIV infections per unit time at calendar time s. Bacchetti (1990) has estimated the infection rate curve (Figure 1.5) for gay men in San Francisco from survey data on seroconversion times. This estimate of $g(s)$ reaches a peak of about 490 infections per month in the last half of 1981. The squares in Figure 1.5 represent monthly AIDS incidence counts, which lag well behind the peak of the infection curve. We define *AIDS incidence* to be the number of AIDS cases that develop in a defined population per unit time. The infection curve in Figure 1.5 indicates that rates of infection were much lower in the last half of the 1980s than when the epidemic was at its peak, but even in 1988, the rate of infection among gay men in San Francisco was about 300 per year.

The HIV infection curve is closely related to the *HIV incidence rate*, which is the ratio of the infection curve at calendar time s to the number of uninfected people in the population at that time. If a population is large and stable and if the HIV infection rate is comparatively small, then the HIV incidence rate is approximately

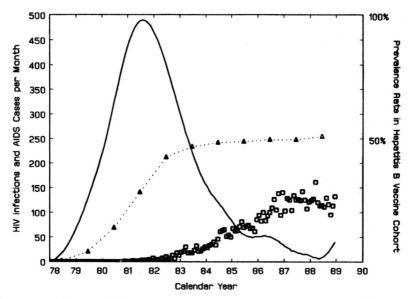

Figure 1.5 The monthly infection rate (solid line) and monthly AIDS incidence (squares) in San Francisco, as estimated by Bacchetti (1990). The plot of HIV prevalence rate (percent) for homosexual and bisexual men participating in hepatitis B vaccine trials in San Francisco (triangles) is derived from data in Hessol, Lifson, O'Malley, et al. (1989).

proportional to the infection curve. The HIV incidence rate measures the instantaneous risk of infection for an uninfected individual, whereas the HIV infection rate measures the instantaneous rate of infection in the population.

The HIV infection curve and HIV incidence rate give the most immediate and direct measures of trends in the epidemic and ultimately determine HIV prevalence and AIDS incidence. Information on HIV incidence would therefore be of immense benefit for planning and monitoring prevention activities. Unfortunately, it is very difficult to measure HIV infection rates directly except in selected cohorts which may not be representative. One can hope to learn something about the HIV infection curve and HIV incidence rate indirectly by studying trends in the prevalence of HIV infection, trends in AIDS incidence, and transmission models that predict the infection curve from theoretical assumptions about infectivity, rates of risky behavior, and mixing patterns among subpopulations.

The *cumulative number infected* to time t is

$$G(t) = \int_{-\infty}^{t} g(s)\,ds. \tag{1.1}$$

For example, the cumulative number infected in San Francisco through 1988 is estimated from Figure 1.5 as $G(1989.0) = 22{,}030$.

The *prevalence*, $c(t)$, is the number of people alive and infected with HIV at calendar time t. In a closed population (no immigration or emigration), the prevalence is the cumulative number infected less the number of infected people who died through calendar time t. For example, assuming there were 3262 deaths among HIV-infected people in San Francisco through 1988 (Lemp, Payne, Rutherford, et al., 1990), the prevalence at the beginning of 1989 would be $22{,}030 - 3262 = 18{,}768$.

If one further assumes that the probability of surviving u time units beyond the date of infection, $\mathcal{J}(u)$, is independent of calendar time of infection, then the prevalence is given by

$$c(t) = \int_{-\infty}^{t} g(s)\mathcal{J}(t - s)\,ds. \tag{1.2}$$

At the beginning of the epidemic, most infected people will survive to t, so that the prevalence will nearly equal the cumulative number infected, as follows from equation (1.2). Over longer periods of time, improvements in the treatment of HIV infection may alter $\mathcal{J}$, as may secular changes in the age distribution of those infected. Moreover, the prevalence will be altered by patterns of immigration and emigration unless each emigrant is matched by a corresponding immigrant. These factors are not accounted for in equation (1.2).

It is useful to distinguish patients with AIDS and AIDS-free patients with advanced immunodeficiency from other people with prevalent HIV infection in order to estimate the resources needed for health care.

We define the *prevalence rate* as $c(t)/N(t)$, where $N(t)$ is the number alive in the population at time t in a general population. It may be difficult to estimate $N(t)$. For example, it is difficult to obtain reliable data from a representative sample to determine the number of men who engage in male-to-male sex in the United States, or even in a city such as San Francisco, where surveys have been conducted within high risk census tracts (Winklestein, Lyman, Padian, et al., 1987). However, it is relatively easy to compute the prevalence rate in a well defined cohort that is followed longitudinally. Seroprevalence rates in a cohort of gay men in San Francisco (Hessol, Lifson, O'Malley, et al., 1989) who were being studied to evelute whether vaccination could prevent Hepatitis B, increased rapidly in 1980, 1981 and 1982 (Figure 1.5), as one would expect if the infection rate curve estimated by Bacchetti (1990) were correct. In fact, that infection curve was estimated, in large measure, from seroconversion data in the Hepatitis B cohort.

In some settings, seroprevalence surveys provide the most reliable means for tracking the epidemic. For example, samples of blood from all newborns in a given state of the United States provide a direct measure of the HIV burden on newborns and childbearing women. In developing countries, where effective systems for monitoring AIDS incidence are not in place, seroprevalence surveys provide the most useful information for gauging the extent of HIV infection.

In the United States, AIDS incidence data have proved extremely useful for monitoring the AIDS epidemic. Quarterly AIDS incidence in the United States, corrected for reporting delays, are shown for all AIDS cases and for each of the major risk groups (Figure 1.1). Because the logarithm of AIDS incidence is plotted, straight lines would indicate exponential growth of the epidemic. In fact, these loci exhibit curvature indicative of subexponential growth, almost from the very beginning of the epidemic. For example, the slope of the locus for all AIDS cases was about 1.0/yr for 1982, corresponding to a doubling time of $\log(2)/1.0 = .69$ years, whereas the doubling time increased to about 1.0 years in 1984. Transmission models provide several explanations for such subexponential growth, including diffusion of the epidemic from groups with high rates of risky behavior to groups with lower rates of risky behavior. Note that the preponderance of cases occurred among homosexual men and intravenous drug users (IVDUs). By December 31, 1991, the percentages in various risk groups of the 206,392 AIDS cases reported to CDC were: homosexual men (57.3%), IVDU's (22.2%), homosexual men who use intravenous drugs (6.4%), patients with hemophillia (0.8%), persons infected by heterosexual contact (5.8%), recipients of blood transfusions (2.1%), pediatric AIDS cases (1.7%) and patients infected by other or undetermined risk factors (3.7%). Further details on AIDS surveillance and precise definitions of those risk groups are published regularly in *HIV/AIDS Surveillance* (see, e.g., CDC, 1992).

Because incubation times are long and variable, the AIDS incidence curve is smoothed and distant reflection of the infection curve, as illustrated in Figure 1.5. In a closed population with negligible mortality from causes unrelated to HIV, the *AIDS incidence*, $a(t)$, is related to the infection rate curve, $g(s)$, and the incubation density, $f(u)$, by

$$a(t) = \int_{-\infty}^{t} g(s)f(t-s)ds. \qquad (1.3)$$

For some risk groups, such as recipients of blood transfusions, mortality may be appreciable before AIDS onset, in which case equation (1.3) is not accurate. In principle, provided f is known, one should be able to learn something about the infection curve by finding that estimate of $g(s)$ that best fits the observed AIDS incidence series, $a(t)$, in equation (1.3). This deconvolution process is called "back-calculation." It turns out that back-calculation yields useful information on the infection curve up to perhaps five years before the end of the AIDS incidence series but that back-calculated estimates of the infection curve closer to the end of the AIDS incidence series are very uncertain. We have implicitly assumed that the incubation distribution is constant in calendar time in equation (1.3). Provision must be made for secular trends in the incubation distribution that arose from changes in the definition of AIDS and from the use of treatments capable of retarding the onset of AIDS, particularly after 1987. Back-calculated extimates of the infection curve have been used to estimate seroprevalence from relationships like equation (1.3) and to project AIDS incidence. Indeed, back-calculation yields comparatively reliable projections of AIDS incidence, unless sudden changes in the surveillance system or new methods of treatment supervene.

The number of persons living with AIDS (AIDS prevalence) and the corresponding *AIDS prevalence rate*, which is obtained by dividing by the population size, are important indicators of the need for health services. Projections of AIDS prevalence can be obtained from projections of AIDS incidence by taking the survival distribution after AIDS diagnosis into account. If $S_A(u; s)$ is the probability that a person diagnosed with AIDS in calendar year s survives beyond year u, then the number of persons living with AIDS in a closed cohort at calendar time t is

$$\int_{-\infty}^{t} a(s)S_A(t - s; s)ds.$$

1.4 WORLDWIDE SCOPE OF THE EPIDEMIC

The World Health Organization (WHO) has developed a program of world-wide AIDS surveillance. As of January 1, 1991, 314,611 AIDS cases have been reported to WHO from 179 countries and territories (WHO, 1991). Table 1.2 gives the distribution of reported AIDS cases by continent. Countries that have reported 1000 or more cases are also listed. Although the largest number of reported cases comes from the United States, the fraction of cumulative cases from the United States has fallen from 56% in 1989 to 49% in 1990. As of January 1, 1992, the numbers of reported AIDS cases had increased to 129,066 in Africa;

2

Risk Factors for Infection and the Probability of HIV Transmission

2.1 INTRODUCTION

In this chapter, we describe several types of observational studies that were used to define behaviors and other factors associated with increased risk of HIV infection and AIDS. Careful interview of individual patients with AIDS identified the major modes of transmission. Case-control studies comparing patients with AIDS to subjects without AIDS further delineated behaviors and other factors associated with increased risk of AIDS. When assays for antibody to HIV became available in 1984, investigators classified populations into seropositive people with prevalent HIV infections and seronegative people. The prevalent seropositives were compared to seronegatives to define risk factors for infection in prevalent case-control studies. A fourth type of study to define risk factors for infection was derived from longitudinal follow-up of cohorts of initially seronegative individuals. Such studies could identify factors associated with increased risk of incident seroconversion. In addition, cohort studies provided estimates of the probability of seroconversion in a specified time interval (Section 3.5.1). In Sections 2.2 and 2.3 we discuss the strengths and weaknesses of these designs and some of the findings from such studies.

Studies of the types just mentioned were applied to determining factors affecting risk of infection among homosexual or bisexual men, intravenous drug users (IVDUs), patients with hemophilia, and heterosexuals. In these case-control and cohort studies, there is usually little information on the precise time or times when exposure to HIV occurred. For example, an individual may have no idea whether or not a given sexual partner is infected. However, in other types of studies, the date or dates of exposure to HIV are more precisely defined. For example, a hospital worker will often know the precise date on which he or she may have been inadvertently stuck by a contaminated needle, and recipients of blood transfusions that are later found to have been contaminated can be studied to determine what proportion of the recipients became seropositive. Such studies can be described as cohort studies with point exposures. We review data from such studies for blood transfusion recipients, hospital and laboratory workers and children born to seropositive mothers in Section 2.4.

Another type of study that provides information on the extent of exposure to an individual who is known to be infected is called a partner study. Partner studies involve subjects who have engaged in monogamous sex with an infected partner and who have no other identified risk behaviors. Ideally, the date of seroconversion of the infected partner is known, as is the frequency and type of sexual contacts between the subject and the infected partner. Such data can be used to study behaviors associated with transmission and to estimate the probability of transmission per partnership and the probability of transmission per sexual encounter. Partner studies are discussed in Section 2.5.

2.2 STUDIES OF AIDS PATIENTS

An enormous amount of epidemiologic information was obtained by carefully interviewing and studying individual patients with AIDS. Such studies of a few patients with *Pneumocystis carinii* pneumonia and Kaposi's sarcoma (CDC, 1981a; CDC, 1981b; Gottlieb, Schroff, Schanker, et al., 1981; DeWys, Curran, Henle, and Johnson, 1982) identified the essential immune deficiency, indicated that homosexual men were at high risk, and suggested that a transmissible agent such as cytomegalovirus might be responsible. Masur, Michelis, Greene, et al. (1981) found a deficit in cell-mediated immunity in 11 males with *Pneumocystis carinii* pneumonia and noted that 5 of these patients were intravenous drug users. Thus, within a few months of the first reports (CDC, 1981a) studies of individual AIDS patients provided information used to define the "acquired immune deficiency syndrome" (CDC, 1982a) and identified the two largest exposure groups in the United States, gay men and IVDUs.

Studies of individual patients quickly expanded the list of known risk groups. AIDS was found among Haitians who denied exposures to intravenous drugs and male-to-male sex (CDC, 1982b), in an infant who received multiple blood transfusions (CDC, 1982c), and among patients with hemophilia (CDC, 1982d). By September 1982, the Centers for Disease Control was reporting (CDC, 1982a) the proportions of AIDS cases that fell into the following risk groups: gay men (75%), IVDUs without a history of male-to-male sex (13%), Haitians (6%), persons with hemophilia A (0.3%) and others (5%). These categories are hierarchical because to be classified in a later category a patient must not fall into any of the preceeding categories.

Early reports of heterosexual transmission to the female sexual partners of men with AIDS in the United States (CDC, 1983) were confirmed by reports of AIDS among black African males and females with no history of drug abuse or homosexual sex (Clumeck, Mascart-Lemone, De Maubeuge, et al., 1983; Clumeck, Sonnet, Taelman, et al., 1984) and by similar reports of heterosexual transmission to females and to males in the United States (Redfield, Markham, Salahuddin, et al., 1985). Likewise, immunodeficiency was reported among infants whose mothers were at high risk of AIDS or had already developed immune deficiency (CDC, 1982e; Oleske, Minnefor, Cooper, et al., 1983; Rubinstein, Sicklick, Gupta, et al., 1983).

By January 1984, the Centers for Disease Control was reporting AIDS cases in the risk categories shown in Table 1.1 (CDC, 1984), except that gay intravenous drug users were not broken out as a separate category. Pediatric AIDS was and continues to be reported separately.

The epidemiologic evidence that AIDS could be transmitted by sexual contact, through blood or blood products, and perinatally strongly implicated a transmissible agent. Additional support for this concept came from studies designed to determine whether individuals with AIDS had had sexual contact with other patients with AIDS. Seventeen cases of AIDS were reported in Los Angeles County, California, and 2 in Orange County, California, between June 1, 1981, and April 12, 1982 (CDC, 1982f). All 8 of the survivors were interviewed to determine their sexual partners in the preceding 5 years, and histories of sexual contacts were obtained from friends of 7 of the 11 AIDS patients who had died. Nine of the 15 AIDS patients for whom interview data were available were found to have had sex with other AIDS patients within the previous 5 years, including 7 from Los Angeles County who had had sex with other AIDS patients in Los Angeles County and 2 from Orange County who had had sex with the same non-Californian ("patient 0" in Auerbach, Darrow, Jaffe and

Curran, 1984). This non-Californian was also linked to several patients with AIDS in New York.

Such extensive clustering seems unlikely to have occurred by chance and is suggestive that a sexually transmitted infectious agent can cause AIDS (CDC, 1982f). However, it is not easy to determine how unusual a cluster is because it is not clear just how to define the clustering event. Is it that the two cases of AIDS in Orange County both occurred in men exposed to the same AIDS patient ("patient 0") who lived outside California? Is it that 9 of 15 patients with interviews had had previous contact with other AIDS patients? We consider the probability that 7 of the 11 AIDS patients in the interview data in Los Angeles County should have had sex with 1 of the 18 other AIDS patients in southern California. If we assume, as in the appendix to Auerbach, Darrow, Jaffe and Curran (1984), that each of these 11 patients had 610 sexual partners in the preceeding 5 years and that these partners were chosen at random from among 250,000 homosexual males in southern California, then the chance that a given patient would have contacted another identified AIDS patient from southern California is approximately $610 \times 18/250,000 = 0.044$. From the binomial distribution, the chance that 7 or more of these 11 patients would have contacted another AIDS patient is only

$$\sum_{x=7}^{11} (0.044)^x (0.956)^{11-x}(11!)/(x!)(11-x)! = 6 \times 10^{-8}.$$

However, the mere existence of an unusual cluster of cases is not proof of a sexually transmitted infectious agent. Auerbach, Darrow, Jaffe, and Curran (1984) compared AIDS cases who had had sex with other AIDS cases ("linked" AIDS case) to "unlinked" AIDS cases. "Linked" AIDS cases were more promiscuous, but they also used more nitrite inhalants than "unlinked" AIDS cases. Thus non-sexual activities, such as drug abuse, may have contributed to the apparent clustering of AIDS.

The success of studies on individual AIDS patients in defining the major risk categories and suggesting an infectious etiology well before HIV had been isolated is due in part to the rarity of AIDS-defining conditions such as *Pneumocystis carinii* pneumonia and Kaposi's sarcoma. Because such conditions are rare, cases are highly informative. Had the only effect of HIV been to increase the risk of developing a common cancer, such as colon cancer, it is likely that several years would have elapsed before the problem was even recognized and that studies of individual cases would have been much less revealing.

Instead, cases would need to have been compared to non-cases to identify possible risk factors. In the next section, we describe such comparative studies, which were useful in identifying specific behaviors and other factors that modified the risk of HIV infection and AIDS among members of the various risk groups shown in Table 1.1. A more extensive discussion of the epidemiology in each of these risk groups is given in the book edited by Kaslow and Francis (1989) and in the review of modes of transmission by Friedland and Klein (1987).

2.3 CASE-CONTROL AND COHORT STUDIES TO IDENTIFY RISK FACTORS

2.3.1 Measures of Risk

The degree of increased risk associated with a specific behavior or other factor is often measured as the relative risk or relative odds of infection comparing those with the factor to those without the factor. We define these terms more precisely in what follows. Suppose that two uninfected cohorts ($i = 1$ or 2) are followed from calendar time $t_0 = 0$ to a later calendar time, t. Let $H_i(t)$ be the cumulative distribution function of times to infection, $h_i(t) = dH(t)/dt$ be the density function and $k_i(t) = h_i(t)/\{1 - H_i(t)\}$ be the hazard function for cohort i. These terms are defined and illustrated in texts on survival analysis, such as the books by Kalbfleisch and Prentice (1980) and by Cox and Oakes (1984). Section 4.2 also gives examples.

To determine whether those in population $i = 2$ are at higher risk than those in population $i = 1$, one can estimate the relative risk (relative hazard) $rr(t) = k_2(t)/k_1(t)$. Estimates of the relative risk may be obtained by following the cohorts to determine when incident HIV infections occur and dividing the incidence rate estimates in population $i = 2$ by those in population $i = 1$ (chapter 5 in Breslow and Day, 1987). Relative risks can also be obtained from time-matched case-control studies comparing cases of new HIV infection at time t with controls chosen from among subjects who are not infected at time t (Liddell, McDonald and Thomas, 1977; Prentice and Breslow, 1978).

It is often assumed that the relative risk remains constant over time. Then the common relative risk $rr(t) = \theta$ can be estimated by use of the proportional hazards model (Cox, 1972), as discussed by Liddell, McDonald and Thomas (1977) and by Prentice and Breslow (1978).

It may not be possible to follow cohort members closely to determine precisely when incident HIV infection occurs. Instead, cohort members are surveyed for prevalent infection at a single time t. The relative odds of infection

$$ro(t) = H_2(t)\{1 - H_1(t)\}/H_1(t)\{1 - H_2(t)\} \tag{2.1}$$

can be estimated either from the cohort data or from case-control data. In the latter instance, $ro(t)$ is estimated as the odds of being in population $i = 2$ among a random sample of infected subjects (the "cases") divided by the odds of being in population $i = 2$ among a random sample of uninfected subjects at time t. This design is called a prevalent case-control design. For values of t small enough that $H_i(t)$ is small, the relative odds is approximately equal to $H_2(t)/H_1(t)$, which is nearly equal to the relative risk $rr(t)$. Thus, prevalent case-control studies can yield estimates of the relative risk provided the cumulative incidence of infection is small. For large t, however, the relative odds is approximately

$$\{1 - H_1(t)\}/\{1 - H_2(t)\} = \exp\left[-\int_0^t \{k_1(u) - k_2(u)\}du\right].$$

Under the proportional hazards assumption, $k_2(t) = \theta k_1(t)$, and provided $H_1(\infty) = H_2(\infty) = 1$, the relative odds tends to 0, 1 or ∞ as t increases, according as θ is <1, 1 or >1 respectively. Thus one can anticipate differences between relative risk estimates and relative odds estimates in populations with large HIV prevalences.

Some case-control studies have compared prevalent AIDS cases with AIDS-free controls. Some of these controls may have been infected, so it is clear that the relative risk of AIDS need not equal the relative risk of infection. If we ignore mortality, immigration, emigration and the possibility that the incubation distribution, F, changes in calendar time, then the cumulative risk of developimg AIDS by time t in population i is

$$H_{Ai}(t) = \int_0^t h_i(s)F(t - s)ds. \tag{2.2}$$

The relative odds of AIDS $roA(t)$ can be computed by substituting H_{Ai} for H_i in equation (2.1).

To see how the relative risk of infection, the relative odds of infection and the relative odds of AIDS may differ, we assume that the hazards of infection remain constant at $k_2(t) = 0.1$ per year and $k_1(t) = 0.05$ per year. Then the true relative hazards of infection at years 1, 3 and 5 are 2, 2 and 2, whereas the corresponding relative odds of infection are 2.05, 2.16 and 2.28. Assuming the incubation distribution of AIDS is Weibull, with $F(t) = 1 - \exp(-0.0021t^{2.516})$, as in Brookmeyer and

Goedert (1989), the corresponding relative odds of AIDS are 1.92, 1.78 and 1.66. Thus, the relative odds of AIDS are attenuated toward unity, compared to the relative risk and relative odds of infection.

An additional problem is that relative risks of infection and relative odds of infection can change rapidly as the epidemic develops (De Gruttola and Mayer, 1988; Koopman, Simon, Jacquez, et al., 1988) and are affected by mixing patterns among high and low risk subgroups of the population (Koopman, Simon, Jacquez, et al., 1988; Koopman, Longini, Jacquez, et al., 1991). Thus relative risks and relative odds are not as stable and reliable as summaries of risk for HIV infection as they are for other illnesses, such as heart disease and cancer.

To see why relative risks for HIV may be unstable or misleading consider an uninfected individual (individual "2") who establishes μ_2 new sexual partnerships per year. Suppose the chance that a selected partner is infected is $\psi_2(t)$. Suppose further that individual "2" engages in behaviors that produce a chance β_2 of infection per partnership with an infected partner. Compared to another uninfected individual ("1") with parameters μ_1, β_1 and $\psi_1(t)$, the relative hazard of infection is

$$\mu_2\beta_2\psi_2(t)/\mu_1\beta_1\psi_1(t). \tag{2.3}$$

The relative hazard will vary in time unless $\psi_1(t) = \psi_2(t)$.

Suppose individual "2" only selects partners from among a homogeneous randomly mixing cohort of individuals with parameters μ_2 and β_2, and likewise for individual "1." Since the prevalence of infection in such randomly mixing homogeneous cohorts grows exponentially in the initial phases of the epidemic (see equation 9.6), the relative risk (2.3) becomes

$$(\mu_2\beta_2 y_2/\mu_1\beta_1 y_1) \exp\{(\mu_2\beta_2 - \mu_1\beta_1)t\} \tag{2.4}$$

where y_2 and y_1 are the initial prevalences in cohorts $i = 2$ and $i = 1$. This relative risk increases in time if $\mu_2\beta_2 > \mu_1\beta_1$.

More generally, individuals "1" and "2" may be selecting partners from various subgroups with different HIV prevalences. Suppose that individual "2" selects partners exclusively from a subpopulation with low prevalence whereas individual "1" selects partners exclusively from a population with high prevalence. Then the relative risk (2.3) will seriously underestimate the ratio $\mu_2\beta_2/\mu_1\beta_1$, which describes the relative risk that would pertain if both individuals "1" and "2" selected the same types of partners.

If one is interested in studying factors that affect the probability of transmission per partnership, β, one must control for the frequency of formation of new partnerships, μ, and for the chance that a chosen partner will be infected $\psi(t)$, as is evident from equation (2.3).

We now discuss some findings from studies of risk factors for transmission. These studies rely on relative risks and relative odds to characterize the strength of association with a risk factor.

2.3.2 Risk Factors for Transmission Among Homosexual Men

Winkelstein, Padian, Rutherford, and Jaffe (1989) review studies of factors affecting the chance of transmission among homosexual men. The earliest studies compared patients with AIDS to controls without AIDS. Marmor, Friedman-Kien, Laubenstein, et al. (1982) conducted a case-control study based on 20 histologically confirmed cases of Kaposi's sarcoma among homosexual men seen at the New York University Medical Center between March 1979 and August 1981 and on 40 controls matched to cases on age and race and selected from the Manhattan practice of a physician treating homosexual men. Risk was associated with level of sexual activity in the previous year, with a history of mononucleosis and of sexually transmitted diseases, and with the use of "recreational drugs." A multivariate logistic model included numbers of previous sex partners and lifetime exposures to amyl nitrite. Despite the suggestion from the multivariate regression that exposure to nitrites might have an etiologic role for Kaposi's sarcoma, the authors cautiously concluded that "amyl nitrite use may have been a surrogate for another causal variable, such as overall drug use or exposure to a sexually transmitted oncogenic virus." Subsequent studies on these cases (Marmar, Friedman-Kien, Zolla-Pazner, et al., 1984) identified receptive anal-genital intercourse with ejaculation and "fisting" (insertion of the hand or the fist into the partner's rectum) as important risk factors. Amyl nitrite was no longer needed in a multivariate model that included detailed information on these two sexual behaviors and cytomegalovirus titre, suggesting that the univariate associations with drug use might be an artifact of multicollinearity with risky sexual behaviors. A larger case-control study of cases with Kaposi's sarcoma and cases with *Pneumocystis carinii* pneumonia (Jaffe, Choi, Thomas, et al., 1983) identified a large number of sexual partners, syphilis, and exposure to feces during sex as associated with increased risk. Thus, even before the isolation of HIV, there was good evidence in homosexual men associating AIDS with large numbers of sexual partners and with anal receptive sex.

These case-control studies on AIDS patients had the great advantage that they could be performed quickly. However, as discussed in Section 2.3.1, the relative odds of developing AIDS is not the same as the relative odds of infection because many control subjects without AIDS were nonetheless infected. Moreover, factors affecting survival after infection and factors affecting AIDS diagnosis, such as access to advanced diagnostic facilities, might influence the odds of having AIDS but not the odds of becoming infected. Case-control studies on AIDS patients are also difficult because it may be hard to elicit a reliable history of sexual exposures at the time of infection, which may have preceeded the onset of AIDS by many years. These difficulties are accentuated if the patient is severely ill or has neurologic complications.

Another difficulty, which applies not only to case-control studies of AIDS patients but to all the designs that were used, was that various possible exposures, such as the use of nitrites and various sexual behaviors were highly correlated. This "multicollinearity" makes it difficult to identify which of several correlated behaviors are, indeed, risk factors, and which are merely incidential correlates of risky behavior. Logistic regression analyses cannot provide unequivocal answers to such questions, and indeed, multicollinearity is a cause of difficulty of interpretation in many types of regression analyses (Mosteller and Tukey, 1977). In such circumstances, it usually makes sense to select variables for modelling transmission in accordance with plausible pathophysiologic mechanisms, rather than purely on the basis of observed statistical associations.

The identification of HIV and the development of serologic assays in 1984 made it possible to compare prevalent seropositive cases with seronegative controls. Several studies based on prevalent seropositive cases (Goedert, Biggar, Winn, et al., 1984; Melbye, Biggar, Ebbesen, et al., 1984; Stevens, Taylor, Zang, et al., 1986; Moss, Osmund, Bacchetti, et al., 1987; Chmiel, Detels, Kaslow, et al., 1987; Winkelstein, Lyman, Padian, et al., 1987; Darrow, Echenberg, Jaffe, et al., 1987) confirmed the importance of number of sexual partners, receptive anal intercourse with ejaculation, rectal douching and rectal trauma as risk factors for seropositivity. The study by Melbye, Biggar, Ebbesen, et al. (1984) emphasized that travel to areas with high rates of seroprevalence—such as New York City, San Francisco, and Los Angeles—was also an important risk factor for Danish homosexuals. Other factors associated with risk for seropositivity have been observed, including a history of venereal disease, and previous sexual contact with a person who developed AIDS. These observations form the basis of prevention efforts in the homosexual community to reduce promiscuity and unprotected receptive anal intercourse.

Studies of incident HIV infection are costly and time-consuming because they require following initially seronegative individuals to determine when seroconversion occurs. Over 2000 initially serone- gative members of the Multicenter AIDS Cohort Study were re- examined at 6 month intervals to determine serologic status and to inquire about sexual behaviors in the preceeding 6 months. The relative risk of incident seroconversion was about 15 for those who had engaged in receptive anal intercourse in the preceeding 12 months compared to cohort members who had avoided anal-genital sex (Kingsley, Detels, Kaslow, et al., 1987; Detels, English, Visscher, et al., 1989). Men who participated both in receptive and insertive anal sex had a relative risk of about 32. These relative risks are higher than the relative odds of receptive anal intercourse found in the earlier case- control comparisons of seroprevalent cases with seronegative controls. In those seroprevalence studies, the odds ratios were usually near 7. This disparity cannot be explained by the mathematical difference between relative risks and odds ratios, which would tend to produce larger odds ratios than relative risks. One possible explanation is that the information on sexual behavior near the time of infection is much more reliable in the longitudinal study of incident seroconversions than in seroprevalence studies. Even if interviews at the time of the cross- sectional seroprevalence surveys yielded accurate information on sexual behavior in the preceeding year, they would not necessarily yield a precise indication of sexual behaviors at earlier times when infection may have occurred. Misspecification of risk behaviors at the time of infection can attenuate the relative risk. It is also possible, however, that members of the Multicenter AIDS Cohort Study who continued to engage in receptive anal intercourse, despite education efforts to promote safer practices, chose partners with a higher prevalence of infection than the partners of men who eschewed anal- genital sex. Such prevalence differences could increase the relative risk in the cohort study (equation 2.3), although one would expect a similar phenomenon to have occurred among participants in seroprevalence studies. It is a limitation of all these studies that the prevalence of HIV in the partners of study subjects is unknown.

2.3.3 Risk Factors in Parenterel Drug Users

Friedland (1989) reviewed the epidemiology of HIV infection among parenteral drug users. Most parenteral drug users are intraven- ous drug users, although some parenteral drug users inject other sites. Clearly identified risk factors for HIV infection include the frequency of drug injections, the frequency of sharing injection equipment with others, and the proportion of injections that use equipment that is also used by two or more other people, as in "shooting galleries." Other factors include nonwhite race and proximity to New York City, which are associated with high HIV prevalence in the drug using community in the United States.

Nicolosi, Leite, Molinari, et al. (1992) found that the seroconversion rate among intravenous drug users attending treatment centers in northern Italy decreased from 4.9 per person-year in 1987—1988 to 2.1 per person-year in 1989—90. From 1987 to 1990, the proportions of drug users who were sharing syringes when initially entered into treatment programs decreased, as did the proportions who continued to share syringes while in treatment follow-up. Further studies on intravenous drug users who seroconverted indicated that having sex with an HIV-positive partner adds to the high risk of seroconversion associated with sharing syringes (Nicolosi, Leite, Musicco, et al., 1992). It was also found that young subjects (<20 years old) and those who had been using drugs for fewer than 2 years were at increased risk of seroconversion.

2.3.4 Risk Factors in Heterosexuals

As mentioned in Section 2.2, strong evidence for heterosexual transmission of HIV came from studies of individuals who denied other known risk behaviors and from clusters of AIDS cases associated with a single infected individual (Clumeck, Taelman, Hermans, et al., 1989). Some of the strongest evidence for male-to-female and female-to-male heterosexual transmission comes from partner studies (Section 2.5). Haverkos and Edelman (1989) reviewed the epidemiologic evidence for heterosexual transmission, both in Africa, where it is a dominant mode of transmission, and in the United States.

Case-control studies in the United States suggest that the primary risk factors for heterosexual transmission are factors that determine the probability that the sexual partner is infected. In particular, risk factors for males in sexually transmitted disease clinics (Quinn, Glasser, Cannon, et al., 1988; Chaisson, Stoneburner, Lifson, et al., 1990) included whether or not the female partner was a potential drug user and nonwhite race. Risk factors for females in these clinics included whether or not the male partner was a potential drug user or a bisexual male. Other risk factors included indicators of sexual promiscuity such as a positive serology for syphillis among men and women, and prostitution among women. Genital warts and positive serology for syphillis remained predictive of HIV infection even after controlling for the type and number of sexual partners, suggesting that abrasion of the mucosa by venereal disease facilitates HIV transmission.

More direct information on factors affecting the risk of heterosexual infection has been obtained from studies of the sexual partners of individuals who are known to be infected. Such studies are called "partner studies" (Section 2.5), and the person known to be infected is called the "index case." A study of 368 female partners (Lazzarin, Saracco, Musicco, et al., 1991) demonstrated an increased risk of HIV transmission to the female if the male index case had fewer than 400 CD4+ T-cells per microliter or if the female partner had genital warts or vaginitis. Behaviors that increased the chance of transmission included frequent sexual contact and anal sex. Frequent use of condoms was protective. Those exposed for 1 to 5 years had a greater chance of infection than those exposed for less than one year. Other partner studies have also found that risk is increased if the index case is severely immunodeficient (Goedert, Eyster, Bigger, and Blattner, 1987; European Study Group, 1989), if anal intercourse is practiced (European Study Group, 1989; Padian Shiboski and Jewell, 1990), if the female partner has a history of sexually transmitted diseases (European Study Group, 1989), and if condoms are not used (Padian, Shiboski, and Jewell, 1990).

The partner study reported by Padian, Shiboski, and Jewell (1991) found only one case of female-to-male transmission among 72 couples (1.4%), compared to 61 infected female partners in 307 couples (20%) with male index cases. Thus the rate of male-to-female transmission was much higher than the rate of female-to-male transmission. However, 19 of 159 (12%) of male partners were infected, compared to 82 of 404 (20%) of female partners in the Multicentric European Partner Study (De Vincenzi, 1992). The higher rates of female-to-male transmission in this study compared to the finding of Padian, Shiboski, and Jewell (1991) may reflect a different distribution of cofactors that promote transmission, unacknowledged risks among male partners, and random variation in both studies.

2.3.5 Risk Factors for Transmission from Blood Products

People in the United States are at low risk of exposure to HIV through blood transfusions, because the chance that a donor is infected is small, especially since the initiation of HIV screening programs and educational programs to deter blood donations from people with risk factors for HIV exposure (Chapter 6). Even before these prevention efforts, the chance that a transfusion recipient in the United States would receive infected blood was small (Peterman and Allen, 1989). Nonetheless, 4636 transfusion-related cases of AIDS had been reported to CDC by the end of 1991. Of these cases, 477 were incident in 1991.

Patients with hemophilia were at much higher risk because clotting factor concentrates were made from pools of plasma derived from 2000 to 20,000 donors (Peterman and Allen, 1989). Fifty-five percent of the members of a cohort of 1219 hemophiliacs from treatment centers throughout the United States were found to be infected by 1988 (Goedert, Kessler, Aledort, et al., 1989). The very first infections occurred at the end of 1978, based on stored sera. However, the hazard of infection was highest between 1981 and 1985. In 1985 and 1986, methods for screening donors and methods to inactivate HIV, such as heat treatment of clotting factor concentrates, dramatically reduced the chance of infection (CDC, 1987a). Nonetheless, the toll of AIDS cases continues to mount as previously infected patients become ill. As of December 31, 1991, the CDC had received reports of 1876 AIDS cases in patients with clotting disorders. This number represents a substantial fraction of the approximately 14,000 patients with hemophilia in the United States (Peterman and Allen, 1989).

The risk of infection was related to the type and severity of hemophilia. Of those with type A hemophilia (factor VIII deficiency), 64% became infected, but the proportion infected increased from 25% for those with mild disease to 46% for those with moderate disease to 76% for those with severe disease (Goedert, Kessler, Aledort, et al., 1989). This dose-response relationship between disease severity, which determines the clotting factor requirements, and the chance of infection was also seen for other types of hemophilia. However, other forms of hemophilia were associated with lower overall risk than type A hemophilia.Thirty-one percent of patients with type B hemophilia (factor IX deficiency) were infected, and 14% of patients with other forms of hemophilia were infected.

Even though it is clear that the risk of infection depended on the type and amount of clotting factors received, it has not been routinely possible to determine which lots of clotting factors infected particular patients. Indeed, a study comparing "exposed" lots, to which an infected donor who later developed AIDS had contributed, with "unexposed" lots revealed no difference in infectivity (Jason, Holman, Dixon, et al., 1986).

2.4 RISKS FROM POINT EXPOSURES

The following observations characterize the probability of infection from well defined point exposures.

2.4.1 Recipients of Contaminated Blood

Several investigators have traced the recipients of blood transfusions that were later found to have come from infected donors. For example, Ward, Deppe, Samson, et al. (1987) traced 201 recipients of blood from 32 infected donors. Of those recipients, 114 had died before the study, 12 refused to be tested for HIV, 3 had other risk factors for HIV infection and 13 had relocated. Of the remaining 59 recipients, 39 (66%) had positive serology for HIV. Some donors seemed to be more infectious than others, and recipients seemed to be more likely to become infected if they received blood close to the time the donor developed AIDS. Thus the variability of the estimate of 66% infected is probably somewhat larger than indicated by the binomial standard error $100\{(.66 \times .34)/59\}^{1/2} = 6.2\%$. Smaller studies found that 6 (67%) of 9 tested recipients (Menitove, 1986) and 5 (38%) of 13 tested recipients (Kakaiya, Cable, and Keltonic, 1987) were infected.

Each of these estimates may be biased if those recipients who died previously or those who refused to be tested had different infection rates from those who agreed to be tested.

2.4.2 Health Care Workers and Medical Researchers

Among 860 health care workers who were exposed to the blood of infected patients by needle stick injuries or cuts with a sharp object, 3 were subsequently shown to seroconvert from seronegative to seropositive. One other subject was found to be seropositive 10 months after the injury, but no antecedent sample was available (Marcus, 1988). Based on binomial sampling, the chance of infection is $4/860 = 0.46\%$, with a one-sided upper 95% confidence limit of 0.90%.

Of 103 health workers exposed to infected blood by contact with mucous membranes or nonintact skin, none were observed to seroconvert. The estimated risk is 0% with an upper one-sided 95% confidence limit of 2.9%.

Medical researchers working with concentrated virus are subject to occupational risk even in the absence of exposure through sharp objects. One of 99 laboratory workers who handled concentrated virus was found to be infected with an HIV-1 strain that was genotypically "indistinguishable" from a strain used in the laboratory (Weiss, Goedert, Gartner, et al., 1988). This worker denied all known risk behaviors for HIV infection, took usual laboratory precautions, and did not recall any episode of direct exposure to skin or mucous membranes. The corresponding HIV infection rate was 0.48 per 100 person-years exposure with an upper 95% confidence limit of 2.30 per 100 person-years. To reduce this risk, further laboratory precautions were recommended, including vigorous decontamination of work surfaces, adherence to procedures for using and changing gloves, and the use of goggles, face shields or face masks to discourage hand contact with the mouth, eyes, ears or nose.

2.4.3 Perinatal Transmission

Several investigators have estimated the probability of transmission of HIV from an infected mother to her infant in prospective cohort studies. A central problem is that a mother's antibodies to HIV are present in the blood of her infant initially. Thus, serologic tests cannot be used to determine whether the infant is infected initially, and there is some variation in the literature as to how to define whether the infant is infected.

Goedert, Mendez, Drummond, et al. (1989) defined the infant as infected if HIV antibodies remained present at 15 months or if earlier clinical "signs of HIV-1 disease" were present. They determined that 16 (29%) of 55 infants were infected. The Italian Multicentre Study (1988) reported that 29 (32.6%) of 89 children of infected mothers who had been followed for more than 15 months were considered to be infected. The remaining 60 children were seronegative and free of symptoms. Blanche, Rouzioux, Moscato, et al. (1989) defined infants as infected if antibodies to HIV persisted to 18 months of age. They found that 32 (27%) of 117 infants were infected. If one defines as infected the 9 additional children who did not have antibodies to HIV at 18 months, but who did have clinical evidence of HIV infection—such as hepatomegaly, splenomegaly, adenopathy, hypergamma-globulinemia, or decreases in CD4 + T-cells—the percentage infected is 35%. Ryder, Nsa, Hassig, et al. (1989) demonstrated increased mortality in the children of HIV infected mothers in Zaire, and, in a randomly selected subset of 92 children who were followed for 12 months, 36 (39%) were found to have "evidence of perinatally acquired infection."

The European Collaborative Study (1991) defined children as infected if the infant remained seropositive at 18 months or if AIDS or an HIV-related death occurred before then or if HIV virus was cultured or if HIV antigen was detected in two samples. Of 419 children with at least 18 months of potential follow-up, infection was demonstrated in 48 (11.4%). However, 47 additional infants were lost to follow-up within 18 months and were still seropositive when last examined. Of these, 20 were older than one month. If these 20 remained seropositive at 18 months, the estimated rate of infection would increase to 16%. The low estimates of the probability of transmission in this study, compared to other studies, may result in part from the fact that children with thrush and hepatosplenomegaly, for example, would not be counted as being infected in this study. It is also possible that the women in this study had less advanced HIV disease or other factors that reduced the chance of transmission.

One methodologic issue concerns the proper analysis of infants who were lost to follow-up or who died of diseases unrelated to HIV. Suppose that 100 infants are born more than 15 months before the end of follow-up. Of these, suppose 10 develop clinical evidence of AIDS within 15 months, 20 are lost to follow-up after they first become seronegative and before age 15 months, 15 are still seropositive but free of clinical disease when lost to follow-up before 15 months, 15 remain clinically well but are HIV antibody positive when tested at 15 months, and 40 remain clinically well and are antibody negative when tested at 15 months. Suppose, further, that one of the 20 infants who was lost to follow-up shortly after being found to be seronegative reverts to seropositivity at 15 months, and that 6 of the 15 infants who were seropositive when lost to follow-up remain seropositive at 15 months. If the definition of "infected" is evidence of clinical disease within 15 months or continued seropositivity at 15 months, the true proportion infected in this study is $p = (10 + 1 + 15 + 6)/100 = 0.320$.

One method of analysis (Blanche, Rouzioux, Moscato, et al., 1989) excludes infants whose potential follow-up is less than 15 months and who are lost to follow-up without clinical evidence of infection before 15 months of age. In the present example, all infants have a potential follow-up of at least 15 months because they are all born more than 15 months before the study ended. Thus, the estimate is $\hat{p} = (10 + 15)/65 = 0.385$. This procedure is unbiased only if excluded patients have the same risk of infection as other patients. In the present example, this estimate is upwardly biased, because those infants who were lost to follow-up have a lower probability of being infected, $(1 + 6)/(20 + 15) = 0.200$, than other infants.

An alternative method of analysis is to regard infants who become seronegative without clinical disease as uninfected, even if the infant is lost to follow-up before 15 months (Goedert, Mendez, Drummond, et al., 1989; European Collaborative Study, 1991). "Indeterminant" infants, who are free of clinical disease but seropositive when lost to follow-up, are excluded. In the present example, this procedure leads to the estimate $\hat{p} = (10 + 15)/85 = 0.294$. This estimate is biased downward, because the proportion of "indeterminant" infants who are infected is higher than the proportion of other infants who are infected and because one of the infants who were seronegative when lost to follow-up was, in fact, infected.

This example indicates the desirability of obtaining complete data on serostatus at 15 months (many investigators prefer 18 months). Additional methodological work might lead to improved estimates by modelling the probability of infection as a function of the last antibody level observed before loss to follow-up. Tsai, Goedert, Orazem, et al. (1992) develop nonparametric procedures for estimating the distribution function of times to clinical disease among infected infants and for using information from those who are lost to follow-up to estimate the probability of transmission. However, these methods depend on the assumptions that the probability of transmission and the times to onset of clinical disease are the same among those who are lost to follow-up as among other cohort members.

A small proportion of infants may have become infected from nursing (Van de Perre, Simonon, Msellati, et al., 1991; Pizzo and Butler, 1991). Such transmission would be difficult to distinguish from transmission in utero or during birth in routine follow-up studies.

Investigators have tried to establish the diagnosis of infection early by attempting to culture HIV virus from blood samples and by searching for HIV genetic material with the polymerase chain reaction (PCR) assay. However, the sensitivities of these two assays are limited, especially in the first few weeks following birth (Rogers, Qu, Rayfield, et al. 1989; Comeau, Harris, McIntosh, et al. 1992).

De Grutolla, Tu, and Pagano (1992) used a different approach to estimate the probability of transmission. In New York City, newborns have been screened since December 1987 to determine HIV serostatus. Although the data collected contain no information to identify individual children, the numbers of seropositive children born each month are known. The numbers of children who develop AIDS and their dates of birth are also available from an AIDS registry for New York City. De Grutolla, Tu and Pagano linked these two types of information and used statistical methods that also accounted for the period before newborns were screened for HIV seropositivity and for AIDS reporting delays. They estimated that the probability that an infant born to an infected mother would develop AIDS within 10 years was 26% with a 95% confidence interval (13%, 39%). The point estimate 26% tends to underestimate the probability of infection because not all children who developed AIDS were reported and not all infected children develop AIDS within 10 years. Indeed, one of the most striking findings of this analysis is that the risk of developing AIDS persists well into childhood.

2.5 SEXUAL TRANSMISSION AND PARTNER STUDIES

2.5.1 General Considerations

In the last section, the risks of infection from well defined point exposures were considered. In this section, risks of infection from sexual transmission are quantified using epidemiological studies called "partner studies." Partner studies can provide unique epidemiological data for studying sexual transmission because it is known if an individual was exposed to an infected partner, and the numbers of contacts between the partners may also be known.

The objective of partner studies is to estimate the probabilities of transmission that are associated with various types of sexual behaviors. The partner study is based on individuals who are known to be HIV infected (the index cases), and their partners (the susceptible partners). The index case is the potential source of infection for his or her susceptible partner. Information is collected on the infection status of the susceptible partner and factors that may affect the probability of transmission. An important factor that affects this probability is the number of sexual contacts between the index case and the susceptible partner that occur subsequent to the infection of the index case. Additional factors that could affect the transmission probability include type of sexual behavior, use of condoms, degree of immunosuppression of the index case and presence of other sexually transmitted diseases or conditions such as genital ulceration.

Ideally, a partner study would be conducted prospectively. In a prospective study, the index case and the susceptible partner would be followed to determine the numbers and types of contacts. The susceptible partner would be serially tested for HIV infection in order to determine if and when infection occurs.

However, nearly all partner studies are conducted retrospectively. In a retrospective study, the current infection status of the susceptible partner is determined, but, if the partner is infected, it is usually not possible to determine *when* the partner was infected (or seroconverted).

Attempts are made to ascertain the calendar time of infection of the index case and the subsequent history of the partnership including the numbers and types of contact, as well as any other high risk behaviors that occurred outside the partnership. The prospective partner study has a number of advantages over the retrospective study. First, information on numbers and types of contacts are more reliable because they are not subject to recall errors. Second, the time when the susceptible partner became infected is determined, unlike the retrospective study in which only the current infection status (yes or no) is determined.

There are several examples of retrospective studies of HIV transmission. The Transfusion Partner Study involved partners of patients with transfusion-associated HIV infection (Peterman, Stoneburner, Allen, et al., 1988). The study involved spouses (susceptible partner) who had sexual contact with the infected transfusion recipient (the index case). Serum samples were obtained for HIV serological testing. Spouses of the index patient were interviewed to determine the numbers and types of sexual contact they had with the index case subsequent to the transfusion. Spouses who were at risk of infection through another source (e.g., intravenous drug use, or high risk sexual behavior outside the partnership) were excluded. The Transfusion Partner Study is unique because the date of infection of all the index cases could be determined.

The Hemophilia Partner Study involved the female partners of HIV infected patients with hemophilia (Ragni, Kingsley, Nimorwicz, et al., 1989). Stored serum samples from patients with hemophilia were tested to determine the date of HIV seroconversion. The date of seroconversion was estimated as the midpoint of the interval between the dates of the last seronegative and first seropositive sample. Information was collected about sexual behaviors following the seroconversion of the index case, as well as the health status of the index case (e.g., CD4+ T cell count).

The California Partner Study involved female sexual partners of HIV infected men (Padian, Marquis, Francis, et al., 1987). The men (the index cases) were either bisexual, intravenuous drug users, hemophiliacs or recipients of blood transfusions. Attempts were made to ascertain the date of infection of the index case from interviews. However, when the index case was infected through sexual transmission, the calendar time of infection could only be approximated (Jewell and Shiboski, 1990). Women such as intravenuous drug users, who were at risk of infection from sources outside the partnership, were excluded.

There are a number of other partner studies that have provided valuable information about heterosexual transmission of HIV. Lazzarin, Saracco, Musicco, Nicolosi, and the Italian Study Group on HIV Heterosexual Transmission (1991) carried out a cross-sectional study of women who were partners of HIV infected men. They estimated that about 28% of the women were seropositive. Similar results on male-to-female transmission were obtained by the European Study Group (1989). De Vincenzi (1992) reported that HIV transmission from female-to-male transmission occurred in 12% of partnerships in the Multicenter European Partner Study.

A major objective of the partner study is to estimate the infectivity parameter, γ, and to identify covariates that affect infectivity. The infectivity is the probability of viral transmission from a given contact between the partner and the index case (Wiley, Herschkorn, and Padian, 1989). If information on numbers of contacts cannot be ascertained, or, if such information is unreliable, it is possible only to estimate the probability of transmission per partnership rather than per contact.

In Section 2.5.2, statistical methods are outlined for estimating infectivity under the simplifying assumption that infectivity is constant across partnerships. More complex models that account for heterogeneity in infectivity are described in Section 2.5.3. Additional topics are considered in Section 2.5.4. Jewell and Shiboski (1992) review statistical considerations in the design and analysis of partner studies of HIV transmission.

2.5.2 Statistical Methods for Partner Studies

Data collected in a retrospective partner study include the current infection status of the susceptible partner and the estimated number of contacts between the partners. The number of contacts refers to the contacts that occurred between the time the index case was infected and the time of ascertainment of the infection status of the susceptible partner. For the ith partnership, let

$$Y_i = \begin{cases} 1 & \text{if susceptible partner is infected} \\ 0 & \text{if susceptible partner is not infected} \end{cases}$$

and let K_i be the number of sexual contacts between the ith index case and his or her partner. We assume that the susceptible partner was at risk of HIV infection only through contact with the index case. Methods to relax this assumption are considered briefly in Section 2.5.4.

The simplest statistical model assumes that each contact produces an independent chance of infection and that the probability of transmission on each contact is the constant, γ. Under these assumptions, the probability that the susceptible partner is infected after K contacts, $p = P(Y = 1 | K \text{ contacts})$, is

$$p = 1 - (1 - \gamma)^K. \tag{2.5}$$

If one had an estimate of p, then the infectivity parameter could be estimated by solving (2.5):

$$\hat{\gamma} = 1 - (1 - \hat{p})^{1/K}. \tag{2.6}$$

For example, data from the California Partner Study is summarized in Table 2.1 where the numbers of contacts have been grouped into intervals. There were 21 partnerships who reported between 200 and 299 contacts, and in 8 of these partnerships the susceptible female became infected. Thus, an estimate of p after 250 contacts (the interval midpoint) is $\hat{p} = 8/21 = .381$ and from (2.6) it follows that an estimate of the infectivity is

$$\hat{\gamma} = 1 - (1 - .381)^{1/250} = .0019.$$

This estimate of infectivity was based only on a single column in Table 2.1. A better estimate would be based on all the data. This is best done using a generalized linear model. By twice taking logs of equation (2.5) one obtains

$$\log\{-\log(1 - p)\} = \log\{-\log(1 - \gamma)\} + \log K. \tag{2.7}$$

The parameters in model (2.7) can be estimated using the data collected on N partnerships (Y_i, K_i) $i = 1, \ldots, N$. This can be done with the generalized linear interactive modeling system (GLIM) (Payne, 1986) by specifying (*i*) binomial error, (*ii*) a complementary log-log link and (*iii*) inclusion in the linear predictor of both an offset term, $\log K_i$, and an intercept term, β_0. The intercept term, β_0, is related to infectivity by the equation, $\beta_0 = \log\{-\log(1 - \gamma)\}$. Using this methodology on the California Partner Study, Jewell and Shiboski (1990) estimated the intercept as $\hat{\beta}_0 = -6.9$, the corresponding infectivity parameter was

$$\hat{\gamma} = 1 - \exp\{-\exp(\hat{\beta}_0)\} = .0010.$$

The crucial assumption in this approach is that the infectivity γ is a constant both across partnerships and from contact to contact within a partnership. A generalization of model (2.7) is

$$\log\{-\log(1 - p)\} = \log\{-\log(1 - \gamma)\} + \beta_1 \log K. \tag{2.8}$$

Table 2.1 Grouped Data from California Partner Study

	Number of Contacts									
	0–9	10–49	50–99	100–199	200–299	300–399	400–599	600–799	800–1499	1500–2170
Female partner infected	2	6	2	3	8	3	8	2	2	2
Female partner not infected	22	20	18	18	13	7	6	9	6	2
N	24	26	20	21	21	10	14	11	8	4
$\hat{p}$	.08	.23	.10	.14	.38	.30	.57	.18	.25	.50

Model (2.8) allows the coefficient of log K, which is called the slope parameter, β_1, to be arbitrary. This is in contrast to model (2.7) where the slope β_1 was forced to be 1.0. When β_1 is not equal to 1.0, the probability of transmission changes from one contact to the next. In particular, the conditional probability of infection on the jth contact given that the individual is not infected after the $(j-1)$st contact is not constant as j varies. If $\beta_1 > 1$, this conditional probability of infection increases monotonically with j. If $\beta_1 < 1$, the conditional probability of infection decreases monotonically with j. There are analogies with the analysis of survival data: Equation (2.8) defines a discrete time Weibull survival model, where the number of contacts plays the role of time (Kalbfleisch and Prentice, 1980) and β_1 is the shape parameter. The conditional probability of infection on contact j given that no infection has occurred before contact j is analogous to the usual hazard function for survival time data.

Jewell and Shiboski (1990) fit model (2.8) to the California Partner data, and obtained $\hat{\beta}_1 = .22$, which suggests that the conditional probability of infection decreases with increasing contacts. The results of fitting models (2.7) and (2.8) are displayed in Figure 2.1. Figure 2.1 suggests that the simpler model (2.7) underestimates infection risk at lower numbers of contacts.

Two explanations have been suggested why model (2.7) or model (2.5) may not adequately describe data from the California Partner Study. The first explanation is that the infectivity varies across partnerships. Transmission may occur more easily in some partnerships than in others, perhaps because of confounding variables such as condom use, or the presence of genital ulcers. These factors cause heterogeneity in infectivity. The susceptible partners in partnerships with high infectivities becomes infected after only a few contacts and are removed from the "at risk" population. This leaves a disproportionate number of susceptible partners in partnerships with low infectivity and creates the appearance of a decreasing per contact risk of infection with increasing contacts. Values of β_1 less than 1.0 reflect this decreasing hazard. These are precisely the same "frailty selection" effects observed in estimating hazards of survival in heterogeneous populations (Vaupel and Yashin, 1985). Models to account for heterogeneity in infectivity are described in Section 2.5.3.

A second explanation for the lack of fit of model (2.7) to the California Partner Study is measurement error in the number of contacts subsequent to infection of the index case. This error could reflect either failure to accurately identify the time when the index case was infected or failure to remember the rate at which contacts occurred

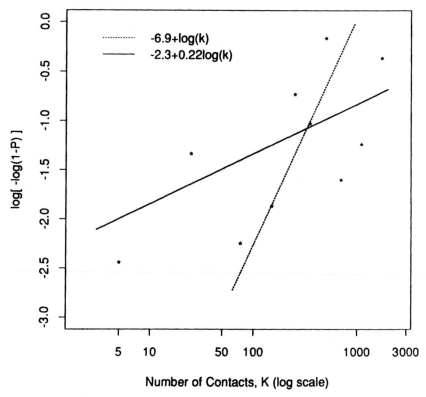

Figure 2.1 Graphs of the fitted regression lines using model 2.7 and model 2.8 from the California Partner Study. (Source: Jewell and Shiboski, 1990.)

after the index case was infected. If random measurement error is ignored, the estimated regression coefficient on $\log K$ will be attenuated toward 0. The lack of fit of model (2.7) is likely due to a combination of both measurement error in the number of contacts, and, heterogeneity in infectivity.

Models (2.5) and (2.7) are based on the assumption that each contact provides an independent constant chance of infection, γ. Alternatively, one can estimate $P(K)$, the probability that infection occurs at or before the Kth contact, non-parametrically. Because $P(K)$ is a distribution function, it must be monotonic non-decreasing. Thus, the nonparametric estimator must maximize the likelihood subject to this constraint (Kaplan, 1990). Ayer, Brunk, Ewing, et al. (1955) developed a simple algorithm known as the "pool-adjacent violators algorithm" to obtain the maximum likelihood estimate of $P(K)$. Jewell and Shiboski (1990) discussed this algorithm and applied it to the

California Partner Study. Here, the algorithm is illustrated (Table 2.2) on the Grouped California Partner Study data in Table 2.1. The basic steps are as follows: (1) Compute the column proportions; (2) Pool the $(K - 1)$ and Kth columns together if $\hat{P}(K - 1) > \hat{P}(K)$ and recompute the proportions; (3) Reinspect the proportions (in the possibly reduced number of categories) and again pool adjacent categories together if $\hat{P}(K - 1) > \hat{P}(K)$; (4) Continue until $\hat{P}(K)$ is nondecreasing. The results in Table 2.2 show that the nonparametric estimate of the probability of transmission with fewer than 10, 200 and 1500 contacts are 0.08, 0.16, and 0.36, respectively. For comparison, the model (2.7) yielded $\hat{\gamma} = .0010$ and from equation (2.5) one obtains $\hat{P}(10) = 0.01$, $\hat{P}(200) = 0.18$ and $\hat{P}(1500) = 0.78$. Model (2.7) leads to an underestimate of risk for small numbers of contacts and to an overestimate for large numbers of contacts. Kaplan (1990) suggests a goodness of fit procedure to compare a parametric model like model (2.7) with the nonparametric maximum likelihood estimate.

2.5.3 Models for Heterogeneity in Infectivity

The assumption that infectivity is a constant across partnerships is an oversimplification. Infectivity may depend on covariates such as condom use, concommittant sexually transmitted diseases and type of contact. We outline two approaches for modelling heterogeneity in

Table 2.2 Illustration of Algorithm to Compute Nonparametric Maximum Likelihood Estimate $\hat{P}(K)$ Using the Data in Table 2.1

Number of Contacts	Iteration		
	(1)	(2)	(3)
0–9	.08	.08	.08
10–49	.23 ⎫		
		.17 ⎫	
50–99	.10 ⎭		.16
100–199	.14	.14 ⎭	
200–299	.38		
		.35	.35
300–399	.30		
400–599	.57		
		.40 ⎫	
600–799	.18		.36
800–1499	.25	.25 ⎭	
1500–2170	.50	.50	.50

infectivity. The first approach incorporates known covariates into the statistical model. The second approach accounts for heterogeneity through a random effects model.

Covariate Modelling of Infectivity

Suppose we have a vector of known covariates, $\mathbf{X}$, for each partnership. The covariates could describe either the index case or the susceptible partner (e.g., presence or absence of genital ulceration) or characteristics of the partnership (types of contacts). We model infectivity as a linear function of the covariates using a complementary log-log link function:

$$\log(-\log(1 - \gamma)) = \mathbf{aX}. \tag{2.9}$$

Model (2.9) generalizes model (2.8). The regression coefficients $\mathbf{a}$ describe how the infectivity depends upon the covariates. Model (2.9) can be fit in GLIM by incorporating the covariate $\mathbf{X}$ as part of the linear predictor. Jewell and Shiboski (1990) used model (2.9) to analyze the California Partner Study. They found that anal intercourse, nonmenstrual bleeding and failure to use condoms increased risk of HIV transmission. Results from other partner studies are presented in Section 2.3.4.

Random Effects Model for Infectivity

If available covariates do not explain the observed heterogeneity in infectivity, a random effects model may be useful. The parameter, γ, the infectivity for a given partnership, is considered to be a random variable drawn from a probability density, $f(\gamma)$. Suppose the ith partnership had K_i contacts. The probability of transmission is

$$p_i = P(Y_i = 1) = \int_0^1 [1 - (1 - \gamma)^{K_i}] f(\gamma) d\gamma. \tag{2.10}$$

The objective is to estimate the parameters of the probability density $f(\gamma)$. This is done by maximizing the likelihood function

$$L = \prod_{i=1}^N (p_i)^{Y_i} (1 - p_i)^{1 - Y_i}, \tag{2.11}$$

where expression (2.10) is substituted for p_i. For example, Wiley, Herschkorn and Padian (1989) suggested a beta distribution for γ:

$$f(\gamma) = \frac{\Gamma(a + b)}{\Gamma(a) \cdot \Gamma(b)} \gamma^{a-1} (1 - \gamma)^b,$$

where a and b are the parameters of the beta distribution. Note that $E(\gamma) = a/(a + b)$ and variance$(\gamma) = ab/(a + b)^2(a + b + 1)$, with

$a > 0$, $b > 0$. Wiley, Herschkorn, and Padian (1989) show that when γ has a beta distribution, expression (2.10) reduces to

$$P(Y_i = 1) = 1 - \prod_{j=0}^{K_i} \frac{b+j}{a+b+j}, \qquad (2.12)$$

which is called a beta binomial distribution.

An alternative random effects model is to assume partnerships are drawn from a mixture of two subpopulations. For example, a proportion of partnerships, π_0, have infectivity γ_0 and the remaining proportion, $\pi_1 = 1 - \pi_0$, have infectivity γ_1. Under this mixture model, expression (2.10) becomes

$$P(Y_i = 1) = \{1 - (1 - \gamma_0)^{K_i}\}\pi_0 + \{1 - (1 - \gamma_1)^{K_i}\}\pi_1 \qquad (2.13)$$

Wiley, Herschkorn, and Padian (1989) applied these models to the Transfusion Partner Study. An unusual feature of the data is that it appears that the likelihood of infection does not increase with increasing numbers of contacts. For example, among husbands of wives infected by transfusion, the mean number of contacts were 67 and 180 for the seropositive and seronegative husbands respectively. Similarly among wives of husbands infected by transfusion, the mean number of contacts were 82 and 156 for the seropositive and seronegative wives respectively. The question is whether this anomalous observation could be explained by heterogeneity in infectivity. Wiley, Herschkorn, and Padian (1989) used both the beta binomial model (2.12) and a special case of the mixture model (2.13) where a proportion of partnerships was assumed to have zero infectivity (i.e., γ_1 was set to 0.0), to analyze the data on the 59 male index cases and their female partners. The estimates obtained from the mixture model were:

$$\hat{\pi}_0 = 0.189 \qquad \hat{\gamma}_0 = 1.0$$
$$\hat{\pi}_1 = 0.811 \qquad \hat{\gamma}_1 = 0.0$$

The beta binomial model yielded similar results. When the simple model (2.7) was fit to this data, $\hat{\gamma} = .00139$. However, a likelihood ratio test indicated that the mixture model and the beta binomial model fit the data considerably better than equation (2.7). Shiboski and Jewell (1992) also analyzed data from the Transfusion Partner Study data using a generalization of model (2.8). They found that the estimated slope $\hat{\beta}_1$ was negative, and that this could not be explained by heterogeneity or random measurement error. They suggested that it could be due to unknown covariates.

2.5.4 Additional Topics

Estimating the Probability of Transmission Per Contact as a Function of Time

The methods outlined in the preceeding sections have been extended to address a number of other situations and questions. Shiboski and Jewell (1992) were concerned with estimating infectivity as a function of time since infection of the index case, $\gamma(t)$. The function $\gamma(t)$, called the infectivity curve, defines the probability of transmission per contact at time t following the infection of the index case. Important questions concern the temporal evolution of the infectivity curve, $\gamma(t)$. Some biological theories suggested that infectivity is highest shortly after the time of seroconversion, and again shortly before the onset of symptoms or AIDS diagnosis. The shape of the infectivity curve has an impact on epidemic growth (Section 9.3). In order to estimate the infectivity curve, information or assumptions are required not only about the total number of contacts that occurred by calendar time T but also about when the contacts occurred. Suppose we are dealing with "long-term partnerships" (Shiboski and Jewell, 1992), that is partnerships in existence at the time of the index case's infection. A simple assumption is that the contacts occur according to a homogeneous Poisson process. Under this assumption the K contacts are distributed uniformly over the interval $[0, T]$. Suppose contacts occur according to a homogeneous Poisson process with constant rate μ. Then, the probability the susceptible partner becomes infected before T time units (time is measured from when the index case became infected) is

$$P(\Upsilon = 1) = 1 - \exp\left\{ -\int_0^T \gamma(t)\mu \, dt, \right\}$$

as shown by Shiboski and Jewell (1992). Parametric models for $\gamma(t)$ could be fit to the data by inserting the above expression in the likelihood function (2.11). Note that if the value assumed for μ is too large, $\gamma(t)$ will be correspondingly underestimated because only the product $\gamma(t) \cdot \mu$ is identifiable. Moreover, the estimate of $\gamma(t)$ depends on the assumption that contacts follow a homogeneous Poisson process. For example, if contacts occur at an increasingly slower rate, perhaps due to onset of symptoms, the assumption of homogeneity may incorrectly suggest declining infectivity. A more general model postulates that contacts occur according to a nonhomogeneous Poisson process with intensity $\mu(t)$, leading to the previous expression for $P(\Upsilon = 1)$ with $\mu(t)$ replacing μ. If $\mu(t)$ was not completely specified, it would be possible to estimate only the product of the infectivity curve and the contact rate, $\mu(t) \cdot \gamma(t)$, because one could not distinguish between declining infectivity and declining contact rates (Shiboski and Jewell, 1992). However, if the shape of $\mu(t)$ were known, the shape of $\gamma(t)$ could be estimated. Even so, if the assumed scale of $\mu(t)$ were incorrect, so would be the estimate of $\gamma(t)$.

Estimating the Probability of Infection per Partnership

In some studies information may be collected on numbers of partners rather than numbers of contacts. In such situations it is not possible to estimate the infectivity per contact, but it may be possible to estimate infectivity per partner. For example, Grant, Wiley, and Winkelstein (1987) analyzed data from the San Francisco Men's Health Study. The study consisted of men who were initially seronegative, and who were followed 6 months for evidence of seroconversion. Data were collected on the numbers of partners each man was exposed to. The statistical model assumed partners were selected at random from a pool in which the probability a partner is infected, f, is known. Then if the ith individual reports n_i partners during the 6-month period, the probability that this individual seroconverted (here we ignore the time lag between infection and seroconversion) is

$$1 - (1 - \gamma_p f)^{n_i},$$

where γ_p is the probability of transmission from an infected partner (i.e., the per partner infectivity). This expression could be substituted for p_i in the Bernoulli likelihood (equation (2.11)). Using this method, Grant, Wiley, and Winkelstein (1987) estimated the infectivity per partner for exposure to unprotected anal sex to be $\gamma_p = .102$ (95% confidence interval $.043 - .160$). These investigators also attempted to glean information about the infectivity per contact by making various assumptions about the number of contacts each individual had with each reported partner. For example, if three contacts per partner are assumed, the estimated infectivity per contact was .0351.

The methods described in Section 2.5.2—2.5.3 are applicable when the susceptible partner is at risk for infection only through contact with the index case. De Gruttola, Seage, Mayer, and Horsburgh (1989) developed statistical methods that are applicable when the susceptible partner is also at risk of infection from a source outside the partnership. An additional parameter is introduced for the probability of infection from a source outside the partnership.

Magder and Brookmeyer (1993) considered the situation in which the partner who was the source of the infection (the index case) is unknown. Suppose both partners are infected and both partners are at risk of infection from sources outside the partnership. Then the direction of transmission is uncertain and, furthermore, the possibility that both partners were infected from sources outside the partnership cannot be ruled out. Madger and Brookmeyer use other covariates such as a history of intravenous drug use or numbers of previous sexual partners to assist in identifying the partner who was the source of infection (index case). The approach requires modelling the probability of infection from outside the partnership and the probability of transmission within the partnership simultaneously. Based on efficiency calculations, Magder and Brookmeyer (1993) conclude that the method will only be successful if one can identify a covariate that is highly predictive of the risk of infection from outside the partnership.

Implications for High Risk Behaviors
Estimates of infectivity are useful for quantifying risks associated with various behaviors. For example, a number of investigators have calculated the probability of infection as a function of numbers of partners and contacts per partner. The motivating question was, "Is it riskier to have more partners with fewer contacts per partner, or, alternatively, fewer partners with correspondingly more contacts per partner?" Assuming constant infectivity as in model (2.5), the probability an individual would be infected after c contacts with each of N partners is

$$p = \sum_{j=0}^{N} P(j \text{ of } N \text{ partners infected}) \ P(\text{infection} | j \text{ partners}$$
infected)

$$= \sum_{j=0}^{N} \binom{N}{j} f^j (1-f)^{N-j} \{1 - (1-\gamma)^{c \cdot j}\}, \tag{2.14}$$

where, as before, f is the probability that a randomly chosen partner is infected. Wiley and Herschkorn (1988) and Eisenberg (1989) show that having n contacts with one partner is less risky (lower probability of becoming infected) than having the same number of contacts but divided among more than one partner. However, surprisingly, if the infectivity γ is low, the number of partners does not significantly effect this risk. Wiley and Herschkorn (1988) suggest that the "perils of promiscuity" emerge as the infectivity increases. However, they caution that these conclusions are based on a model that does not account for heterogeneity in infectivity.

Equation (2.14) can be refined to account for heterogeneity in infectivity. For example, consider a mixture model where a proportion π of partnerships have infectivity 1.0 and the remaining proportion have infectivity 0.0. Then f in equation (2.14) should be replaced by (πf). Under this model, and assuming $f = .10$ and $\pi = .189$, the probability of infection for an individual who had 10 contacts with one partner is .019, compared to .174 for an individual who had one contact with each of 10 partners. Thus the risk associated with large numbers of partners becomes greater when infectivity varies among partnerships (see also Eisenberg, 1991).

2.5.5 Summary

Estimates of infectivity derived from partner studies are uncertain and subject to a number of important sources of error. One source of error is measurement error in the number of contacts between the index case and the susceptible partner. If the exact date of infection of the index case is unknown, it is impossible to precisely estimate the relevant numbers of contacts. Furthermore, considerable uncertainty and complexity is introduced if either the susceptible partner is at risk of infection from another source, or if it is unclear which partner was in fact the index case. A number of crucial assumptions underlie the statistical models used to estimate infectivity. These include assumptions of independence of the chance of transmission across contacts, constancy of infectivity and the form of the models used to account for heterogeneity and temporal evolution in infectivity.

The large uncertainties in infectivity are illustrated by the wide range of estimated transmission probabilities found in various studies and by various methods of analysis and modelling assumptions (Table 2.3). The probability of transmission per partnership is, of course, larger than the probability of transmission from a single contact with an infected partner (Table 2.3). Although precise quantitative estimates of transmission probabilities are unavailable, some qualitative conclusions can be drawn from these data. There is evidence for heterogeneity in infectivity among partnerships. Overall the probability of HIV transmission from a single contact with a randomly selected infected partner is believed to be less than 0.20 and could be as low as .001. Male to female transmission appears to be more efficient than female to male transmission although there is considerable uncertainty in both the per partner and per contact transmission probabilities (Padian, Shiboski, and Jewell, 1991; De Vincenzi, 1992). A number of factors appear to affect heterosexual transmission proba-

Table 2.3 Summary of Some Estimates of Infectivity from Sexual Transmission

I.	Transmission probability from a single contact with an infected partner	
	Heterosexual transmission	
	Male to female (California Partner Study)	$.001^a-.03^b$
	Male to female (Transfusion Partner Study)	$.001^a-.189^b$
	Homosexual transmission	$.008^c-.032^c$
II.	Per partnership transmission probability from a relationship with an infected partner	
	Heterosexual transmission	
	Male to female	$.20^d, .27^e, .28^f$
	Female to male	$.01^d-.12^g$
	Homosexual transmission	
	San Francisco Men's Health Study	$.10^h$

[a]Wiley, Herschkorn, and Padian (1989), assuming constant infectivity model (2.5); see also Jewell and Shiboski (1990).

[b]Wiley, Herschkorn, and Padian (1989), assuming a mixture model.

[c]DeGruttola, Seage, Mayer, and Horsburgh (1989); refers to receptive anal intercourse.

[d]Padian, Shiboski, and Jewell (1991).

[e]European Study Group (1989).

[f]Lazzarin, Saracco, Musicco, Nicolosi, and Italian Study Group on HIV Transmission (1991).

[g]De Vincenzi (1992).

[h]Grant, Wiley, and Winkelstein (1987); refers to receptive anal intercourse.

bilities (see also Section 2.3.4). Condom use reduces risk of transmission substantially. Several studies have demonstrated that severe immunodepression in the male "index case" increases the risk of transmission to a female partner. Other factors, such as anal sex, bleeding during sex, and the presence of genital lesions increase the risk of transmission to female partners. As mentioned in Section 2.3.2, unprotected receptive anal intercourse greatly increases the risk of transmission among homosexual men.

3

Surveys to Determine
Seroprevalence and Seroincidence

3.1 INTRODUCTION

The introduction and licensing of reliable assays to detect HIV in 1985 prompted studies to determine seroprevalence. Some studies used sera stored in previous years, but most studies relied on new samples available in a variety of settings, such as clinics for sexually transmitted diseases. Valuable and comprehensive reviews of such data (CDC, 1987b, 1989a) give detailed references for studies of homosexual and bisexual men, intravenous drug users, patients with hemophilia and other persons known to be at risk. Table 3.1 contains selected seroprevalence data for the major risk groups of homosexual men and intravenous drug users as well as data for female prostitutes and patients with hemophilia. It is clear that seroprevalence rates among gay men increased rapidly in San Francisco and New York in the first half of the 1980s and that seroprevalence rates varied by city. Such geographic variation is even more pronounced for intravenous drug users and female prostitutes. Patients with severe hemophilia A, who required large amounts of clotting factor, tended to seroconvert earlier and in larger proportions than patients with less severe clotting disorders.

Despite the huge variability in these seroprevalence estimates, they provided a completely new perspective on the magnitude of the epidemic. In June of 1986, when 21,517 cases of AIDS had been reported to the CDC, seroprevalence data were used to estimate an HIV prevalence in the United States of between 1 and 1.5 million (Public Health Service, 1986). The shocking disparity between numbers of AIDS cases and estimated HIV prevalence reflects the long

Table 3.1 Selected Seroprevalence Rates (%) in the United States, 1978–86

	1978	1979	1980	1981	1982	1983	1984	1985	1986
Homosexual Men									
New York City						61		65	
Washington, D.C.					53			44	
San Francisco									
Hepatitis B Cohort[a]	0.3	4.1	13.8	28.1	42.4	46.7	48.4	48.8	49.6
Random Sample from High Risk Census tracts[b]					22.8		48.6	49.4	
Boston							21		
Intravenous Drug Users									
New York City					46		68		
New Jersey									
<5 miles from Manhattan							59		
100 miles from Manhattan							2		
Boston							42		
Chicago							11		
San Francisco							9		
New Orleans								1	
Female Prostitutes									
Northern New Jersey									57
Miami									19
Atlanta									1
Hemophilia Patients[c]									
Severe Hemophilia A	0	0	0	12	34	59	68	72	73
Other Clotting Disorders	0	0	0	0	0	10	15	25	29

Notes: Unless noted by letters a, b, or c, these estimates are taken from Goedert and Blattner (1988), who provide primary references. The letters a, b, and c refer respectively to Hessol, Lifson, O'Malley, et al. (1989); Winkelstein, Samuel, Padian, et al. (1987); and Goedert, Kessler, Aledort, et al. (1989).

incubation distribution of HIV infection. This large estimate of HIV prevalence made extrapolated projections of 270,000 cumulative AIDS cases through 1991 seem plausible (Public Health Service, 1986; Morgan and Curran, 1986). Although these estimates of seroprevalence may have been a little high, and although the cumulative AIDS incidence through 1991 turned out to be 206,392 (CDC, 1992a), these initial Public Health Service estimates were remarkably prescient and provided a useful framework for public health planning and allocation of resources.

In addition to providing important information on the magnitude of the epidemic, seroprevalence studies suggested strategies to prevent further infections. For example, the alarming rates of infection among female prostitutes in some locations indicated a need for informing the public, offering testing and counseling services to female prostitutes, and encouraging the use of condoms.

Although data from selected populations such as those in Table 3.1 helped define the magnitude of the HIV epidemic and suggested strategies for prevention, such data are not ideally suited for estimating HIV prevalence in the general U.S. population (Sections 3.3 and 3.4). It is difficult to know if members of a selected population are representative of the general population or even of a subclass of the general population. For example, homosexual males in clinics for the treatment of sexually transmitted diseases, where a selected sample might be obtained (see Table 3.6), may have different HIV prevalence rates from other homosexual males. This problem is called "selection bias." Furthermore, the information on what proportions of the general population correspond to various subclasses, such as homosexual men, is uncertain, which compounds the difficulty of estimating prevalence in the general population from data on subclasses. For these reasons, it is attractive to consider the use of representative sampling methods to try to estimate seroprevalence in the general population.

In principle, a representative survey sample avoids sampling bias and is an ideal approach for estimating seroprevalence in the general population. However, this method depends on being able to identify all members of the population under study in order to set up a rigorous probability sampling plan. In addition, those sampled must agree to provide a specimen for determination of HIV status. In Section 3.2, we discuss representative sampling to estimate HIV prevalence rates in a defined population. Even studies based on representative sampling are subject to potentially serious biases. The most serious bias, "nonresponse bias," occurs when the very people who are most likely to be infected refuse to participate in the study. In Section 3.3 we review efforts to estimate seroprevalence rates in selected populations, and in Section 3.4 we consider methods to combine such estimates to obtain estimates of prevalence for the United States. In many instances, nearly everyone in these selected populations will provide a blood sample, so that nonresponse bias is less an issue, but, as mentioned previously, it is often unclear just how to relate these selected populations to the general population in the United States.

An even more challenging goal is to estimate trends in seroincidence rates (Section 3.5). We discuss how such rates have been estimated for selected cohorts using survival methodology and for other populations by studying a series of cross-sectional seroprevalence surveys.

Because back-calculation (Chapter 8) provides information on the infection curve, it can also be used to estimate seroincidence rates, cumulative numbers infected, and HIV prevalence rates (Rosenberg, Biggar, Goedert, and Gail, 1991; Brookmeyer, 1991; Rosenberg, Gail, and Carroll, 1992). It is helpful to compare seroprevalence estimates obtained by back-calculation with estimates obtained by survey methods, because these two approaches are based on completely independent data sources (Chapters 8 and 10).

3.2 ESTIMATING SEROPREVALENCE RATES FROM REPRESENTATIVE (PROBABILITY-BASED) SAMPLES

3.2.1 Defining the Population and Survey Approach

The best survey strategy depends on the nature of the population for which one desires to estimate HIV prevalence and prevalence rates. One such population might be all persons living in the United States in 1990. Another might be gay men between ages 25 and 54 in 19 defined high-risk census tracts of San Francisco. Another might be all intravenous drug users in California in 1990. A fourth might be all women who had live births in the state of New York in 1990. In order to obtain a representative or exhaustive sample from such populations, one must be able to identify all members of the population and define a sampling mechanism that selects each member of the population with a known probability. Because the blood of practically every newborn in New York State is now assayed for antibodies to HIV (Novick, Glebatis, Stricof, et al., 1991) and because maternal antibodies to HIV are found in the blood of newborns, one has an exhaustive sample of the population of women who had live births. Hence, the seroprevalence rate is known without error in this population, except perhaps for a few technical failures and for minor imperfections in the assay itself.

Winkelstein, Lyman, Padian, et al. (1987) estimated the number of gay men aged 25 to 54, and the HIV seroprevalence among these men, in 19 high-risk census tracts of San Francisco. They sampled residential blocks within each tract, the number of blocks sampled being proportional to tract size, and the probability of block selection proportional to block size. Then they sampled households within blocks, the number of households sampled being inversely proportional to block size. Finally, all single men aged 25 to 54 living in the sampled households were invited to participate in a study to determine their sexual practices and serostatuses. This sampling procedure implied that each single man age 25 to 54 who lived in a household in these 19 census tracts had the same chance to participate in the survey. If all those who were offered the chance to participate had done so, a truly representative sample of responses would have been obtained. However, 645 (36.9%) of the 1750 sampled men refused to participate, and 71 (4.1%) were not studied for other reasons. If the 1034 (59.1%) men who did participate were nonrepresentative of the 1750 who were sampled, estimates of the proportions engaging in various homosexual practices and estimates of the seroprevalence among gay men could be biased. Such bias is termed *nonresponse bias*, because it arises when the nonrespondents have different measured characteristics from the respondents.

It is hard to obtain a representative sample of intravenous drug users in California because one does not know how to identify and contact them. Some are in prison. Some have no fixed address. If one took a representative sample of people living in households and asked them to identify themselves as drug users or not, it is likely that many would give false information. Thus it is difficult to set up a procedure to obtain a representative probability-based sample for this population. Instead, one usually studies selected subpopulations, such as intravenous drug users in treatment programs, and tries to use data from such selected subpopulations to make informed judgements about what the rates might be in the general population of intravenous drug users (Section 3.3).

To estimate HIV prevalence in the United States, one could imagine obtaining a representative sample, but the issue of nonresponse bias and other problems reduce the attractiveness of this approach. We discuss these issues in connection with a representative survey conducted in Dallas between September and December of 1989 (CDC,

1991a). Partly on the basis of this pilot study, officials at the Centers for Disease Control decided not to attempt to obtain a representative sample from the United States at present (CDC, 1991a).

Instead, as described in Section 3.3, survey estimates for the United States have been obtained by dividing the entire population into exclusive and exhaustive strata. Samples in selected subpopulations are used to estimate seroprevalence rates in these strata, and the HIV prevalence in the entire United States is estimated as a sum over strata of the product of the number of persons in each stratum times the corresponding estimated seroprevalence rate (Section 3.4). Some of the difficulties of interpreting these data are indicated in Section 3.4.

To summarize, the choice of the target population for which seroprevalence estimates are required is an important determinant of the survey strategy. If members of the population can be identified and contacted, a rigorous procedure for representative probability-based sampling can often be developed. Although such representative sampling is ideal in principle, one may face uncertainties from nonresponse bias and other difficulties (Section 3.2.2). If it is hard to identify or contact the members of the target population, or if it is thought that available adjustment procedures cannot adequately control for nonresponse bias, one may be forced to abandon the representative sampling approach. An alternative approach is to base estimates on samples from selected subpopulations and stratification techniques (Section 3.4). However, these latter estimates are not protected by random sampling from the target population and are subject to selection biases of unknown magnitude.

3.2.2 General Problems in Estimating Seroprevalence in the United States by Representative Sampling

Public health officials began studies to determine the feasibility and reliability of a representative survey to estimate seroprevalence in the United States in late 1987. A pilot study to test survey methods was planned for July 1988 in Washington, D.C. However, opposition by community leaders and District of Columbia public health officials caused the cancellation of this pilot study. In a second attempt, officials from the National Center for Health Statistics worked closely with community leaders and public health officials in Allegheny County, Pennsylvania, where a pilot household survey was carried out in January 1989. In this survey, 263 (85%) of 308 eligible persons provided questionnaire data and a blood sample. This result encouraged officials to carry out a larger "pretest" survey in Dallas, in final preparation for a national survey.

These experiences demonstrated the importance of obtaining the cooperation of local officials and the public in order to carry out a survey on sensitive issues related to HIV disease. In addition, public health officials identified four potential sources of bias that could affect the pretest survey in Dallas and the subsequent national survey (Massey, Ezzati, and Folsom, 1989). We discuss these potential biases for a survey design like that used in the Dallas "pretest."

Coverage Bias

The survey is based on sampling households. Therefore, individuals who are institutionalized for crimes, drug treatment or mental illness and homeless persons are not represented. Thus, the survey suffers from *coverage bias* if the aim is to estimate HIV prevalence among all people in the target population, including those who do not live in households. The major impact of undercoverage is on intravenous drug users (IVDUs). If, for example, only half of IVDUs are covered by the household survey, and if IVDUs constitute 25% of all persons with HIV infection, the coverage bias would amount to $0.25 \times 0.5 \times 100 = 12.5\%$.

Assay Errors

The HIV assay with Western blot confirmation is very reliable (Chapter 6). Assuming a sensitivity of 0.92, a specificity of 0.9999, and an HIV prevalence rate of 0.005, the probability of a positive test result is $0.005 \times 0.92 + 0.995 \times (1 - 0.9999) = 0.0046 + 0.0001 = 0.0047$. Thus the net effect of *assay errors* would be to underestimate HIV prevalence by $100 \times (0.0050 - 0.0047) = 0.03\%$, which is 6% of the true prevalence in this example.

False Information about Risk Behaviors

If all sampled persons gave a blood sample, there would be no need to inquire about risk behaviors in order to estimate HIV prevalence. An important motivation for gathering information on risk behavior, in addition to its value for understanding how HIV infection spreads (Chapter 9), is to try to impute the missing HIV serostatus of those sampled individuals who refuse to provide a blood sample. If persons who refuse to provide blood often falsely deny behaviors that put them at high risk of HIV infection, such as male-to-male sex or use of intravenous drugs, this approach to imputing HIV prevalence may lead to serious underestimates of prevalence.

Nonresponse Bias

The major problem facing this survey is nonresponse bias, which arises when the true seroprevalence in the sampled individuals differs from that of those sampled individuals who do not provide blood, the nonrespondents. Suppose that a fraction, f, refuse to provide blood, that π_1 is the seroprevalence among responders and that $\pi_0 = \rho\pi_1$ is the seroprevalence among nonresponders. The quantity ρ is the relative risk of seropositivity of nonresponders compared to responders. Then the seroprevalence in the entire population is

$$\pi = (1 - f)\pi_1 + f\pi_1\rho, \tag{3.1}$$

and the ratio of true seroprevalence to that in respondents is

$$\pi/\pi_1 = \{1 + f(\rho - 1)\}. \tag{3.2}$$

Note that this ratio is one if everyone responds ($f = 0$) or if $\rho = 1$. The condition $\rho = 1$ means that nonresponders and responders have the same seroprevalence rates so that respondents are representative of the entire population.

Hull, Bettinger, Gallaher, et al. (1988) studied nonresponse bias among patients in a New Mexico clinic for sexually transmitted diseases. These patients were invited to be tested for HIV under conditions of anonymity. The patient could obtain his or her result by calling the clinic one week later and giving an identification number. Persons who were HIV positive were asked to return to the clinic, where their serostatus would be revealed and counseling offered. The investigators also tested previously stored sera used for syphilis assays to determine the HIV serostatus of those who refused to be tested. These latter tests were performed in a blinded manner so that test results could not be identified with particular patients. Nonresponse rates, f, for men were small (Table 3.2), but the relative risk ρ was 8.8 for black and Hispanic men, 7.4 for homosexual men, 5.3 for all men and 2.7 for white men. The corresponding ratios of true prevalence to prevalence among respondents were 2.63, 2.02, 1.75 and 1.22. In particular, the true prevalence rate for all men was 1.75 times the rate observed in male respondents to the survey. It is noteworthy that even among admitted homosexual men, nonrespondents had a much higher seroprevalence than respondents. Possibly, nonresponding homosexual men tended to engage in very risky behaviors, such as receptive anal intercourse, in greater proportions than responders. Possibly some nonresponders who already knew they were symptomatic or HIV-positive refused testing. If similar differences obtained among nonre-

Table 3.2 Nonresponse Bias Among Men in a New Mexico Clinic for Sexually Transmitted Diseases

	Patients Accepting Testing HIV+/Total Tested (%)	Patients Refusing Testing HIV+/Total Tested (%)	Nonresponse Rate (f)	Relative Risk of Infection (ρ)	Ratio of Population Prevalence to Prevalence in Responders (π/π_1)
All	8/782 (1.02)	9/167 (5.39)	.177	5.26	1.75
Homosexual men	5/90 (5.56)	7/17 (41.2)	.159	7.41	2.02
White men	5/338 (1.48)	2/50 (4.0)	.129	2.70	1.22
Hispanic and black men	3/430 (0.70)	7/114 (6.14)	.210	8.80	2.63

Source: Based on data in Hull, Bettinger, Gallaher, et al. (1988).

spondents and respondents in the Dallas pretest survey or the national survey, nonresponse bias would dominate the sources of error.

Several strategies are used to minimize nonresponse bias, as discussed for the Dallas pretest survey (Section 3.2.3). First, every effort is made to encourage participation and prevent nonresponse. Second, nonrespondents are approached repeatedly to obtain the needed information and blood samples. However, there may be restrictions on how vigorously one can pursue such data from nonrespondents. Finally, one can attempt to impute the serostatus of nonresponders who never provided a blood sample. Using data from responders, one first constructs a model that predicts the probability of being seropositive conditional on a set of demographic variables, risk factors and other covariates. One then applies such models to nonrespondents to impute their serostatus. The basic assumptions in this procedure are: (1) conditional on available covariates, the nonrespondents have the same probability of being seropositive as the respondents, and (2) the probability model is valid for responders. Both of these assumptions are questionable, and failure of these assumptions may lead to incomplete corrections for nonresponse bias. If these adjustment procedures fail to correct fully for nonresponse bias, there is said to be "residual nonresponse bias."

3.2.3 The Dallas "Pretest" Survey

The target population for the Dallas household survey included all people in Dallas County who lived in identifiable housing units and who were between the ages of 18 and 54. The estimated target population had 954,423 people, of whom about 267,000 were married men, 203,000 were unmarried men, 286,000 were married women and 199,000 were unmarried women (Research Triangle Institute, 1990). The basic survey strategy was to oversample households in census blocks where HIV prevalence was thought to be high or medium (Table 3.3). Classification of census blocks into high, medium or low risk geographic strata was based on AIDS incidence rates, syphilis rates and other factors (Massey, Ezzati, and Folsom, 1990). Within each geographic stratum, household sampling was balanced so as to have the same racial composition as for Dallas County as a whole.

Only 15 seropositive samples were detected among 1374 individuals who gave blood (Table 3.3). An estimate of the prevalence in the entire population is obtained by weighting the stratum-specific prevalence rates by the fractions that each stratum represents in the entire population. This estimate is $2.558 \times 0.0773 + 0.916 \times 0.2165 + 0 \times 0.7062 = 0.396\%$. In a population of 954,443, this corresponds

Table 3.3 Dallas Survey Data Within Geographic Risk Strata

Geographic Strata	Identified Eligibles[a]	Provided Blood and Questionnaire[a]	Number HIV+	Percent HIV+	Distribution of Risk Strata in the Population (%)
High risk	480	391	10	2.558	7.73
Medium risk	676	546	5	0.916	21.65
Low risk	568	437	0	0.000	70.62
Total	1724	1374			100.0

Percent of eligibles with blood and questionnaire data   79.7%

Note: Population HIV prevalence (%) from the sum of products in last two columns is 0.396%
[a]Derived from exhibits 4.4 and 4.5 in Research Triangle Institute (1990).

to 3780 infections. Note, however, that $1374/1724 = 79.7\%$ of eligible subjects provided blood. If the remaining 20.3% had higher HIV prevalence, the estimate of 0.396% prevalence would be too low. There was, in fact, further potential for nonresponse bias, because of 2141 occupied houses in the original sample, only 2061 (96%) were allowed to be screened to identify eligible subjects.

The first strategy used to reduce nonresponse bias was to try to minimize nonresponse rates by careful training of interviewers, enlisting the support of community leaders, offering $50 for participation, and providing strict assurances of anonymity. Nonetheless, 4% of sampled household units were not allowed to be screened for eligible subjects, and 22% of the identified eligibles did not provide blood initially.

A second strategy was to try to obtain questionnaire data and blood from initial nonrespondents. However, community leaders would not allow every nonrespondent to be recontacted. Instead, a sample of 175 nonrespondents was recontacted. Of these, 87 were offered $100 to provide questionnaire data only, and 88 were offered $175 to provide both questionnaire data and blood. Twenty-three of those recontacted provided blood and questionnaire data, and 64 provided questionnaire data only. This recontact survey was called the Quality Assessment Study (QAS), and QAS data are included in Table 3.3. Thus the 20.3% of nonresponders in Table 3.3 included $88 - 23 = 65$ people who would not give blood even when recontacted and offered $175.

There is reason to believe that nonresponders have higher seroprevalence rates than responders. For example, 8.42% of never-married men who responded to the initial questionnaire reported having had male-to-male sex since 1978, compared to 46.71% of initially nonrespondent men who provided QAS questionnaire data (exhibit 4.17, Research Triangle Institute, 1990). There are two reasons why the relative risk for infection among never married men may be even higher than the relative risk for male-to-male sex, $.4671/0.0842 = 5.5$. First, those who refused to provide QAS data ("ultimate nonresponders") may have higher proportions engaging in male-to-male sex. Second, nonrespondents who report homosexual behavior may have higher seroprevalence rates than respondents who report homosexual behavior, as was found in the study (Table 3.2) of Hull, Bettinger, Gallagher, et al. (1988). Similarly, 2.83% of men admitted using intravenous drugs since 1978 on the initial survey, compared to 12.25% on the QAS survey (exhibit 4.15, Research Triangle Institute, 1990).

The previous calculation of 0.396% infected is partly adjusted for nonresponse bias because nonresponders in the high risk geographic stratum are assumed to have a seroprevalence of 2.488%, whereas nonresponders in the low-risk stratum are assumed to have a seroprevalence of 0.000%. Nonetheless, there is every reason to suspect residual nonresponse bias. For example, even conditional on being in the high risk geographic stratum, it is likely that nonresponders have a higher seroprevalence than responders.

A more elaborate "fully adjusted" correction for nonresponse bias was carried out as described by Horvitz, Folsom, Ezzati and Massey (1992). Those investigators assume that nonresponse is ignorable among women, perhaps because earlier adjustments for women produced minimal changes in prevalence estimates (Massey, Ezzati, and Folsom, 1990). Of 845 sampled males, 91 provided neither data on risk factors nor blood specimens, either in the initial survey or in the QAS survey. For these 91 males, a risk factor category was first imputed, and then, conditional on that category, a probability of being HIV-positive was imputed. For 36 other sampled males who had provided questionnaire data but no blood specimens, it was only necessary to impute HIV status.

Risk behaviors for males age 18 to 54 were classified into eight nonbaseline risk categories and one baseline category (Table 3.4). The nonbaseline categories included 12 of the 13 HIV-positive men in the survey. Logistic regression was used to estimate the probability that an individual fell into one of these nine risk categories, based on the following independent variables: age, race, sex, marital status, geographic stratum (high, medium or low risk), mention of survey information sources, mention of objections to the survey, and attitude toward the QAS survey. This logistic model was estimated from the 754 males who had completed the questionnaire. Then the model was used to assign probabilities that nonrespondents belonged to particular risk categories, leading to imputed estimates of numbers of nonrespondents in each category (Table 3.4). Of the 64,868 persons who are estimated to be nonresponders in a hypothetical complete census of all 469,409 males age 18 to 24 in Dallas County, 48,192 are imputed to have no risk factors (Table 3.4).

It was assumed that any male who had not provided blood and who did not fall into one of the eight nonbaseline risk categories in Table 3.4 was seronegative. The probability of being seropositive was computed from a logistic model based on the number of male partners since 1978, receptive anal intercourse, and the use of intravenous drugs since 1978. This model was obtained by analyzing data from the 86 males with blood samples who had at least one of the nonbaseline risk factor

Table 3.4 Estimated Sizes of Risk Groups and "Fully Adjusted" HIV Prevalence Rates in Dallas County, Classified by Responses to the Initial Survey and QAS Survey

Risk Group	Receptive Anal Sex	Number of Male Partners	IVDU	Initial Respondents (Male) Population Size[a]	% HIV+[a]	QAS-Respondents (Male) Population Size[a]	% HIV+	Nonrespondents (Male) Population Size[a]	% HIV+[a]	Dallas County Population Size[a]	Number HIV+[a]
1	Yes	10+	No	3646	33.05	1078	18.81	2776	24.82	7500	2097
1	Yes	5–9	Yes	168	0.00	0	0.00	0	0.00	158	0
3	Yes	5–9	No	951	9.43	3987	11.50	1187	11.50	6125	684
4	Yes	1–4	No	4831	3.89	140	4.86	803	4.86	5774	234
5	No	10+	No	1145	0.00	0	0.00	473	3.17	1618	15
6	No	1–4	Yes	1595	0.00	0	0.00	71	2.67	1666	2
7	No	1–4	No	5786	0.00	2505	0.50	6140	0.50	14,431	43
8	No	0	Yes	10,238	2.46	6425	0.74	5226	1.07	21,889	356
9	No	0	No	333,217	0.00	28,829	0.00	48,192	0.00	410,238	0
Total males age 18–54				361,577		42,964		64,868		469,409	
HIV prevalence rate (%)					0.48		0.17		1.49		0.73
Females age 18–54 (615 infected)										485,014	0.127
Total population										954,423	0.42
Number infected										4047	
95% confidence-interval on number infected										2200–7500	

[a]Imputed as described in Section 3.2.3 and by Horvitz, Folsom, Ezzati, and Massey (1992).

combinations in Table 3.4. Of these 86 men, 12 were seropositive. Summing probability-weighted individual estimates of the probability of HIV infection yielded estimated numbers of nonrespondents who were infected in each risk category and, hence, model-based seroprevalence rates, not only for respondents, but also for nonrespondents (Table 3.4). In some categories, the imputed seroprevalence rate is higher among nonrespondents than initial respondents and QAS respondents, but, surprisingly, the seroprevalence rate for nonrespondent males in the first category was 24.82%, which is less than found among initial respondents, 33.05%. The overall imputed seroprevalence rate is 1.49% for nonrespondents, compared to 0.48% for initial respondents and 0.17% for QAS respondents.

This imputation procedure yielded a "fully adjusted" prevalence rate of 0.42% for the entire population (Table 3.4). The corresponding number infected was 4047, with 95% confidence interval 2200–7500. This "fully adjusted" value is only slightly higher than the prevalence rate 0.396% obtained from geographic risk stratum specific rates (Table 3.3).

There are several reasons to suspect that the procedures used to produce Table 3.4 may have failed to account for nonresponse bias completely. First, even conditional on factors such as age, race and sex used to model the chance of a given risk behavior, the "ultimate nonresponders" who failed to provide QAS questionnaire data and the nonresponders who were never recontacted probably had higher proportions with various risk behaviors than responders. Yet responders were used to model the probability of falling into a given risk category. Second, even conditional on risk behavior category, it is likely that those who failed to provide blood, including the $88 - 23 = 65$ QAS "ultimate nonresponders," have higher seroprevalence rates than those who provided blood, just as in Table 3.2. Thus, even if the logistic model correctly describes the probability of HIV infection given risk behaviors among those who provided blood, it may not do so among those who did not provide blood. Third, it is questionable whether that logistic model is reliable even for describing risk of infection among those who provided blood, because it is based on only 12 seropositive males. The results in Table 3.4 also seem anomalous because the estimated seroprevalence among QAS responders, 0.17%, is less than among initial responders, 0.48%, and the estimated rate among nonresponders, 1.49% is only $\rho = 1.49/0.48 = 3.1$ times that in initial responders. Finally, by the end of 1989, about 1/58th of all AIDS cases in the United States had been reported from Dallas. If the epidemic in Dallas was typical, then a "fully adjusted" estimate of 4047 cases infected in Dallas would correspond to $4047 \times 58 = 234,700$ infections nationally, which is much smaller than national estimates based on selected surveys (Section 3.4) and back-calculation (Chapter 8).

For these reasons, we present a sensitivity analysis to explore plausible ranges of nonresponse bias (Table 3.5). We consider a range of relative risk factors ρ in equation 3.2 that seem to be consistent with data presented in the National Household Seroprevalence Survey Feasibility Study Final Report, Volume 1 (Research Triangle Institute, 1990) and with data in Table 3.2. Unfortunately, because we have no definite information on nonresponders, it does not seem appropriate to restrict the range of ρ to smaller values. We also consider the possibly that the seroprevalence in the low risk geographic stratum was 0.1% or 0.2%. These possibilities are quite consistent with chance, because if the true rate were 0.2%, the chance of observing no seropositives among the 437 members of the low risk stratum (Table 3.3) would be approximately $\exp(-437 \times 0.002) = 0.42$. Even moderate relative risks of $\rho = 5$ are consistent with 7000 to 9000 infections, and higher numbers infected are also plausible (Table 3.5).

It might be objected that women are not subject to nonresponse bias, even though a similar fraction of eligible women failed to give blood (14%) as men (18%) (Exhibit 4.5, Research Triangle Institute, 1990). However, because only 2 of the 15 seropositive results occurred among women, the results in Table 3.5 would be little reduced by assuming women were not subject to nonresponse bias.

Results like those in Table 3.5 are also subject to random variation. Confidence intervals were obtained by Horvitz, Folsom, Ezzati, and Massey (1992) from design weights. If we apply the same ratios of

Table 3.5 Sensitivity Analysis to Account for Potential Nonresponse Bias on the Estimated Number infected in Dallas

Assumed Prevalence in the Low Risk Geographic Stratum	ρ			
	1	2	5	10
0.000	3780	4547	6848	10,685
0.001	4457	5362	8076	12,600
0.002	5125	6166	9287	14,489

Note: The quantity ρ is the relative risk of infection in nonresponders, compared to responders, used in equation (3.2). The table assumes a nonresponse rate $f = 0.203$ in equation (3.2). In that equation, the prevalence rates in responders $\pi_1 = 0.396\%$, 0.467%, and 0.537% correspond respectively to the assumptions that seroprevalence in the low risk stratum in Table 3.3 is 0.0%, 0.1% and 0.2%.

confidence interval limits to estimated values as in Table 3.4, we get a rough idea of stochastic uncertainty. For example, this procedure puts a 95% confidence interval of (4400—15,100) about the estimate 8076 in Table 3.5. The sensitivity analysis therefore indicates that the survey is consistent with substantially more infections than the "fully adjusted" confidence interval of 2200—7500.

Rosenberg, Gail and Massey (1992) estimated the number alive and infected in Dallas County on January 1, 1990, by back-calculation (Chapter 8). One back-calculation procedure employed AIDS incidence data only through mid-1987, before zidovudine was in wide use. The back-calculated "plausible range," which takes uncertainty in the incubation distribution into account, was 7500—14,600 infected. A second back-calculation method used AIDS incidence data through 1990 and took treatment and changes in the AIDS surveillance definition into account. Rosenberg, Gail and Carroll (1992) describe the model used. This method yielded a plausible range of 7500—20,000 infected. Both these results are substantially higher than the "fully adjusted" range 2200—7500 found from the survey (Table 3.4). The back-calculated estimates might be upwardly biased if the incubation distributions used were too slow or if the infection curve was decreasing rapidly between 1986 and 1990 (see Rosenberg, Gail, and Pee, 1991 and Chapter 8). On the other hand, the "fully adjusted" survey estimate may be too small if there is residual nonresponse bias (Table 3.5). For these reasons, Rosenberg, Gail, and Massey (1992) concluded that an intermediate range of 6000—11,000 infected, was reasonable and consistent both with the survey information and with back-calculation.

Partly because of these uncertainties associated with nonresponse bias, it was decided not to attempt a national representative survey to estimate HIV seroprevalence at present (CDC, 1991a). Instead, resources were used to support a family of surveys in selected populations (Section 3.3). It can be argued that the procedures used to adjust for nonresponse bias in the Dallas pretest survey, such as those leading to Table 3.4, would perform better in the national survey, because much more data would be available to estimate the imputation models. Other ways to strengthen such a survey have been described (Research Triangle Institute, 1990, Chapter 6).

3.2.4 Group Testing to Preserve Anonymity

Gastwirth and Hammick (1990) proposed that blood samples be pooled into batches before assaying so as to increase the confidence of study subjects that their HIV serostatus would remain anonymous. Presumably, increasing subjects' confidence in anonymity through group testing would increase participation rates, though this concept has not been verified empirically. The proposal also has cost advantages, because only those batches that are screened as positive with relatively inexpensive enzyme immunoassays (Chapter 6) need be confirmed using more expensive procedures like the Western blot.

The maximum likelihood estimate of prevalence with groups of size $k = 10$ has high statistical efficiency, compared to testing individuals ($k = 1$), provided the prevalence is low. For prevalences 0.1%, 1%, 5%, and 20%, the ratios of the variance of the estimate based on individual testing to the variance based on batch testing are 99.7%, 98.1%, 88.0%, and 50.4%, respectively (table 1, Gastwirth and Hammick, 1989). Thus, group testing would be highly efficient in a general population like Dallas County, where prevalence rates are well below 5% (Table 3.3). However, statistical efficiency would be lost by group testing homosexual men in a clinic for sexually transmitted diseases, where prevalences are higher (Table 3.1).

This design has not been used in seroprevalence surveys. There might be practical problems in deciding which specimens will be batched together and in convincing a subject in a particular household that his or her blood will, in fact, be pooled with other bloods. Most representative surveys employ multistage cluster samples. The theory in Gastwirth and Hammick (1989), which was based on simple random sampling, would need to be extended to account for clustering.

Group testing has also been proposed as a way to reduce screening costs in settings where anonymity is not desired (see Section 6.3).

3.2.5 Randomized Response Design

Randomized response (Warner, 1965) is a sampling procedure designed to yield unbiased estimates of the proportion of a group of people with a given sensitive characteristic, without ever knowing precisely whether that characteristic was present in any particular individual. This procedure was proposed as a possible means to determine what proportion of persons falsely denied risk behaviors for HIV infection (Massey, Ezatti, and Folsom, 1989). The subject would flip two coins and hide the outcomes. If one coin came up "heads" and the other "tails," the subject would truthfully answer the question: "Have you falsely denied being gay, bisexual or injecting street drugs?" If both coins were "heads," the subject would say "yes"; if both coins were "tails," the subject would say "no." If subjects followed these rules, the probability of a false denial of risk behavior, p, could be estimated, because the probability of answering "yes" would be $0.5p + 0.25$. Yet the interviewer would not know whether any particular subject had answered the sensitive question.

Perhaps because this design requires that subjects be somewhat sophisticated, willing to play the game, and willing to provide the true answer when a "head" and "tail" are observed, the procedure was not attempted in Dallas County.

3.3 SURVEYS OF SELECTED SUBPOPULATIONS

Staff at the Centers for Disease Control, other federal agencies, state and local health departments, and a variety of private health organizations are carrying out seroprevalence surveys and monitoring trends in a number of special subpopulations (Table 3.6). In 1987, staff from the Centers for Disease Control initiated joint programs to coordinate and standardize data collection methods, assay methods and data management and analysis methods among the various participating agencies (Pappaioanou, Dondero, Petersen, et al., 1990). The resulting surveys in Table 3.6 are known as the "family of HIV seroprevalence surveys." Ongoing surveys of populations 1, 2, 3, 4, and 5 in Table 3.6 were established in 46 metropolitan areas throughout the Unite States and territories, and the serostatus of newborns is being monitored in 44 states and territories. The aims of this program are to guide prevention and control activities by studying HIV prevalence trends and levels in various populations and to obtain some information useful for estimating national seroprevalence rates.

Blinded, anonymous testing of blood from all participants is used in most of these surveys, so there is little potential for nonresponse bias. Even in clinics that provide voluntary confidential testing to facilitate counseling, blood is drawn for anonymous testing. Therefore, some persons at high risk may avoid such clinics. Also, blood donors and applicants for military service are advised that their blood will be screened. It is thought that persons at high risk for infection tend not to donate blood or apply for military service ("self-deferral"). The degree of such selection bias is hard to quantify. The potential for selection bias is present in every component of the family of surveys. Even the nearly exhaustive sampling of blood from newborns does not preclude selection bias for estimating seroprevalence in women of childbearing age, because the probability of having a live birth may be related to HIV infection status.

People at clinics for sexually transmitted diseases (STD), people in

Table 3.6 Sentinel Populations in the Family of HIV Seroprevalence Surveys

Type of Population	Point of Access	Risk of Exposure to HIV
1. Persons with sexually transmitted disease (STD): homosexual men males without other risk females without other risk	State and local STD clinics	increased
2. IVDUs	Drug treatment centers	increased
3. Persons treated for tuberculosis (TB)	State and local tuberculosis clinics	increased
4. Women seeking family planning, prenatal care and abortion services	Clinics	all levels
5. Hospital patients admitted for non HIV related conditions	Hospitals	all levels
6. Primary care patients	Centralized clinical laboratories throughout U.S.	all levels
7. Primary care patients	Network of 242 primary care physicians	all levels
8. Childbearing women	Neonatal screening programs	all levels
9. American and Alaskan Natives	Indian Health Service clinics	
10. Job Corps entrants	Dept. of Labor screening program	all levels
11. University students	University health clinics	all levels
12. Prisoners	Prisons and jails	all levels
13. Homeless persons	Health clinics	all levels
14. Civilian applicants for military service	Dept. of Defense screening program	reduced by self-deferral
15. Blood donors	Blood collection agencies	reduced by self-deferral

[a]The range refers to the range of the median values over metropolitan areas unless otherwise indicated.

[b]CDC (1991b).

[c]St. Louis, Rauch, Petersen, et al. (1990).

[d]Gwinn, Pappaioanou, George, et al. (1991).

[e]St. Louis, Conway, Hayman, et al. (1991).

[f]Gayle, Keeling, Garcia-Tunon, et al. (1990).

[g]CDC (1989a).

[h]Department of Defense (1992). Data through March, 1992.

Table 3.6 (Continued)

Number of Metropolitan Areas	Number of Clinics	Seroprevalence (%)		References
		Median	Range[a]	
34	95	3.2	15–61	b
43	104	1.1	0.3–6.5	b
43	104	0.7	0.0–11	b
40	61	3.9	0.0–44	b
18	35	5.9	0.4–36	b
38	146	0.2	0.0–1.7	b
21	26	0.7	0.1–7.8	c
39 states/territories		0.07	0.0–0.58	d
52 states/territories		0.23	0.0–1.11	e
9 universities		0.0	0.0–0.9	f
16 populations with compulsory tests		0.8	0.0–17	g
52 states/territories		Black males 0.37; Hispanic males 0.18; White males 0.05; Black females 0.14; Hispanic females 0.09; White females 0.02		h
50 Red Cross Centers		Males 0.04; Females 0.01		b

treatment for drug abuse, and people in treatment for tuberculosis are at high risk of HIV infection (Table 3.6).

Categories 4–13 in Table 3.6 represent populations at all levels of risk. For example, the seroprevalence in newborns ranges from 0.00% to 0.58% among 39 states (Table 3.6), and within Massachusetts, levels range from 0.8% for inner-city hospitals to 0.09% for suburban and rural hospitals (Hoff, Berardi, Weiblen, et al., 1988). Tremendous variation is also seen among women in clinics for family planning and prenatal care, among patients being treated for non-HIV related illness in "sentinel" hospitals, in prison populations, and among university students (Table 3.6).

The armed forces have been screening civilian applicants since 1985 (Brundage, Burke, Gardner, et al., 1990). Overall seroprevalence rates have declined gradually from about 0.15% in 1986 to 0.11% in 1989 to 0.07% in 1991 (Department of Defense, 1992). These rates are much higher in urban areas of the Northeast, and, as of March 1992, about 2.1 times higher in men than women. The ratio of rates for black, Hispanic, and non-Hispanic white groups is 6.9 : 3.4 : 1.0 for men and 7.1 : 4.6 : 1.0 for women. Such racial differences have been seen in other populations (table 10, CDC, 1989a). Seroprevalence increases almost linearly with age from 16 to 30 among military applicants. Increasing prevalence with age is also found in sentinel hospitals and patients at STD clinics (figure 8, CDC, 1987b). It is thought that homosexual men and intravenous drug users are aware of the military's screening program and often decide not to apply. Such "self-deferral" would tend to make prevalence rates lower in military applicants than in age and race-matched populations from the same geographic regions.

Active programs to discourage persons at elevated risk of HIV infection from donating blood (Chapter 6) also increase self-deferral and account for the very low seroprevalences among blood donors (Table 3.6).

3.4. ESTIMATING NATIONAL SEROPREVALENCE FROM SURVEYS OF SELECTED SUBPOPULATIONS

Stratification is used to estimate national seroprevalence from surveys in selected subpopulations. The entire population is stratified into mutually exclusive and exhaustive subpopulations ($i = 1, 2, \ldots I$), and the prevalence rate, p_i, in each subpopulation is estimated from a variety of surveys of members of that subpopulation. However, in most cases it is not possible to obtain a representative probability-based sample of the subpopulation of interest. If the size of each subpopulation, n_i, is known, the national prevalence is

$$T = \sum_{i=1}^{I} n_i p_i, \tag{3.3}$$

and the national prevalence rate is $P = T/N$, where $N = \Sigma_{i=1}^{I} n_i$.

The Public Health Service (1986) used this method to estimate that 1–1.5 million people were infected in June 1986 (Table 3.7), at a time when only 21,517 cases of AIDS had been reported. Such an estimate is subject to considerable uncertainty. First, estimated prevalence rates in a given selected population are subject to selection bias. Second, there is enormous variability in prevalence rates for a given subpopulation from one sample to the next (Section 3.3). Thus it is not clear what estimate of p_i to use. Third, it is not clear exactly how to define relevant subpopulations. For example, it is difficult to define risky homosexual behavior and to estimate the size of the homosexual risk groups. The extimates of n_i in Table 3.7 were based on studies of male sexual behavior published by Kinsey, Pomeroy, and Martin (1948), which may be outdated. Estimates of the numbers of intravenous drug abusers are also uncertain, despite national surveys and innovative capture-recapture studies used to estimate the prevalence of drug abuse (Woodward, Bonett, and Brecht, 1985). Finally, in 1986, there was very little information on other risk groups. For these reasons, the

Table 3.7 Public Health Service Estimates of HIV Prevalence in the United States, 1986

Subpopulation	Estimated Size	Estimated Prevalence Rate (%)	Estimated Number Infected
Exclusively homosexual	2.5×10^6	15–20	375,000–500,000
Other homosexual contact	$2.5–7.5 \times 10^6$	10	250,000–750,000
Weekly IVDU	7.5×10^6	30	225,000
Less frequent IV drug use	7.5×10^5	10	75,000
Persons with hemophilia	1.4×10^4	70	10,000
Other Groups (transfusion, infants, other heterosexuals)	not available	not available	not available
Total			935,000–1,560,000
Rounded total with allowance for other groups			1,000,000–1,500,000

Note: Adapted from table 13 in CDC (1987b).

estimated HIV prevalence is uncertain. The broad range in Table 3.7 reflects uncertainty in the prevalence rate for exclusively homosexual men and uncertainty in the number of men who engage in occasional male-to-male sex.

A reevaluation of the breakdown in Table 3.7 (Table 14 in CDC, 1987b) yielded a slightly smaller estimate of 945,000–1,402,000 infected. The subpopulation totals were: exclusively homosexual men ($5.00-6.25 \times 10^5$), other homosexual contact ($1.25 - 3.75 \times 10^5$), weekly IVDU (2.25×10^5), occasional IV drug user (10^4), persons with hemophilia (10^4), heterosexuals without specified risk factors ($142 \times 10^6 \times 0.021\% = 3 \times 10^4$), and other groups, such as heterosexual partners of persons at high risk, heterosexuals from Haiti and central Africa, and transfusion recipients ($0.45 - 1.27 \times 10^5$).

Another type of stratification is based on age, sex, and race. If age, race, and sex-specific HIV prevalence rates, p_i, were available, these could be combined to estimate national prevalence from equation (3.3), where n_i would be the number of people in a given age, race and sex stratum.

There are two main difficulties in using data from the family of surveys (Table 3.6) to obtain such estimates. First, because of potential selection bias it is not clear just how the rates found in a particular type of survey relate to the corresponding age, sex, and race-specific rates in the general population of the United States. For example, even though efforts are made to exclude people with HIV-related illnesses from the survey in sentinel hospitals, stratum-specific rates from such a survey are probably higher than corresponding national rates (Dondero, St. Louis, Petersen, et al., 1989). It is not possible to quantify such selection biases at present. A second difficulty is that various surveys cover only limited age, race or sex ranges, and, in some surveys, protection of anonymity requires that race information not be collected.

Dondero, St. Louis, Petersen, et al. (1989) proposed a technique to extrapolate national rates from a limited range of age, sex, and race-specific seroprevalence rates. For example, civilian applicants to the military are between ages 17 and 35. Using age and race-specific seroprevalence rates from civilian applicants, and weighting these rates in proportion to their numbers in the U.S. population, Dondero, St. Louis, and Petersen (1989) calculated U.S. prevalence rates of 0.27% for males and 0.07% for females in the age range 15–34. They also estimated the corresponding numbers infected in this age range for each sex in the United States. For example, about 27,000 women were estimated as infected. From data in sentinel hospitals, they determined that 6.7% of all HIV infections occur in women aged 15 to 34, a number very close to the proportion of all AIDS cases that occur in women aged 15 to 34. National estimates for all infections were therefore estimated from the data on female applicants to the military as 27,000/0.067 = 402,000. These numbers were taken from graphs in Dondero, St. Louis, Petersen, et al. (1989) and are therefore approximate.

Dondero, St. Louis, Petersen, et al. (1989) used similar techniques to obtain national estimates of prevalence from six types of surveys. National estimates of about 200,000 from male military applicants and 400,000 from female military applicants were considered too small because of selection biases from self-deferral. Estimates of about 1,900,000 from sentinel hospitals were assumed to be too large because some illnesses may be HIV-related, even though the connection is not obvious. In addition, sentinel hospitals tend to be located in urban areas where prevalence rates are often elevated. Estimates of 2,200,000 for male Job Corps applicants and even larger numbers for female Job Corps entrants were considered to be too large because Job Corps applicants are not excluded from entry on the basis of sexual orientation, drug use or an HIV screening program, and Job Corps entrants overrepresent people from urban and low socioeconomic backgrounds. The estimate of about 1,600,000 from male prisoners was also assumed to be too high. Childbearing women yielded an estimate of about 825,000 and ambulatory patients an estimate of about 1,200,000.

Dondero, St. Louis, Petersen, et al. (1989) concluded that the "bulk of the data, however, appear consistent with a true figure lying somewhat above 800,000 and somewhat below 1.5 million," but they emphasized that biases are "incompletely understood." Data from the family of surveys should be considered in connection with other independent estimates (Section 3.3; Chapter 8; Chapter 10) in arriving at national estimates of HIV prevalence. The Centers for Disease Control (1990a) sponsored a workshop for such a purpose in October of 1989, and CDC staff concluded that survey estimates of 0.8–1.2 million infected by June 1989 were consistent with independent estimates of 0.65–1.4 million from back-calculation (Chapter 8).

3.5 ESTIMATING HIV INCIDENCE FROM SURVEY DATA

Seroincidence can be estimated directly by studying selected cohorts (Section 3.5.1), and indirectly by studying seroprevalence trends (Section 3.5.2) and by back-calculation (Chapter 8). Seroincidence data give the most immediate insight into needs for prevention activities, progress in prevention activities, and the likely course of the HIV epidemic and AIDS incidence more than 5 years hence. Despite the public health importance of HIV incidence rates and the multiplicity of approaches to estimating HIV incidence rates, there is even greater uncertainty in estimates of HIV incidence than of seroprevalence and of future AIDS incidence. The uncertainty is especially severe for the present and immediate past few years, where seroincidence trends are most useful.

3.5.1 Longitudinal Follow-up of Selected Cohorts

Selected cohorts of homosexual men, patients with hemophilia, intravenous drug users and heterosexual partners of infected companions have been followed longitudinally to estimate rates of new infection (Table 3.8). Because cohorts are usually defined in special subpopulations, because people who are willing to participate in long term follow-up studies may not be typical, and because the medical care and advice given to people in long term follow-up may modify the subsequent risk of infection, one must be cautious in generalizing findings from cohort studies. Nonetheless such studies provide some of the best information on HIV incidence trends.

Suppose a cohort of N uninfected individuals was assembled on $s_0 =$ January 1, 1977 and followed closely. Then standard survival methods (Kalbfleisch and Prentice, 1980; Cox and Oakes, 1984) could be used to estimate $H(t)$, the probability that a cohort member becomes infected within t years after s_0. The density $h(t) = dH(t)/dt$ and the hazard $k(t) = h(t)\{1 - H(t)\}^{-1}$ can also be estimated. Then the infection rate curve (Chapter 1) at calendar time $s = t + s_0$ would be given by $g(s) = Nk(t)\{1 - H(t)\} = Nh(t)$.

If subjects were followed at regular intervals, as in the Multicenter AIDS Cohort Study (Kingsley, Zhou, Bacellar, et al., 1991), then the hazard rate $k(t)$ corresponding to a given calendar period $s = t + s_0$ could be estimated as the number of seroconversions in a time interval centered on s divided by the person-years at risk accumulated during the interval, and "Poisson regression" could be used to study factors affecting $H(t)$ (Kingsley, Zhou, Bacellar, et al., 1991).

In some cohorts there are irregular gaps between serial HIV assay measurements. The likelihood contribution for a subject who was seropositive when first assayed at calendar time $s = t_1 + s_0$ is $H(t_1)$. For a subject who was seronegative when last tested at calendar time $s_2 = t_2 + s_0$, the likelihood is $1 - H(t_2)$. A person who seroconverted

Table 3.8 Annual Percentage Seroconverting Among Seronegatives in Selected Cohorts

	1978	1979	1980	1981	1982	1983	1984	1985	1986	1987	1988	1989
Homosexual Men												
Hepatitis B Cohort in S.F.[a]	0.3	3.8	10.1	16.6	19.8	7.4	3.3	0.7	1.5	0.0	2.6	
S.F. Men's Health Study[b]					18.4[b]	18.4[b]	18.4[b]	4.2	4.2			
Washington, D.C.[c]					18.8[c]	18.8[c]	10.7	4.9	4.0			
Baltimore/Washington[d]							7.0	4.8	1.2	1.0	0.3	0.3
Chicago[d]							12.0	2.5	1.0	0.8	0.2	1.8
Pittsburgh[d]							6.0	1.8	1.2	1.5	0.6	0.6
Los Angeles[d]							8.6	1.7	1.4	1.0	1.0	0.5
Patients with Hemophilia												
Severe Type A[e]	0.0	5.0	10.5	11.8	26.7	36.4	20.0	10.7	0.0	0.0	0.0	
Other Clotting Disorders[e]	0.0	0.0	2.0	2.0	4.2	6.5	7.0	10.0	0.0	0.0	0.0	
IVDUs in Bronx[f]							19.0					
IVDUs in northern Italy[g]										6.1	4.1	2.2
Heterosexual Partners of												
Infected Partner												
Of hemophiliacs[h]							16.0[h]	16.0[h]				
Of general partner[h]							36.2[h]	36.2[h]				

[a]Hessol, Lifson, O'Malley, et al. (1989).
[b]Winkelstein, Samuel, Padian, et al. (1987). Data were grouped from 1982–1984.
[c]Table 12 in CDC (1987b). Data were grouped in 1982–1983.
[d]Kingsley, Zhou, Bacellar, et al. (1991).
[e]From Figure 1 in Goedert, Kessler, Aledort, et al. (1989).
[f]Table 12 in CDC (1987b).
[g]Nicolosi, Leite, Molinari, et al. (1992).
[h]Table 12 in CDC (1987b). Data were grouped in 1984–1985.

between the date last tested negative, $s_1 = t_1 + s_0$ and the date first tested positive, $s_2 = t_2 + s_0$, contributes $H(t_2) - H(t_1)$ to the likelihood. The distribution $H(t)$ can be estimated non-parametrically from this likelihood for interval-censored data (Turnbull, 1974). Goedert, Kessler, Aledort, et al. (1989) assumed $k(t)$ was piecewise constant over calendar years and estimated $k(t)$ parametrically from the likelihood. Smoother estimates of $k(t)$ have been obtained by representing $k(t)$ as a spline model (P. S. Rosenberg, 1992, personal communication). If subjects continue in follow-up beyond seroconversion to determine when AIDS develops, the information can be used both to estimate the hazard of seroconversion, $k(t)$, and the AIDS incubation distribution (Chapters 4 and 5).

If one assumes $k(t) = k(s - s_0)$ is constant over calendar year s, then the annual hazard for year s, $k(s - s_0) \equiv k_s$, is related to the probability p_s that an individual who is uninfected at the beginning of year s will be infected by the end of year s by $1 - p_s = \exp(-k_s)$. If p_s is small, $p_s \doteq k_s$, where k_s is expressed in units of years^{-1}. If p_s is expressed in percent, k_s is nearly equal to p_s, provided k_s has units per 100 person-years. In most studies, p_s was estimated by actuarial methods and expressed in percent (Table 3.8).

It is clear that rates of seroconversion peaked in the early 1980s for selected cohorts of homosexual men in San Francisco and Washington, D.C. (Table 3.8), but appreciable annual rates of seroconversion continue to occur in Baltimore/Washington, Chicago, Pittsburgh, and Los Angeles in 1989 (Table 3.8). If the annual seroconversion rate is 1% among exclusively homosexual men, and if 2.5×10^6 men are at risk (Table 3.7), such data would indicate that perhaps 25,000 new infections continue to occur each year among homosexual men. It is, of course, questionable whether the seroincidence trends observed in these selected cohorts reflect the current infection rates in smaller cities or rural locations, or whether participants in these cohort studies have unusually low or high rates of seroincidence, even when compared to other homosexual men in the same cities.

The cessation of risk among patients with hemophilia in 1986 reflects active screening programs to detect HIV contamination and methods of treating coagulation products to inactivate HIV. Screening programs and educational programs have also dramatically reduced the risk from blood transfusions (Chapter 6). Seroconversion rates among the partners of infected patients with hemophilia (Table 3.8) indicate that male-to-female heterosexual transmission poses a very substantial threat (Chapter 2). The susceptible partners of patients with hemophilia are thought to have little risk of exposure from drugs or promiscuous sex, which may explain why partners of infected companions in other studies exhibit higher rates of seroconversion (Table 3.8).

Decreasing rates of seroconversion seen among people in treatment for drug abuse in northern Italy (Table 3.8) coincide with a decreasing frequency of sharing syringes (Nicolosi, Leite, Molinari, et al., 1992).

McNeil, Brundage, Wann, et al. (1989) measured the incidence of seroconversion between October 1985 and October 1987 among 171,974 U.S. Army personnel who had been tested for HIV two or more times and who were initially seronegative. Recent analyses (personnel communication from Dr. John McNeill, 1991) indicate that the rate of seroconversion was 0.49×10^{-3} per person-year from November 1985 to October 1987 and that the rate dropped to 0.29×10^{-3} per person-year from November 1988 to October 1989. Standardization of the combined data from November 1985 through October 1989 for age, race and gender yielded an estimate of 22,000 new infections per year in the United States in the age range 17–39 years. However, many analysts believe that rates of new infection are lower among military personnel than among comparable age, race and gender-specific groups in the general population of the United States. Some reasons for this belief are: (1) seropositive applicants for military service and applicants who admit to homosexual behavior or intravenous drug use are not inducted; (2) military personnel are informed of the risks of HIV infection and are subjected to serial HIV testing; (3) military personnel are often stationed in geographic regions where the prevalence of HIV is low; (4) proscriptions against homosexual behavior may cause some people at high risk to leave military service.

3.5.2 Serial Seroprevalence Surveys of a Cohort

We have seen that HIV incidence can be estimated from longitudinal follow-up of the members of a well-defined cohort (Section 3.5.1). If one studied such a cohort periodically to determine the seroprevalence rates (proportions infected) at successive time points but did not retain information on individual cohort members, it might still be possible to infer the HIV incidence rate from equation (1.2). To do so, one would need to know how long infected cohort members survive and remain in follow-up. If deaths and other types of loss to follow-up are negligible, the seroincidence rate can be estimated from the slope of the seroprevalence rate curve (equation 1.2).

Brundage, Burke, Gardner, et al. (1990) proposed using serial seroprevalence rates on birth cohorts of applicants for military service to estimate HIV incidence rates. Of course they were not able to exhaustively sample each birth cohort, so they had to assume for this calculation that (1) applicants for military service are representative of other members of their birth cohort, regardless of infection status, and (2) for the period of the study, the chance that infected individuals will die is negligible.

Under these assumptions, the slope of the plot of seroprevalence against time yields estimates of the HIV seroincidence rate for each birth cohort. Brundage, Burke, Gardner, et al. (1990) found that most such slopes ranged from 0.2×10^{-3} to 0.4×10^{-3} per year. Older cohorts tended to show the largest seroincidence rates.

If one applied the rate of 0.3×10^{-3} per year to the 116,852,000 residents of the United States between the ages of 14 and 44 (U.S. Bureau of the Census, 1991, page 15), one would estimate about 35,000 infections annually. However, this estimate is subject to two important sources of bias that act in opposite directions. Because applicants for military service have a larger representation of men, blacks and Hispanics than the entire U.S. population, and because these groups have elevated seroprevalence rates, it is likely that there is a bias tending to overestimate seroincidence in the U.S. population.

A more serious potential bias that acts in the opposite direction is "self-deferral." People who engage in homosexual behavior, intravenous drug abusers, and people who have other reasons to suspect they are infected are increasingly aware that they will be screened for HIV and asked about risk behaviors when applying for military service. Self-deferral is the preferential tendency of such people not to apply for military service. If this tendency to self-deferral increases in calendar time, observed seroprevalence rates may remain stable or even decline, despite increasing seroprevalence in the general population, leading to serious underestimates of seroincidence rates (Brundage, Burke, Gardner, et al., 1990). Some infected people in the birth cohort will die of HIV disease and others may preferentially decline to apply for military service. Both these factors will lead to underestimates of seroincidence.

3.5.3 Serial Cross-sectional Seroprevalence Surveys

Sometimes one obtains serial seroprevalence data on a dynamically changing population, such as all 21-year-old applicants for military service (Brundage, Burke, Gardner, et al., 1990), or all infants born in a given year. In this setting there is no obvious relationship between serial seroprevalence rates and seroincidence rates, because seroprevalence is largely determined by migrations into and out of the population. For example, the fact that seroprevalence rates among newborns in New York State remained nearly constant in 1988 and 1989 (Novick, Glebatis, Stricof, et al., 1991) does not imply that there are no new infections during this period. Rather, these data indicate a fairly constant number of new infections in successive monthly birth cohorts (see Section 10.4). Likewise, the fact that the prevalence rate has declined slightly from October 1, 1985, to September 30, 1989, among civilian applicants for U.S. military service (Brundage, Burke, Gardner, et al., 1990) does not imply that there are no new HIV infections among such applicants. Rather, successive cohorts of applicants have been infected, though perhaps at decreasing rates. As mentioned above, another explanation is increasing self-deferral of those at highest risk.

4

The Incubation Period Distribution

4.1 INTRODUCTION AND HISTORICAL OVERVIEW

The incubation period is the time between infection and the diagnosis of AIDS. Infected individuals remain seronegative until they develop detectable HIV antibodies, usually within several months (Figure 1.4). This event is called seroconversion. Although we define the *incubation period* as the time from infection to AIDS diagnosis, many studies cannot identify the dates of infection and only provide information about the time from seroconversion to AIDS. However, the time between infection and seroconversion is relatively short (approximate median is 2 months; see Section 4.7) compared to the median of the time from seroconversion to AIDS (approximate median is 10 years). Accordingly, we also use incubation period to refer to the time from seroconversion to AIDS. In fact, many published studies on the incubation distribution implicitly use this latter operational definition.

Incubation periods are extremely variable and some are very long. This chapter is concerned with methodological problems associated with estimating the distribution of incubation periods. We discuss problems in identifying cofactors that alter the incubation period distribution and markers of disease progression in Chapter 5.

An ideal study for estimating the incubation period distribution would be to monitor uninfected subjects closely with repeated HIV antibody tests to determine the date of seroconversion and then to continue following the infected patients to determine the date of AIDS onset. Such ideal data would yield straightforward estimates of the incubation distribution. However, the data that first became available were far from ideal and required special statistical methods to avoid serious misinterpretation.

The first data on the incubation period came from a 1986 study of transfusion-associated AIDS cases (Lui, Lawrence, Morgan, et al. 1986). Transfusion-associated AIDS cases provide unique epidemiological data because the dates of infection can be ascertained as the dates of transfusion with infected blood. However, the 1986 study had a number of limitations because it consisted only of AIDS cases for whom the dates of infection were determined retrospectively. Because this was a study of AIDS cases rather than a study of a cohort of infected individuals, the study provided no information about the proportion of infected individuals who will eventually progress to AIDS, and, more generally, about the probability that a member of an infected cohort would develop AIDS in a given time period. An additional complication is that infected transfusion recipients with long incubation periods would not have been diagnosed by 1986 and are thus selectively excluded from the data set. These and other issues are discussed in Section 4.3.

The limitations of studies which consist only of AIDS cases, such as the transfusion study, called attention to the importance of following cohorts of infected individuals to monitor their immune systems and to determine progression rates to AIDS. One rapid and convenient study design involves assembling a cohort of individuals who are already HIV seropositive but whose dates of seroconversion are typically unknown. These are called prevalent cohort studies. A number of statistical problems arise in the interpretation and analysis of prevalent cohorts (Section 4.4).

Some studies were based on periodic screening of individuals for HIV antibody. Thus, the date of seroconversion could be determined up to an interval defined by the latest screening test that was negative for HIV infection and the earliest screening test that was positive. Examples of these studies include cohorts of hemophiliacs who were patients at hemophilia treatment centers (National Cancer Institute Multicenter Hemophilia Cohort Study (Goedert, Kessler, Aledort, et al. 1989)) and a cohort of homosexual men in San Francisco enrolled in a study of hepatitis B vaccine (Hessol, Lifson, O'Malley, 1989). Sera obtained from periodic follow-up visits on these cohorts had been stored in the 1970s and 1980s. Statistical problems that arise because of the uncertainty in the dates of seroconversion are discussed in Section 4.5.

As mentioned earlier, the ideal study for learning about the incubation period would consist of a cohort of uninfected individuals

who are closely monitored for evidence of infection and then followed
to detect onset of AIDS. A number of such studies got underway in
1984–1985 including the San Francisco Men's Health Study (Winkelstein, Lyman, Padian, et al., 1987), the Multicenter AIDS Cohort
Study (Kaslow, Ostrow, Detels, et al., 1987), and the Sydney Cohort
(Tindall, Swanson, and Cooper, 1990). One limitation of these studies
is the relatively short follow-up times on the identified seroconverters
compared to older cohorts for which stored sera are available, such as
the National Cancer Institute Multicenter Hemophilia Cohort
(Goedert, Kessler, Aledort, et al., 1989) and the San Francisco City
Clinic Cohort of homosexual men enrolled in a vaccine trial against
hepatitis B (Hessol, Lifson, O'Malley, et al., 1989). An additional
complication is that increasingly widespread use of effective treatments
such as zidovudine since 1987 may have altered the incubation period
distribution within these cohorts. Methodological issues associated with
quantifying the effects of treatment on the incubation period are
considered in Chapters 8 and 11.

4.2 MATHEMATICAL MODELS FOR THE INCUBATION
PERIOD DISTRIBUTION

The incubation period distribution, $F(t)$, is the probability that an
infected individual progresses to AIDS within t years of the time of
infection, which we usually take to be the time of seroconversion. That
is, if the random variable U represents the incubation period then
$F(t) = P(U \leqslant t)$. The survival function is $S(t) = 1 - F(t)$ and the
probability density of the incubation period is $dF/dt = F'(t) - f(t)$.
The hazard function $\lambda(t) = f(t)/S(t)$ is the risk of developing AIDS at
time t following infection conditional on not having AIDS just before t.
The hazard function represents the time specific progression rate and
quantifies how the risk of AIDS evolves with time from infection.

The incubation distribution $F(t)$ could be estimated nonparametrically or parametrically (Cox and Oakes, 1984). Below we describe
some useful parametric models for $F(t)$.

Parametric models for the hazard $\lambda(t)$ (which induces a parametric
model for $F(t)$) should be consistent with epidemiological data and
with theoretical considerations of the pathogenesis of HIV infection.
The hazard of progression to AIDS is known to be very small shortly
after infection and then increases. The behavior of the hazard function
after 6 years is uncertain because few untreated patients have been
followed beyond this point. Below we describe a number of parametric
models (functional forms) which may be useful in describing the

incubation period distribution. These models allow for initially increasing hazard functions.

The Weibull Model

The incubation period distribution for the Weibull model has the form $F(t) = 1 - e^{-\lambda t^p}$ $\lambda > 0$, $p > 0$. The hazard function for the Weibull model, $\lambda(t) = \lambda p t^{p-1}$, is monotonically increasing if $p > 1$, monotonically decreasing if $p < 1$, and constant (the exponential model) if $p = 1$. Weibull models with $p > 1$ have been useful for modelling the HIV incubation period and have been consistent with a number of epidemiologic data sets with up to 8 years of follow-up after seroconversion. The Weibull model has been used in studies of the incubation periods among hemophiliacs (Brookmeyer and Goedert, 1989; Darby, Doll, Thakar, et al., 1990), homosexuals (Lui, Darrow, and Rutherford, 1988), and transfusion recipients (Lui, Lawrence, Morgan, et al., 1986; Kalbfleisch and Lawless, 1989; Medley, Anderson, Cox, and Billard, 1987). However, the Weibull model assumes the hazard increases indefinitely and is proportional to a power of time from infection. This assumption may not be accurate in the long term, particularly if a proportion of infected individuals never progress to AIDS.

The Gamma Model

The probability density function for the gamma model has the form

$$f(t) = \frac{\lambda^k t^{k-1} e^{-\lambda t}}{\Gamma(k)} \qquad \lambda > 0; \, k > 0$$

where $\Gamma(\cdot)$ is the gamma function. The gamma model can arise if one hypothesizes that infected individuals must pass through a series of k stages and the hazard function of transition from one stage to the next is the constant λ. When $k > 1$, the hazard function monotonically increases and asymptotically approaches λ. The gamma model has been used in studies of the incubation period among blood transfusion recipients (Medley, Anderson, Cox, and Billard, 1987).

Log-Logistic Model

The incubation period distribution for the log-logistic model has the form

$$F(t) = 1 - (1 + (\lambda t)^\beta)^{-1} \qquad \lambda > 0, \, \beta > 0.$$

If $\beta > 1$, the hazard function increases initially, until it reaches a maximum and then decreases monotonically as $t \to \infty$. The behavior of the hazard function is similar to the lognormal model (the lognormal model assumes that the logarithm of the incubation period follows a normal distribution). The log-logistic distribution was used by Lui, Darrow, and Rutherford (1988) to model the incubation period among homosexual men.

Piecewise Exponential Model

The hazard function is assumed to be constant over prespecified time intervals; that is

$$\lambda(t) = \lambda_i \qquad c_{i-1} \leqslant t < c_i.$$

The piecewise exponential model is very flexible, although one may need a number of intervals and corresponding parameters to accurately represent the rapidly increasing hazard function for the first several years following infection. If $\lambda(t) = 0$ beyond some time t^*, a proportion of infecteds will never develop AIDS.

Staging Models

These models assume infected individuals pass through a series of k stages with the last stage being AIDS. It is usually assumed that HIV disease is progressive so that transitions occur in the direction of advancing disease. The durations in each stage are typically assumed to be independent random variables. The hazard functions of transition may differ from stage to stage and may vary with time since entry in a given stage. A gamma model arises if transition rates are equal and constant across stages.

An application of these ideas arises in modelling the depletion of CD4+ T-cells. Suppose that the time from infection to CD4+ cell depletion (e.g., <200 CD4+ T cells) follows a Weibull model with hazard function $\lambda_1 p t^{p-1}$ and that the time from CD4+ T cell depletion to AIDS follows an exponential model with hazard function λ_2. The assumption, here, is that once the CD4+ T cells have dropped to a low enough level, the individual has a constant hazard λ_2 of developing an AIDS-defining condition. Then the incubation period distribution is given by the convolution of Weibull and exponential models (under the assumption that the durations in the two stages are independent):

$$F(t) = \int_0^t \lambda_1 p s^{p-1} e^{-\lambda_1 s^p} \{1 - e^{-\lambda_2(t-s)}\} ds.$$

If $p > 1$, the hazard for this model is monotonically increasing and asymptotically approaches λ_2, which is similar to the behavior of the hazard function of the gamma model. This model was used by Brookmeyer and Liao (1990a). Longini, Clark, Gardner, and Brundage (1991) considered a multistage Markov model in which infected individuals progress from infection, to seroconversion, to symptomatic (pre-AIDS) HIV disease, to AIDS. The hazard of transition from stage i to $i + 1$ was assumed constant at λ_i (the exponential model). These models are considered again in Section 5.6.

Mixture Model

The model assumes that a certain proportion of infected individuals, α, have incubation period distribution, $F_1(t)$ and the remaining proportion, $1 - \alpha$, have incubation period distribution $F_2(t)$. Then the incubation period distribution for the entire population of infected individuals is a mixture of F_1 and F_2 and is

$$F(t) = \alpha F_1(t) + (1 - \alpha) F_2(t).$$

As a special case, suppose the incubation period distribution $F_1(t)$ follows a Weibull distribution with $p > 1$ and $F_2(t) \equiv 0$. This implies that the proportion $(1 - \alpha)$ of infected individuals never progress to AIDS while the proportion, α, are the "susceptibles" who progress to AIDS according to the incubation period distribution $F_1(t)$. In this example, the hazard function for the mixed population is initially increasing but eventually decreases as the proportion α of susceptibles are removed. Such a model was used by Lui, Darrow, and Rutherford (1988) in a study of the incubation period among homosexual men. Auger, Thomas, and DeGruttolla (1988) used a mixture of two Weibull distributions (i.e., $F_1(t)$ and $F_2(t)$ were assumed to be Weibull models) in a study of the incubation period among maternally infected newborns.

4.3 RETROSPECTIVE DATA ON AIDS CASES

4.3.1 Introduction

Some epidemiological studies of the incubation period have involved only a sample of AIDS cases for whom the dates of infection are determined retrospectively. For example, the 1986 study of blood transfusion-associated AIDS was based on all AIDS cases reported to the CDC with transfusion as the only known risk factor who were diagnosed before 1986. The dates of infection were assumed to be the dates of transfusion with infected blood, which is a reasonable assumption if the AIDS case has no other known risk factors for HIV infection (Lui, Lawrence, Morgan, et al., 1986). A second example concerns a study of pediatric AIDS patients whose only known HIV risk was maternal transmission (Auger, Thomas, and De Gruttola, 1988). In this study it was assumed that the date of birth was the date of infection.

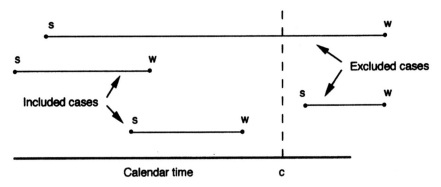

s = Infection date
w = AIDS diagnosis date
c = Case ascertainment date

Figure 4.1 Schematic illustration of a retrospective study of cases (e.g., transfusion-associated AIDS). Only cases diagnosed before calendar time of case ascertainment are included (i.e., $w_i < c$).

In this section we consider the statistical problems associated with the analysis and interpretation of incubation period studies that involve only a sample of cases of disease. Figure 4.1 illustrates the sampling scheme: All AIDS cases diagnosed before some calendar time c are sampled. The data consist of the calendar dates of infection, s_i, and the calendar dates of diagnosis, w_i, for each of N retrospectively ascertained cases. The incubation period for the ith cases is $u_i = w_i - s_i$. The criterion for inclusion in the data set is that $w_i \leqslant c$ or alternatively $u_i \leqslant T_i$, where $T_i = c - s_i$ is called the truncation time for the ith individual. Figure 4.1 indicates the two main problems with the analysis and interpretation of data of this sort. First, since the data involve only AIDS cases it can provide no information about the proportion of infected individuals who eventually develops disease. Second, the sampling scheme tends to capture cases with shorter incubation periods. This bias is a form of length biased sampling, the result of truncation on the right. This bias must be accounted for in the statistical analysis.

4.3.2 Nonparametric Estimation of the Truncated Distribution

A serious limitation of retrospective data on AIDS cases is that incubation periods longer than the maximum truncation time cannot be observed. For example, suppose the analysis consists of all AIDS cases diagnosed by January 1, 1986, and it was found that the earliest calendar time of infection among these cases was January 1, 1977. The maximum truncation time is $T^* = 9$ years. The best we can do, nonparametrically, is to estimate the incubation period distribution conditional on the incubation period being less than 9 years. We call this the conditional incubation period distribution

$$F^*(t) = P(u \leqslant t | u \leqslant T^*)$$

and it is related to $F(t)$ by

$$F^*(t) = F(t)/F(T^*).$$

Only if T^* is sufficiently large and if $F(t)$ is a proper distribution (i.e., all infected patients eventually develop AIDS) will $F(T^*)$ be approximately 1.0. In this case F^* will be a good approximation to F. In general, $F^*(t) \geqslant F(t)$. An important point is that there is no information in the data about the probability of having an incubation period larger than T^*, unless one makes strong parametric assumptions about F.

A simple computational method for finding the nonparametric estimate of the conditional incubation period distribution, F^*, adapts survival and life table techniques for use with right truncated data (Kalbfleisch and Lawless, 1989; Lagakos, Barraj, and De Gruttola, 1988). This involves expressing F^* as the product of conditional probabilities. For simplicity, we assume the incubation distribution is discrete with probability mass at the times $t_1 < t_2 < \cdots, < t_m$. We define the conditional probability p_j to be the probability that the incubation period is equal to t_j given that it is less than or equal to t_j, that is $p_j = P(U = t_j | U \leqslant t_j)$. Then

$$F^*(t_s) = \prod_{j=s+1}^{m} (1 - p_j). \qquad (4.1)$$

A nonparametric estimate of the incubation period distribution is obtained by substituting estimates of $\hat{p}_j$ into equation (4.1). The only cases who can contribute information about p_j are those cases whose truncation times are greater than or equal to t_j and whose incubation periods are less than or equal to t_j. We call these individuals the "risk set" at t_j to emphasize the analogy with life table analyses. The number of individuals in the risk set at t_j is called n_j. Let d_j be the number of individuals with incubation times exactly equal to t_j. Then a nonparametric estimate of p_j is $\hat{p}_j = d_j/n_j$. The non-parametric estimate of $F^*(t)$ is then

$$\hat{F}^*(t_s) = \prod_{j=s+1}^{m} \left(1 - \frac{d_j}{n_j}\right) \qquad s = 1, \ldots, m-1, \qquad (4.2)$$

and $F^*(t_m) = 1.0$. The nonparametric estimate (4.2) applies even when the incubation distribution is not assumed to be discrete, in which case the product is over all distinct observed incubation times. The estimate (4.2) is a step function with jumps at observed incubation times and is analogous to the Kaplan–Meier estimate (1958). An estimate of the variance is given by an adaptation of Greenwood's formula

$$\text{Var}(\hat{F}^*(t_s)) = [\hat{F}^*(t_s)]^2 \cdot \sum_{j=s+1}^{m} \frac{d_j}{n_j(n_j - d_j)}.$$

In small sample sizes, it may happen that $\hat{p}_j = 1.0$, in which case $F^*(t) = 0.0$ (and its variance is not defined) for $t < t_j$. It is recommended that the time axis be grouped into intervals within which events are grouped to avoid this degeneracy.

These methods were applied to transfusion associated AIDS cases who were diagnosed in the United States prior to July 1986. The data are reported in Kalbfleisch and Lawless (1989), and include the calendar dates of infection (transfusion), AIDS diagnosis, and ages at infection on 295 transfusion associated AIDS cases. The earliest calendar date of infection (i.e., transfusion with infected blood) among the 295 cases was March 1978. Thus, the maximum truncation time was $T^* = 102$ months (the time between March 1978 and July 1986). Thus, the best that can be done nonparametrically is to estimate the incubation distribution among incubation periods less than 102 months. Figure 4.2 illustrates the conditional distribution, $\hat{F}^*$, of incubation times among individuals who develop AIDS in less than $T^* = 8.5$ years (102 months) based on the nonparametric procedure given by equation (4.2). In general, $F^*(t) > F(t)$. Thus, incubation periods from $\hat{F}^*$ tend to be shorter than the desired unconditional incubation periods from F. Also shown in Figure 4.2 is the naive estimate of F based on the empirical distribution, $\hat{F}_E$, of the observed incubation times. The estimate $\hat{F}_E$ is the proportion of cases with incubation periods less than or equal to t years. This analysis grossly overestimates the true incubation distribution F (that is, suggests incubation periods are shorter than they really are), because, unlike $\hat{F}^*$, it does not adjust for length biased sampling that arises from right truncation. Both $\hat{F}^*$ and $\hat{F}_E$ reach the value 1.0 at 89 months, which was the largest observed incubation period among the 295 cases. Similar statistical problems arise in the analysis of reporting delays (see Section 7.3.1).

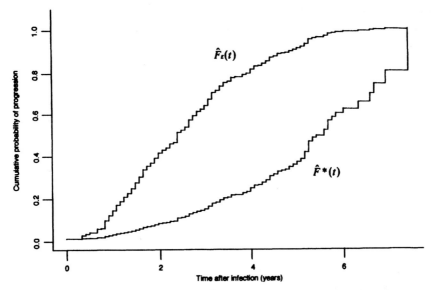

Figure 4.2 Nonparametric estimate $\hat{F}^*(t)$ of the conditional incubation distribution and of the naive empirical distribution function $\hat{F}_E(t)$, based on transfusion-associated AIDS cases.

4.3.3 Parametric Estimation

A parametric approach could be used for the analysis of retrospective data on cases. A parametric model is assumed for F and a likelihood function is used for parameter estimation. An important point is that parametric approaches do not circumvent the main weakness in the data: It is not possible to observe incubation periods longer than the maximum truncation time. While some parametric assumptions permit one to estimate not only F^* but also F, the resulting estimates of F are extremely imprecise and depend strongly on the parametric assumptions (Kalbfleisch and Lawless, 1989).

Unless one is willing to assume that the incubation period distribution is proper or to assume that the proportion who will eventually develop AIDS is known, one cannot obtain F from F^*, even under parametric assumptions (Brookmeyer and Gail, 1988; Kalbfleisch and Lawless, 1989). For example, assume that an unknown proportion, α, of those infected will eventually develop AIDS and that the incubation period distribution among such individuals, $F_1(t)$, has a known parametric form. Retrospective data on cases can be used to estimate $F^*(t) = F_1(t)/F_1(T^*)$, which does not depend on α. Thus, under parametric assumptions, one can estimate $F_1(t)$ but not the desired distribution, $F(t) = \alpha F_1(t)$. Most investigators assume that $F(t)$ is proper (i.e., $\alpha = 1$), in which case parametric models for $F(t)$ can be estimated from $F^*(t) = F(t)/F(T^*)$.

We review a number of different likelihood functions that have been proposed for the parametric analysis of retrospective data on cases. Suppose infections are generated by a point process with infection intensity $g(s; \gamma)$ where γ are unknown parameters. For convenience, the origin of calendar time is taken to be the start of the epidemic (that is, $g(s; \gamma) = 0$ for $s < 0$). The first likelihood function is conditional on N, the number of cases diagnosed prior to calendar time c.

$$L_1 = \prod_{i=1}^{N} \left[\frac{g(s_i) f(u_i)}{\int_0^c g(s) F(c - s) ds} \right]. \tag{4.3}$$

The second likelihood function, which does not condition on N, assumes infections are generated by a nonhomogeneous Poisson process. Then the number of cases diagnosed by calendar time c has a Poisson distribution with mean

$$\mu = \int_0^c g(s) F(c - s) ds.$$

The full likelihood L_2 is then the product of L_1 with the probability of N diagnosed cases by calendar time c,

$$L_2 = \frac{e^{-\mu}}{N!} \prod_{i=1}^{N} g(s_i) f(u_i).$$

The conditional likelihood L_1 allows $g(s)$ to be estimated only up to a proportionality constant, because if $g(s) = \gamma g_o(s)$ then γ would cancel in the numerator and denominator in (4.3) and involve only g_o. Thus, L_1 provides information about the shape of $g(s)$ but not about the absolute rate of infections. On the other hand, L_2 permits estimation of $g(s)$ itself. An advantage of L_1 is that it can be used with only a sample of cases while L_2 assumes that all cases diagnosed by c are ascertained and included in the analysis. Both L_1 and L_2 produce identical maximum likelihood estimates and observed Fisher information matrices for the parameters of F (Kalbfleisch and Lawless, 1989).

A third likelihood function conditions on both N and the calendar dates of infection of the N cases (Lui, Lawrence, Morgan, et al., 1986), namely

$$L_3 = \prod_{i=1}^{N} \frac{g(s_i) f(u_i)}{g(s_i) F(c - u_i)} = \prod_{i=1}^{N} \frac{f(u_i)}{F(c - u_i)}.$$

Several points are worth noting about L_3. First, it does not involve $g(s)$.

This is attractive if interest is focused only on estimating $F(t)$. Second, once we condition on the date of infection s_i, the only variability in the data is from the variability in the diagnosis dates within the window of calendar time $[0, c]$. The narrower the window, the less information is available for estimating F. If accurate parametric assumptions are made on the form of $g(s)$, then inference based on L_1 or L_2 will usually lead to more precise estimates of F than inference based on L_3 (Brookmeyer and Gail, 1988).

4.3.4 Competing Causes of Death

Infected individuals may be subject to appreciable mortality from causes unrelated to HIV. This is especially true of transfusion recipients who tend to be older and sick. If there is significant risk of death from competing causes, the methods of Sections 4.3.2 and 4.3.3 will be biased toward shorter incubation periods. The reason is that the cases who are included in the data are those who are diagnosed with AIDS before death from a competing cause could occur. Thus, these cases tend to have shorter incubation periods.

In the presence of competing causes of death, the parametric methods of Section 4.3.3 do not estimate F, but rather the distribution function, $F_s(t)$, which is the probability of developing AIDS within t time units of infection given that AIDS occurs before death. If the hazard of death, from a competing cause is a constant δ then

$$F_s(t) = \int_0^t f(u)e^{-\delta u} du \bigg/ \int_0^\infty f(u)e^{-\delta u} du.$$

For example, suppose the incubation period distribution follows an exponential distribution $F(t) = 1 - e^{\lambda t}$. Then the parametric methods of Section (4.3.3) estimate $F_s(t) = 1 - e^{-(\lambda + \delta)t}$ rather than $F(t) = 1 - e^{-\lambda t}$. The ratio of the median of F_s to the median of F is

$$\frac{\text{median of } F_s}{\text{median of } F} = \frac{\lambda}{\lambda + \delta}.$$

Thus, if the risk (hazard) of death (δ) is greater than the risk of progression to AIDS (λ), the median incubation time will be underestimated by more than 50%.

The nonparametric methods of Section 4.3.2 are also asymptotically biased in the presence of competing causes of causes and, in this example, estimate the conditional distribution

$$F_s^*(t) = \frac{1 - e^{-(\lambda + \delta)t}}{1 - e^{-(\lambda + \delta)T^*}}$$

rather than

$$F^*(t) = \frac{1 - e^{-\lambda t}}{1 - e^{-\lambda T^*}},$$

where T^* is the maximum truncation time. It follows that $F_s^*(t) \geqslant F^*(t)$.

4.4 PREVALENT COHORT STUDIES

The prevalent cohort study follows individuals who were infected with HIV before enrollment but whose calendar times of infection are unknown. Figure 4.3 is a schematic illustration of the prevalent cohort study. A prevalent sample of infected individuals is taken at calendar time Y. There are three time scales: calendar time (s), time from infection (u) and follow-up time (t).

An important issue concerns the biases inherent in performing analyses on the scale of observed follow-up time, t, instead of the desired, but unobservable scale of time from infection. Specifically, how do estimates derived from prevalent cohorts of the probability of developing disease within t years of follow-up, $F_p(t) = 1 - S_p(t)$ relate to the incubation period distribution $F(t)$?

The proportion of persons in a prevalent cohort who develop AIDS within t years of follow-up, $F_p(t)$, does not in general approximate $F(t)$. Only if the hazard $\lambda(u)$ is constant (an exponential distribution for F) do the two coincide. This follows from the lack of memory property of the exponential distribution, which implies that newly infected indiv-

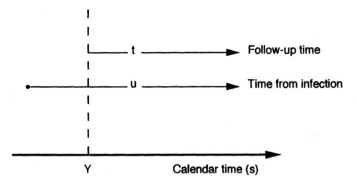

Figure 4.3 Schematic illustration of the prevalent cohort study.

iduals will progress to AIDS at the same rate as individuals who have been infected for some time. If the hazard $\lambda(u)$ is increasing, then individuals in the prevalent cohort will be at greater risk of AIDS than newly infected individuals, that is $F_p(t) > F(t)$. The direction of the bias is reversed for a decreasing hazard. Regardless of shape of the hazard, $F_p(t)$ is a lower bound on the ultimate proportion of infected individuals who will develop AIDS, $F(\infty)$. For example, an early prevalent cohort study yielded an estimate of the cumulative probability of developing AIDS within 3 years of follow-up of $F_p(3) = .36$ (Goedert, Biggar, Weiss, et al., 1986). We now know that the cumulative probability of developing AIDS within 3 years of *infection* is much closer to $F(3) = 0.05$ (see Section 4.5). Nevertheless, the prevalent cohort study indicates that the ultimate proportion of infected individuals who will eventually develop AIDS is at least 0.36, apart from sampling variation.

Brookmeyer and Gail (1987) derived an exact expression for the induced incubation distribution on the observed follow-up time scale, $F_p(t)$, in terms of the probability density of infection times, g^* among cohort members and the true incubation distribution F. They determined the direction of the bias associated with using F_p (based on prevalent cohorts) to estimate F. The following results (Brookmeyer and Gail, 1987) hold for an arbitrary $g^*(s)$:

If the hazard $\lambda(t)$ is constant then $F_p(t) = F(t)$.
If the hazard $\lambda(t)$ is monotonically increasing, then $F_p(t) > F(t)$.
If the hazard $\lambda(t)$ is monotonically decreasing, then $F_p(t) < F(t)$.
If infected individuals are a mixture of a proportion α who eventually develop disease and a proportion 1-α who never develop disease, then $F_p(t) \leqslant \alpha$.

The magnitude of these biases depends not only on the hazard $\lambda(t)$ but also on $g^*(s)$. For example, the bias would be small if the prevalent cohort is assembled near the beginning of the epidemic, in which case the backward recurrence times (i.e., times from infection to the onset of follow-up Υ) would be short.

Some analyses of the data from prevalent cohorts involve imputing the dates of infection. For example, one would postulate a calendar time prior to which infection was unlikely to occur, say time $s = 0$. Then one could impute the infection date as the midpoint of the interval $[0, \Upsilon]$ or the conditional mean with respect to an assumed distribution for g^* (Section 4.5). Alternative methods based on markers or disease progression have also been suggested (Section 5.7).

4.5 STUDIES WITH DOUBLY CENSORED AND INTERVAL CENSORED DATA

4.5.1 Introduction

In some epidemiological studies, it may be possible to ascertain the calendar time of seroconversion or infection up to an interval. For example, consider a cohort of individuals who are periodically screened for evidence of infection (i.e., presence of HIV antibody). Then the calendar dates of seroconversion are within the interval defined by the calendar date of the most recent screening test that was negative for HIV antibody and the earliest screening test that was positive for HIV antibody. Such data are described as "interval censored."

An example of such a study was the National Cancer Institute Multicenter Hemophilia Cohort Study which consisted of hemophiliacs who were regularly seen at hemophilia treatment centers (Goedert, Kessler, Aledort, et al., 1989). Serum samples from each patient visit, some dating back to the mid-1970s, had been stored for reasons unrelated to the HIV/AIDS epidemic. The sera were subsequently tested for evidence of HIV infection, and the individuals in the cohort were followed for onset of clinical AIDS. Another study, the San Francisco City Clinic Cohort Study, involved a cohort of homosexual men enrolled in a study of hepatitis B vaccine (Hessol, Lifson, O'Malley, et al., 1989). Serum samples on these men had also been stored, and the intervals in which seroconversion occurred was determined by testing the sera. The data structure from the two studies are very similar. A complication is that while such studies provide information about the seroconversion date, they provide no information about the infection date. Estimates of the incubation period from such studies have typically ignored the time between infection and seroconversion because it is thought to be short compared to the time from seroconversion to AIDS (Section 4.7).

In some situations, one may not have both a negative and positive screening test on an individual, but, nevertheless, one may be willing to infer an interval of infection based on other considerations. For example, in the hemophilia cohort study, the first available serum sample was positive for a number of hemophiliacs. This pattern resulted primarily from the fact that a number of frozen serum samples were lost because of freezer malfunctions. A reasonable assumption, based on the fact that no hemophilia serum samples were found to be infected before 1978, is that replacement clotting factors in the United States had not been contaminated before January 1, 1978. Thus one could assume that seropositive hemophiliacs with missing early serum samples seroconverted between January 1, 1978, and the individuals' first positive serum sample.

Interval censored dates of infection also arise in cohort studies in which the date of infection is determined from detailed information on sexual exposure history. For example, a Canadian cohort (Coates, Soskolne, Read, et al., 1986) involved 249 homosexual/bisexual men who had sexual contact with individuals who had been diagnosed with HIV disease (the index case). Information on the date of first and last sexual contact with the index case was collected for each individual in the cohort and the calendar dates of infection were assumed to occur within the intervals defined by these two dates. Implicit assumptions are that members of the cohort did not have sexual contact with HIV infected individuals other than the index case, and that the reported sexual behaviors are accurate. Infection intervals ascertained in this way are less reliable than those based on repeated serum samples.

The term *right censored* refers to data for which all that is known is that the event of interest, such as onset of AIDS, had not occurred before a certain time. The term *doubly censored* data refers to time-to-event data for which both the time origin and failure time are censored. For example, in the NCI Multicenter Hemophilia Cohort and San Francisco City Clinic Cohort studies the incubation periods are doubly censored because the date of infection is interval censored and the date of diagnosis of AIDS onset is right censored for those individuals who had not developed AIDS by the time of last follow-up.

A schematic illustration of incubation period studies with doubly censored data is shown in Figure 4.4. A cohort of infected individuals is identified at calendar time $s = 0$. An indicator ε_i is set to 1 if the ith individual had a positive screening test and 0 otherwise. For those individuals with a positive screening test, the calendar time of sero-conversion is known to have occurred in the interval (L_i, R_i) where L_i is the known calendar time of the last (most recent) negative test and R_i is the known calendar time of the first (earliest) positive test. The calendar time w_i is the earlier of the date of the last follow-up and the date of diagnosis of clinical disease. An indicator δ_i is set to 1 if the individual developed clinical disease and 0 if the individual had not developed disease by last follow-up.

4.5.2 Simple Methods Based on Imputed Infection Dates

An ad hoc approach for analyzing doubly censored data is to estimate (impute) the calendar date of infection (or seroconversion) by the

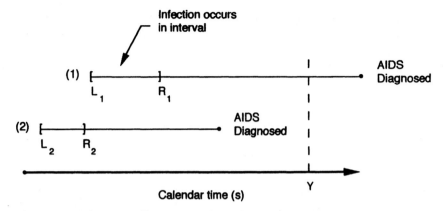

Figure 4.4 Schematic illustration of incubation period studies with doubly censored data. Infection occurs in calendar time interval (L_i, R_i). Figure also illustrates truncation effects in a cohort consisting of individuals who are free of AIDS at calendar time Y: Individual 1 is included in the cohort and individual 2 is excluded (see Section 4.5.3).

midpoint of the interval. The imputed midpoint calendar date of infection is

$$\hat{s}_i = \frac{L_i + R_i}{2}. \tag{4.4a}$$

For individuals who are diagnosed with clinical disease at calendar time w_i without a prior positive screening test the calendar date of infection could be estimated by

$$\hat{s}_i = \frac{L_i + w_i}{2}. \tag{4.4b}$$

Using these imputed times of infection, the incubation periods for individuals diagnosed with disease $(\delta_i = 1)$ is $\hat{u}_i = w_i - \hat{s}_i$. For individuals who did not have disease by last follow-up $(\delta_i = 0)$, the incubation period is right censored with value $\hat{u}_i = w_i - \hat{s}_i$.

Standard survival analysis techniques for right censored data are used in the imputed incubation times. For example, the Kaplan–Meier estimate of the survival function $S = 1 - F$ could be computed from the data $(\hat{u}_i, \delta_i)$. However, such approaches will typically be biased and give incorrect variance estimates. The bias of the estimated incubation distribution resulting from midpoint imputation depends on the width of the intervals, the true incubation period distribution, F, and the probability density of infection times $g^*(s)$ (Law and Brookmeyer, 1992). For example, if the infection density is monotonically increasing, as in the exponential growth phase of simple epidemics (see Chapter 9), then midpoint imputation will tend to underestimate the time of infection and thus overestimate the incubation period. Thus, F is underestimated or equivalently $S = 1 - F$ is overestimated. Table 4.1 shows the asymptotic bias of the Kaplan–Meier estimates of $S = 1 - F$ with different interval widths using midpoint imputation (4.4a–b). The calculations assume an exponential growth model for the infection rate with a doubling time of one year, and the true incubation period distribution is assumed to be Weibull with a 10-year median. The magnitude of the bias by midpoint imputation depends on t. If t is less than the 10th percentile of F, and if the interval widths are large (>4 years) the relative bias (bias/$F(t)$) can be large. However, if the interval width is 2 years or less the bias is small, even for doubling times as fast as 1.0 year.

Midpoint imputation was used in a study of 84 men enrolled in the San Francisco City Clinic Hepatitis B cohort between 1979 and 1980 (Lui, Darrow, and Rutherford, 1988). These men were randomly selected from a larger cohort of homosexual and bisexual men, all of whom had a positive screening test within 12 months of a negative test. Table 4.1 suggests that the bias resulting from midpoint imputation is negligible if the interval widths are less than one year. However, if the study is restricted to individuals with short screening intervals, an implicit assumption is that they have a similar incubation distribution as other members of the cohort.

An alternative imputation method, called *conditional mean imputation* is to estimate the date of infection by the expected infection date given that infection occurred between L_i and R_i. This approach requires an estimate, $\hat{g}^*$, of g^*. Here, g^* is the probability density of infection times

Table 4.1 Asymptotic Bias of Kaplan–Meier Estimate Based on Midpoint Imputation Assuming Exponential Growth in Infections

Quantile of Incubation Distribution	Interval Widths (years)			
	1	2	4	8
.10	.002	.0009	.030	.073
.25	.004	.016	.055	.151
.50	.005	.020	.072	.216
.75	.004	.016	.061	.202
.90	.003	.010	.037	.134

Source: Adapted from Law and Brookmeyer, 1992.

Note: Asymptotic bias is $|S_m(t) - S(t)|$ where $S_m(t)$ is the large sample value of the Kaplan–Meier estimate using midpoint imputation and $S(t) = 1 - F(t)$. Infection rates are assumed to grow exponentially with 1 year doubling time, $g(s) = .6931 \exp(.6931s)$. Incubation distribution is $F(t) = 1 - \exp(-.0021t^{2.516})$.

among individuals infected before the end of the study, say c. Then the imputed infection date is:

$$\hat{s}_i = \frac{\int_{L_i}^{R_i} s \hat{g}^*(s) ds}{\hat{G}^*(R_i) - \hat{G}^*(L_i)},$$

where $\hat{G}^*(t) = \int_0^t \hat{g}^*(s) ds$. When $\hat{g}^*$ is constant (uniform) over the intervals, midpoint and conditional mean imputation are equivalent. An estimate of g^* can be obtained by postulating a parametric model for g. The maximum likelihood estimates of the parameters of the probability density g^* can be estimated from the interval censored data (L_i, R_i) using the likelihood function:

$$\prod_{i=1}^n \{G^*(R_i) - G^*(L_i)\}.$$

4.5.3 Likelihood and Penalized Likelihood Approaches

The parametric approach for analyzing doubly censored data involves joint estimation of both the probability densities of infection times, g^*, and of incubation times, f. Parametric models are postulated for $g^*(s)$ and $f(u)$. We make three assumptions that simplify the construction of the likelihood function. First, we assume a cohort of uninfected individuals is assembled at a fixed calendar time, say $s = 0$. Second, the calendar time of infection is assumed independent of the incubation period. Third, the calendar dates of the screening test are generated by a point process that is independent of both the calendar date of infection and the incubation period.

The likelihood contribution for an individual depends on his disease (δ_i) and infection status (ε_i). For the ith individual with a positive screening test ($\varepsilon_i = 1$), and with clinical disease ($\delta_i = 1$), the likelihood contribution is

$$l_i = \int_{L_i}^{R_i} g(s) f(w_i - s) ds. \tag{4.5}$$

For an individual with a positive screening test ($\varepsilon_i = 1$) who was free of clinical disease at last follow-up ($\delta_i = 0$), the likelihood contribution is (4.5) with the probability density f replaced by the survival function S.

An individual who was diagnosed prior to a positive screening test ($\varepsilon_i = 0$) must have seroconverted in the interval (L_i, w_i). The likelihood contribution is (4.5) with the upper limit of integration R_i replaced by w_i.

Individuals whose last screen was negative ($\varepsilon_i = 0$) and who were

AIDS free at last follow-up ($\delta_i = 0$) contribute approximately $1-G(w_i)$ to the likelihood. This approximation results from assuming that the individual remained uninfected between the last screening test L_i and the last follow-up w_i. Alternatively, these uninfected individuals could be eliminated from the analysis, in which case $g(s)$ in equation (4.5) becomes $g^*(s)$, the density of infection times given that infection occurred before the end of the study. The log likelihood function is $\Sigma \log l_i$. Maximum likelihood estimates can be obtained by maximizing the log likelihood function by Newton-Raphson iteration.

A weakly (semi) parametric approach was considered by Bacchetti and Jewell (1991). A discrete monthly time scale was used for the incubation period distribution and a separate parameter, α_i, was used to represent the discrete hazard for each month i. Here α_i is the probability AIDS develops in month i given that the person was still AIDS free at the beginning of month i after infection. To avoid irregularities that result from trying to estimate a large number of parameters, they used a penalized likelihood function; that is, the log likelihood function is penalized for "roughness." The penalized log-likelihood function is

$$\sum \log l_i - \lambda \sum [(\alpha_i - \alpha_{i+1}) - (\alpha_{i+1} - \alpha_{i+2})]^2, \qquad (4.6)$$

where $\lambda > 0$ is the "tuning" parameter that calibrates the desired smoothness of the estimated hazard function. A completely nonparametric approach to the problem has been given by De Gruttola and Lagakos (1989a). However the completely nonparametric estimate is often numerically unstable, and it is not defined for all values of t.

4.5.4 Application to Hemophilia-associated AIDS

Some of the methods described in Sections 4.5.2 and 4.5.3 are illustrated on a study of 458 hemophilia-associated AIDS cases and analyzed by Brookmeyer and Goedert (1989). These data are from a subset of patients in the National Cancer Institute Multicenter Hemophilia Cohort Study, who were active patients on January 1, 1978, at one of three hemophilia treatment centers (Hershey, New York, and Pittsburgh). Of the 458 hemophiliacs, 296 had a positive screening test for HIV, and 42 of these progressed to AIDS by last follow-up (May 1, 1988). One hundred twenty-two of these hemophiliacs seroconverted before the time of their earliest available serum sample (that is, their first serum sample was positive). It was assumed these individuals seroconverted between January 1, 1978, and R_i. The widths of the 296 seroconversion intervals ($R_i - L_i$) were variable and ranged between 2 months and 7.5 years with a median of 2.3 years. We computed the incubation distributions among hemophiliacs over the age of 20 at seroconversion using three methodologies: midpoint imputation (Section 4.5.2), conditional mean imputation (Section 4.5.2), and joint parametric modeling (Section 4.5.3).

In order to use conditional mean imputation or joint parametric models, parametric models are needed for the distribution of seroconversion times. It had been suggested that the severity of hemophilia (mild, moderate, or severe) was a risk factor for HIV infection. More severe cases of hemophilia receive larger and more frequent doses of replacement clotting factors. Thus, it is plausible that more severe cases of hemophilia were more likely to have been infected and at an earlier calendar time than milder cases. Accordingly, we estimated the cumulative distribution function, G, of calendar times of seroconversion separately for mild, moderate and severe cases of hemophilia. These estimates were based on the interval censored data $[(L_i, R_i), \varepsilon_i]$ using the nonparametric methods of Turnbull (1976) (Figure 4.5). Figure 4.5 displays the nonparametric estimates of the cumulative proportions infected (G) for mild, moderate, and severe hemophilia. The figure shows that severity was a strong risk factor for infection. For example, by January 1, 1985, more than 84% of severe cases of hemophiliacs had

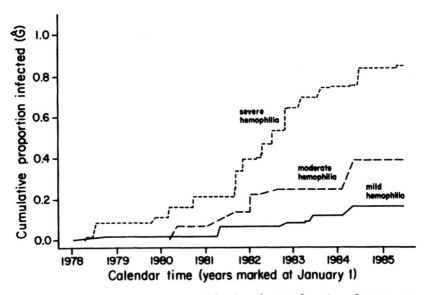

Figure 4.5 Nonparametric estimates of the distribution function of seroconversion times among hemophiliacs by severity of hemophilia: mild (91 hemophiliacs), moderate (55 hemophiliacs), and severe (312 hemophiliacs).

seroconverted compared to only 15% among mild cases. The figure also suggests a burst of infections in the early 1980s. Accordingly, piecewise exponential distributions with jumps in the hazard occurring at January 1, 1981, and January 1, 1983, were chosen to model the infection curves for mild, moderate and severe hemophilia. These three curves were used to impute seroconversion dates using conditional means. We also performed joint parametric modelling using separate piecewise exponential curves for g for the three grades of severity, and a Weibull model for F. The resulting estimates of F are shown in Figure 4.6. There was good agreement among all three estimates (midpoint, conditional mean, and joint parametric modeling).

4.5.5 Truncation Effects

The previous likelihood developed in Section 4.5.3 assumed that a cohort of uninfected individuals was assembled at calendar time $s = 0$. However, this may not always be the case, and special attention must be paid to the sampling criteria for entry into the cohort.

For example, uninfected individuals may enter the cohort at arbitary calendar times, E_i. In the hemophilia example, E_i could refer to the date of birth of hemophiliacs born after calendar time $s = 0$ (taken to

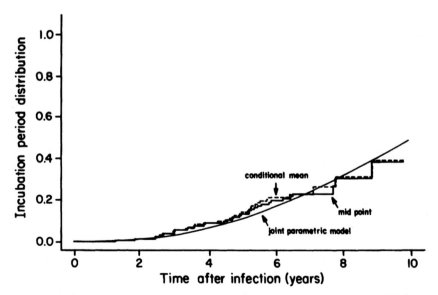

Figure 4.6 Incubation distribution estimates derived from a cohort of hemophiliacs over age 20 at seroconversion using three methodologies: midpoint imputation, conditional mean imputation, and joint parametric modelling.

be January 1, 1978). These hemophiliacs are not at risk of infection for all calendar time and this is accounted for in the analysis by using the truncated density

$$g_i(s) = \frac{g(s)}{1 - G(E_i)} \qquad \text{for } s \geqslant E_i$$

instead of $g(s)$ in equation (4.5).

Another example of truncation effects arises if the cohort consists of a sample of individuals who are free of AIDS at calendar time Υ (see Figure 4.4). The individuals may or may not be infected at time Υ, but must not have been diagnosed with AIDS prior to Υ. Thus in Figure 4.4 individual 1 is included, but individual 2 is excluded. The qualitative effect of this sampling scheme is to selectively exclude those with very short incubation periods since those who develop AIDS prior to calendar time Υ are not eligible. This can be accounted for in the analysis by using the truncated density

$$g_i(s) = \frac{g(s)}{\int_0^{\Upsilon} g(s)S(\Upsilon - s)ds + (1 - G(\Upsilon))}$$

in place of g in equation (4.5). The denominator of this truncated density is the probability of being AIDS free at calendar time Υ which is the probability of being either infected and AIDS free or uninfected at time Υ.

4.6 DECONVOLUTION METHODS (Back-Calculating the Incubation Distribution)

Another approach to estimating the incubation period distribution uses population AIDS incidence data and estimates of the HIV infection rates in the population (Bacchetti and Moss, 1989; Bacchetti, 1990). The expected cumulative AIDS incidence up to calendar time t, $A(t)$, is related to infection rates at calendar times $g(s)$, and the incubation period distribution, by the convolution equation

$$A(t) = \int_0^t g(s) \cdot F(t - s)ds. \tag{4.7}$$

The basic idea is to use data on $A(t)$ and an estimate of $g(s)$ to glean information about F. These methods are closely related to the back-calculation methodology described in Chapter 8, which uses data on $A(t)$ and an estimate of F, to estimate historical infection rates $g(s)$.

The usefulness of this method depends upon the availability of accurate information on the infection rates in the population. This approach has been used successfully in the population of homosexual men in San Francisco, where there is detailed information from epidemiologic surveys on the historical infection rates.

The statistical framework is as follows. Let y_i represent the number of AIDS cases diagnosed in the calendar interval $[t_{i-1}, t_i)$ $i = 1, \ldots, m$. Suppose, N, the cumulative number of infections that occurred before t_m is known, and the probability density of infection times of the N individuals, g^*, is known. Then, $\mathbf{y} = (y_1, \ldots, y_m)$ have a multinomial distribution with sample size N and cell probabilities

$$p_i = \int_0^{t_i} g^*(s) \cdot [F(t_i - s) - F(t_{i-1} - s)]ds,$$

where the incubation distribution $F(t)$ is defined to be 0 for $t \leqslant 0$. In this formulation, g^* and N are assumed known, and a parametric model for F is postulated. Then, apart from an additive constant, the log-likelihood function for the observed AIDS incidence data $(y_1, \ldots, y_m)$ is

$$\text{LL} = \sum_{i=1}^{m} y_i \log p_i + \left(N - \sum_{i=1}^{m} y_i \right) \log \left(1 - \sum_{i=1}^{m} p_i \right). \tag{4.8}$$

The log-likelihood function is maximized over the parameters of F.

Bacchetti (1990) applied these ideas to estimate F from data on AIDS incidence and infection rates in gay men in San Francisco. Using data from three cohorts of gay men in San Francisco, he first estimated $g^*(s)$, the probability density of dates of seroconversion among all those infected before 1989. Semiparametric methods with a penalty function like that in equation (4.6) estimate $g^*(s)$ as a discrete probability mass function on each month from January, 1978, to December, 1988. In order to estimate F from the likelihood (4.8), it was necessary to estimate the total number of infections in gay men in San Francisco before 1989. This was done by rescaling the estimate of 8760 AIDS-free seropositive gay men obtained from a population-based probability sample in the San Francisco Men's Health Study (Winkelstein, Lyman, Padian, et al., 1987). Because the estimate of 8760 pertained to those recruited through September 1984 in an area of San Francisco that had contributed 45.5% of all AIDS cases reported, the estimate was rescaled to $8760/0.455 = 19,253$. Addition of some patients with AIDS who were not included in the original survey estimate and a further rescaling based on $g^*(s)$ to account for infections occurring between October 1984 and December 1988 yielded an estimate of $N = 22,030$. Uncertainties in N are important, because N varies inversely with $\hat{F}$, as is seen by setting $g(s) = Ng^*(s)$ in equation (4.7).

Both the estimation of $g^*(s)$ and N are based on the assumption that the studied cohorts and the population-based sample in one part of San Francisco are representative of the epidemic among all gay men in San Francisco.

To estimate F, a semiparametric model was used that included a separate discrete time hazard for each month. The hazard estimates were smoothed using a penalized likelihood like that in equation (4.6). The hazard of AIDS is negligible for the first several years after seroconversion and then rises sharply (Figure 4.7). There is considerable uncertainty about the shape of the hazard after 7 years, as reflected in the sensitivity of the estimated hazard to the degree of smoothing used.

Two other sources of uncertainty, apart from choice of the tuning parameter (degree of smoothing) are important. First, an assessment of the effects of random variability in estimates of N, $g^*(s)$ and the incubation times themselves yields wide confidence intervals on the estimated hazard after 7 years (figure 6 in Bacchetti, 1990). Continued increases in the hazard after 7 years and slight decreases in the hazard after 7 years both fall within these confidence intervals. Second, the estimate of $g^*(s)$ indicates that the HIV infection rate peaked in late

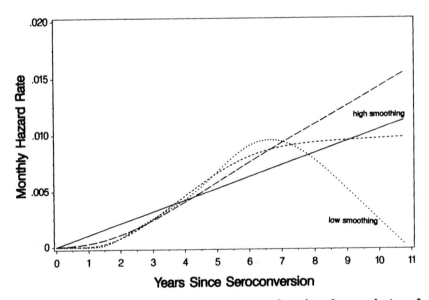

Figure 4.7 Hazard functions of progression to AIDS based on deconvolution of AIDS incidence data in San Francisco with four choices of the smoothing parameter. (Source: Bacchetti, 1990. Reprinted with permission from the *Journal of the American Statistical Association.* Copyright 1990 by the American Statistical Association.)

1981 (see Figure 1.5). Because clinical trials of zidovudine were ongoing in 1986 and because zidovudine and other treatments were introduced in 1987, only 5 or 6 years after the estimated peak infection rates, it is possible that the leveling of the hazard beyond year 7 (Figure 4.7) reflects the effect of treatment (Bacchetti, 1990).

Estimates of the incubation distribution based on equation (4.7) with $g(s)$ assumed known are more precise than analogous back-calculated estimates of the infection curve $g(s)$ with F assumed known (Chapter 8). This is because the sharp peak in the infection curve for San Francisco (Figure 1.5) reduces uncertainty about when infections occurred. In contrast, the incubation distribution, F, is diffuse, making it more difficult to extract information about $g(s)$ by deconvolving equation (4.7).

4.7 DURATION OF THE PRE-ANTIBODY PHASE

The interval between first exposure to HIV and the development of detectable antibodies (seroconversion) is called the pre-antibody phase. The duration of the pre-antibody phase has important implications for the scope of the epidemic because individuals could be infectious even though they test seronegative (no detectable antibodies).

The duration of the pre-antibody phase is uncertain. The major methodological problem with studies of the pre-antibody phase is that the calendar time of first exposure to HIV is often unknown. The most reliable studies are based on patients who acquire HIV infection through blood transfusion and organ transplantation or health care workers exposed to HIV through identifiable accidents, such as needle sticks. In these instances the date of first HIV exposure (infection) can be ascertained.

Horsburgh, Qu, Jason, et al. (1989) analyzed 45 published reports of cases with known infection dates (7 infected by blood transfusion; 8 by organ transplantation; 17 by contaminated factor VIII among hemophiliacs; 7 needle stick injuries; 2 by sexual contact with HIV infected individuals; and 4 related to contaminated needles associated with intravenous drug use). These patients were serially tested for HIV antibody, and thus the date of seroconversion could be ascertained up to an interval (L_i, R_i) where L_i is the time of the last seronegative antibody test and R_i is the time of the first seropositive antibody test, and where these times are measured since the known point of infection. These investigators studied several distributions $F(t)$ for the duration of the pre-antibody phase, including a Weibull model and an exponential model, each with a guarantee time parameter (Longini, Clark, Haber, and Horsburgh, 1989). Models of this type can be fitted by maximizing

$$\prod_{i=1}^{N} [F(R_i) - F(L_i)] \tag{4.6}$$

Horsburgh, Qu, Jason, et al. (1989) reported a median pre-antibody duration of 2.1 months (standard error 0.1 months) and a 95th percentile of 5.8 months, based on an exponential model with a guarantee time of 1 month. This distribution is $F(t) = 0$ for $0 \leqslant t < 1$, and $F(t) = 1 - \exp(-0.625(t - 1))$ for $t > 1$, where t is measured in months.

A caveat concerning these results is that individuals with long pre-antibody durations may have been selectively excluded because the data set included only individuals who were known to have seroconverted within their follow-up time. Strictly, the contribution of the ith individual to the likelihood in equation (4.6) should be divided by $1 - e^{-\lambda T_i}$ where T_i is the maximum period of follow-up for the ith individual. An important point is that this study design involves only seroconverters and thus provides no information about the probability of seroconversion given exposure to HIV. It is only informative about the time to seroconversion following exposure among those individuals who seroconvert.

A second type of study for quantifying the duration of the pre-antibody phase is based on detection of HIV DNA by the polymerase chain reaction (PCR). In these studies, the time of infection was estimated by detection of HIV DNA from serial alliquots of blood. The date of infection is assumed to occur in the interval defined by the last negative and first positive PCR test. Similarly, the dates of seroconversion are assumed to occur in the interval defined by the last negative and first positive HIV antibody test. Thus, the data is interval censored on both the left and the right. Horsburgh, Qu, Jason, et al. (1989) reported the results of such a PCR study based on 39 infected individuals and assumed an exponential distribution for the pre-antibody duration. They estimated that the median duration of the pre-antibody phase was 2.4 months and that 95% of infected individuals had a pre-antibody phase of less than 10.3 months.

In contrast, Wolinski, Rinaldo, Kwok, et al. (1989) reported a median pre-antibody duration of 18 months based on a PCR study. The discrepancy between the Horsburgh and Wolinski studies is partially explained by selection bias in the Wolinski study. The latter study selected individuals from the Multicenter AIDS Cohort Study who seroconverted late in calendar time (in the late 1980s). These individuals are a biased sample and overrepresent the longer pre-antibody durations because individuals with short pre-antibody durations would have been more likely to seroconvert earlier in calendar time and thus not be included in the study (Winkelstein, Royce, and Sheppard (1990); Wolinski, Rinaldo, and Phair (1990)).

4.8 SYNTHESIS OF KNOWLEDGE OF THE INCUBATION PERIOD DISTRIBUTION

The main complexities in the analysis and interpretation of epidemiological studies of the incubation period include uncertainty in the dates of infection and the sampling criteria by which individuals are included in the data set. Synthesizing and comparing estimates across studies is important since the estimates are typically based on various methodologies with different underlying assumptions.

Reviews of studies of the incubation period distribution have been given by Moss and Bacchetti (1989) and by Gail and Rosenberg (1992). Table 4.2 presents several estimates of the incubation period distribution reported from a number of different studies that were selected to show a range of methodologies and populations. These studies include: (a) midpoint imputation for the San Francisco City Clinic Cohort of homosexual men; (b) deconvolution of AIDS incidence data in San Francisco; (c) parametric modeling of a hemophilia cohort; and (d) midpoint imputation for a cohort of intravenous drug users in Italy. Several of these studies have identified a significant age effect. For example Goedert, Kessler, Aledort, et al. (1989) found that hemophiliacs over the age of 30 at infection are at higher risk of progression to AIDS than individuals 19 to 30 years old at the time of infection. Similar results were found among hemophiliacs by Darby, Rizza, Doll, et al. (1989) and in a cohort of intravenous drug users (Mariotto, Mariotti, Pezzotti, et al. 1992; see also Italian Seroconversion Study, 1992). Cofactors such as age are considered again in Chapter 5.

A general picture emerges from Table 4.2. First, the probability of developing AIDS within the first two years of seroconversion is very small, less than .03. Then, the hazard of progression to AIDS begins to rise rapidly so that the cumulative probability of developing AIDS within 7.0 years of seroconversion is approximately .25. The cumulative probability of AIDS approaches .50 at 10.0 years following seroconversion.

A striking feature of Table 4.2 is the similarity of the estimates in columns (a) – (d), especially since the modes of viral transmission are

Table 4.2 Cumulative Probabilities of Progressing to AIDS, $F(t)$

Years Following Seroconversion (t)	SFCC[a] (midpoint)	San Francisco[b] (deconvolution)	Hemophiliacs[c] (joint parametric modeling)	IVDU[d] (midpoint)
1.0		.002	.002	.002
2.0	.010	.009	.012	.015
3.0		.031	.033	.031
4.0	.040	.074	.066	.048
5.0		.135	.113	.093
6.0	.20	.208	.174	.143
7.0		.290	.245	.212
8.0	.37	.371	.325	
9.0		.445	.411	
10.0	.51	.512	.498	
11.0	.54			

[a]San Francisco City Clinic Cohort of homosexual men enrolled in hepatitis vaccine study. Date of seroconversion estimated by midpoint imputation (Hessol, Lifson, O'Malley, et al., 1989).

[b]Deconvolution of AIDS incidence data in San Francisco using epidemiologic surveys to reconstruct the distribution of infection times (Bacchetti and Moss, 1989).

[c]Joint parametric modeling of 458 hemophiliacs with Weibull model for $F(t)$. $F(t) = 1 - \exp(-.0021t^{2.516})$ for hemophiliacs > age 20 (Brookmeyer and Goedert, 1989).

[d]Cohort of 468 seroconverters who were injecting drug users (Italian Seroconversion Study, 1992). Additional details of this study in Rezza, Lazzarin, Angarano, et al. (1989).

different. Mariotto, Mariotti, Pezzotti, et al. (1992) compared the incubation distribution among male homosexuals and intravenous drug users in Italian cities and did not find a significant difference.

Follow-up was restricted to about 10 years after infection in these studies. Thus estimates of the incubation period distribution beyond 10 years, and estimates of the mean incubation period, depend on assumptions about how to extrapolate the incubation distribution or upon assumptions about the validity of parametric models beyond the range of the data. Only additional follow-up on these cohorts will further define the tail of the distribution. However, the use of treatments such as zidovudine in these cohorts may alter the incubation period distribution (see Section 8.6, and Chapter 11). Zidovudine was introduced in 1987 for both AIDS patients and infected individuals without AIDS but with advanced HIV disease. Treatments such as zidovudine, inhaled pentamidine and other therapeutic advances may lengthen the incubation period. Accordingly, there will be little

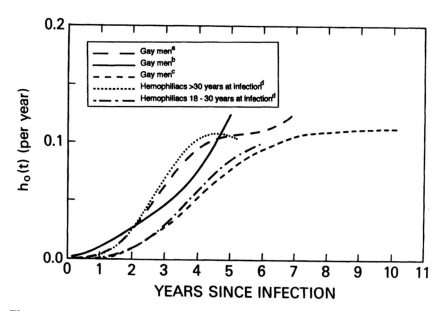

Figure 4.8 Smoothed estimates of the hazard of AIDS using follow-up through January 1, 1987. (Source: Gail and Rosenberg, 1992.)
   Key:
[a]Hessol, Lifson, O'Malley, et al. (1989)
[b]Biggar and the International Registry of Seroconverters (1990), excluding those in curve (a)
[c]Bacchetti (1990)
[d]Goedert, Kessler, Aledort, et al. (1989)

available information on the *natural history* of HIV infection (i.e., no treatment intervention) beyond 10 years.

Gail and Rosenberg (1992) evaluated and synthesized information on the hazard of AIDS following seroconversion from various studies. They attempted to eliminate the possible effects of treatment by restricting follow-up to calendar time before 1987. They obtained smooth hazard estimates by fitting spline models (Figure 4.8) to data from: (1) the San Francisco City Clinic Cohort of homosexual men who participated in hepatitis B vaccine trials (Hessol, Lifson, O'Malley, et al. (1989); (2) a cohort of hemophiliacs who attended hemophilia treatment centers (Goedert, Kessler, Aledort, et al., 1989); and (3) an international registry of seroconverters (Biggar and the International Registry of Seroconverters, 1990). In addition, they included hazard estimates by deconvolving AIDS incidence and infection rate estimates in San Francisco (Bacchetti, 1990), as described in Section 4.6. Each of those studies indicates a rapidly increasing hazard up to about year 5 (Figure 4.8). There is little information about the hazard of progression to AIDS, in the absence of treatment, beyond 6 years.

5

Cofactors and Markers

5.1 INTRODUCTION

This chapter is concerned with statistical issues in studies of cofactors and markers of HIV infections. Cofactors are variables that affect the duration of the incubation period and may explain why some infected individuals progress to AIDS faster than other individuals. Markers are variables that track the progression of HIV infection. Markers are consequences of infection, while cofactors are causal agents rather than consequences of disease progression (Brookmeyer, Gail, and Polk, 1987). An example of a cofactor is age at infection. Some studies have shown that infants and the elderly have shorter incubation periods than other infected individuals. An example of a marker is the number of CD4+ T cells. The CD4+ T cell is the target cell of HIV, and many studies show marked declines of the CD4+ T cell count with progression of HIV disease (Gottlieb, Schroff, Schanker, et al., 1981; Polk, Fox, Brookmeyer, et al., 1987; Goedert, Biggar, Melbye, et al., 1987).

Three general classes of AIDS markers have emerged (Goedert, 1990). Immunological markers include concentrations of CD4+ T cells and CD8+ T cells, levels of serum $beta_2$-microglobulin and serum neopterin, and anergy to cutaneous tests for delayed hyposensitivity. Viral markers include presence or absence of detectable p24 (core) antigen and plasma viremia (detection of infectious HIV in fresh plasma). Clinical markers include weight loss, candidiasis, persistent diarrhea, herpes zoster, fatigue and night sweats, persistent fever, and oral hairy leukoplakia. Some established markers and cofactors of HIV disease are summarized in Table 5.1.

Knowledge of markers and cofactors is important in three broad areas of inquiry. First, markers and cofactors characterize the natural

Table 5.1 Some Established Markers and Cofactors of HIV Disease

I. Markers for Progression to AIDS
    Immunological
        Depressed CD4+ T cells
        Elevated serum Beta-2
            microglobulin
        Elevated serum neopterin
        Cutaneous anergy

    Viral
        Detectable p24 (core) antigen
        Plasma viremia

    Clinical

Weight loss	Night sweats
Oral candidiasis	Persistent fever
Persistent diarrhea	Oral hairy leukoplakia
Herpes zoster	

II. Cofactors
    Age at infection (very young and very old at increased risk)

Note: General reference: Goedert (1990).

history of HIV infection. Cofactors may at least partially explain the wide variability in incubation periods. The evolution of markers with time, such as the CD4+ T cell count trajectory, chronicle the progression of HIV infection. Second, markers and cofactors are useful for designing and analyzing clinical studies of treatment for HIV infection. For example, when comparing two therapies for HIV infected individuals it may be important to stratify or control for cofactors and markers measured at baseline (prognostic factors) to insure the two treatment groups are comparable at baseline. Markers also may be useful surrogate endpoints in clinical trials. Surrogate endpoints are alternatives to traditional clinical endpoints such as AIDS diagnosis or death. The use of surrogate endpoints may shorten clinical studies, but the clinical interpretation of the results may be problematic (Chapter 11).

Third, markers and cofactors may be useful prognostic factors for predicting progression to AIDS and are thus useful in the clinical management of patients. For example, one might wish to withold a potentially toxic treatment in asymptomatic HIV infected patients with CD4+ T cells above 500 cells/μl but aggressively treat an HIV infected patient with fewer than 200 CD4+ T cells/μl.

We begin our discussion with cofactors. Markers are considered in Sections 5.5–5.8. Since the early years of the epidemic, epidemiologists have been searching for cofactors that may explain why some infected individuals progress to AIDS faster than others. Variables that have been investigated as potential cofactors include age at infection, risk or transmission group (e.g., sexual transmission, blood transfusion recipient, intravenous drug use), genetic factors such as human lymphocyte antigen (HLA) type, and behavioral factors such as smoking and alcohol use.

It is useful to distinguish between two types of cofactors, fixed and variable. Fixed cofactors are variables that are fixed at the time of infection. Examples of fixed cofactors include age at infection and transmission (risk) group. Variable cofactors may change values over time and could include conditions not present at the time of the initial HIV infection. An example of a variable cofactor is the number of pregnancies subsequent to HIV infection. In this framework, treatments given to HIV infected individuals could be viewed as variable cofactors. Statistical issues in treatment evaluation are considered in Chapter 11.

The ideal study for learning about cofactors would be a cohort study of newly infected individuals, an incident cohort. For each member of the cohort, information would be ascertained on cofactors, date of infection and date of AIDS diagnosis. Classical survival methods could be used to analyze the data. For example, the Cox proportional hazards model (1972) relates the hazard of progression to AIDS at t years following infection, $\lambda(t)$, to a vector of covariates, $\mathbf{X}(t)$, through

$$\lambda(t) = \lambda_0(t)e^{\boldsymbol{\beta}\mathbf{X}(t)}, \tag{5.1}$$

where $\boldsymbol{\beta}$ are regression coefficients and $\lambda_0(t)$ is an arbitrary nonnegative function, the *baseline hazard*. The vector $\mathbf{X}(t)$ may include both fixed and time-varying covariates measured at time t.

A number of important statistical problems arise in applying classical survival methods to epidemiological studies of cofactors. For example, in prevalent cohort studies, the duration of infection is unknown (Section 4.4), and a potentially serious bias known as *onset confounding* could result if we use follow-up time rather than duration of infection as the underlying time scale t in model (5.1). The evaluation of cofactors from prevalent cohorts is discussed in Section 5.3. Serious potential biases can also arise in analyses of cofactor effects based on retrospective studies of AIDS cases (Section 5.4), such as the studies of transfusion-associated AIDS described in Section 4.3. The most useful information about cofactors has been obtained from cohort studies in which the times of infection are known or confined to lie within a known interval (doubly censored data). Statistical methods for the evaluation of cofactors from doubly censored data are considered in Section 5.2.

5.2 COFACTORS AND DOUBLY CENSORED DATA

In most epidemiological studies of cofactors, the dates of infection will be known only to lie within defined intervals (see Section 4.5). The only exceptions are the transfusion-associated studies of AIDS considered in Section 5.4. If the interval is short, very simple analytic procedures may be satisfactory, such as using the midpoint of the interval as the infection date. A number of epidemiological studies have used this approach. For example, in the National Cancer Institute Multicenter Hemophilia Cohort Study, the date of infection was estimated as the midpoint in time between the last negative and first positive specimens for subjects with previously frozen serum samples (Goedert, Kessler, Aledort, et al., 1989). This study demonstrated a strong association between older age at seroconversion and higher risks of progression to AIDS. A study of hemophiliacs in the United Kingdom also identified these age effects (Darby, Rizza, Doll, et al., 1989). In that study, the dates of infection were imputed as the conditional mean, namely the expected seroconversion date given that seroconversion occurred in a particular interval. We present simple imputation methods and more sophisticated procedures that may be needed if the intervals are wide.

5.2.1 Analytic Procedures

Simple Imputation Methods
The following discussion generalizes Section 4.5.2 to incorporate covariates. We adopt the notation introduced in Section 4.5.2, where (L_i, R_i) is the interval of infection; ε_i is the infection indicator; δ_i is the disease indicator; w_i is the calendar time of last follow-up or AIDS diagnosis.

An ad hoc approach is to impute (estimate) the calendar time of infection by the midpoint of the interval in which infection was known to have occurred (see equations (4.4a) and (4.4b)). This yields imputed (possibly right censored) incubation periods $(\hat{u}_i, \hat{\delta}_i)$. Standard survival analytic techniques are used on the imputed incubation periods. For example, Kaplan–Meier curves could be computed for each level of a fixed cofactor and one could test for differences between the corresponding incubation distributions by a nonparametric procedure such as the logrank test (Cox and Oakes, 1984).

If the probability density of infection times does not depend on the cofactor, X, under investigation, that is $g_x^*(s) \equiv g^*(s)$, the discussion in

Section 4.5.2 suggests the bias of the Kaplan–Meier estimates based on the data $(\hat{u}_i, \delta_i)$ from midpoint imputation will be small for interval widths less than two years (Law and Brookmeyer, 1992). Furthermore, the logrank and other nonparametric tests will have the correct size using midpoint imputed data for testing the null hypothesis,

$$H_o: F_0(t) = F_1(t),$$

where F_0 and F_1 are the incubation distributions for those with $X = 0$ and $X = 1$ respectively. The power of the test will be reduced compared to using known infection times.

However, there are situations where the covariate X may be associated with the calendar time of infection, in which case midpoint imputation can be misleading. In particular, tests of the null hypothesis $H_o: F_0 \equiv F_1$ may not have the correct size (Law and Brookmeyer, 1992). This is illustrated qualitatively by the following example. Suppose the *dose of innoculum*, X, is associated with the risk of infection, and we are interested in determining if X affects the incubation distribution. Examples of such covariates are the level of sexual activity, which is a possible surrogate for the dose of viral innoculum in sexual transmission and the amount of replacement clotting factor received by a patient with hemophilia, which is again a possible surrogate for the dose of viral innoculum. Suppose in truth that X was unrelated to the incubation period but that individuals with $X = 1$ were at higher risk of infection than individuals with $X = 0$. Then, those with $X = 1$ are likely to have been infected earlier than those with $X = 0$, and midpoint imputation could falsely give the appearance that the $X = 1$ subgroup has shorter incubation periods than the $X = 0$ subgroup. A similar difficulty would attend the use of the conditional mean or any other imputation procedure that does not allow for the fact that X is a determinant of when infection occurred. As the intervals widths get smaller and smaller so that the exact dates of infection are known precisely, this type of bias vanishes.

If it is believed that X is associated with calendar time of infection, the following is a sensible alternative to midpoint imputation. The approach is to separately estimate the infection time distribution for each level of X based on the interval censored data $(L_i, R_i, \varepsilon_i)$. Specifically one would assume parametric models for the infection time distributions g_0 and g_1, and obtain estimates $\hat{g}_0$ and $\hat{g}_1$ using techniques for interval censored data. An imputed incubation period is then computed from the estimates of the conditional mean infection time:

$$\hat{s}_i = \frac{\int_{L_i}^{R_i} s\hat{g}_X(s)\,ds}{\hat{G}_X(R_i) - \hat{G}_X(L_i)}.$$

The key feature of this equation is that the imputation procedure depends on X. Standard survival analyses are then applied to the imputed incubation times. This is the approach used by Darby, Rizza, Doll, et al., (1989).

Joint Parametric Modelling

If the interval widths are large, simple imputation methods may not be satisfactory, and more formal parametric modelling may be required. The methods of Section 4.5.3 can be generalized to allow the distribution of calendar time of infection to depend upon covariates X_1, and the incubation period distribution to depend on covariates X_2 (Brookmeyer and Goedert, 1989). Some of the same covariates may be common to both X_1 and X_2. Brookmeyer and Goedert (1989) referred to this approach as a two-stage regression model, where stage 1 was a model for calendar time of infection and stage 2 was a model for the incubation period given that infection occurred.

The probability density of infection at calendar time s is called $g^*(s; X_1, \alpha)$ where α is a vector of unknown parameters. The probability density of incubation periods is called $f(t; X_2, \beta)$ with survivorship function $S(t; X_2, \beta) = 1 - F(t; X_2, \beta)$ where F is the distribution of incubation periods and β is a vector of unknown parameters. It is assumed that conditional on the covariates X_1 and X_2, the calendar time of infection is independent of the incubation period. The validity of this assumption would be suspect if either the virulence of the virus changes over time, or if there are additional cofactors, such as the use of effective treatments, that are not included in X_2. It is also assumed that the frequency and timing of screening serum samples to determine when infection occurred are independent of both the calendar date of infection and the incubation period. Under these assumptions, the likelihood function is constructed as outlined in Section 4.5.3.

5.2.2 Application to Hemophilia Cohort

These methods were applied to the National Cancer Institute Multicenter Hemophilia Cohort Study (Brookmeyer and Goedert, 1989). The data derived from 458 patients with hemophilia (see Section 4.5.4 for the study design). Covariates (X_1) that were thought to affect risk of infection included hemophilia treatment center, hemophilia type, and severity of hemophilia. Covariates (X_2) that were thought to affect the incubation period included age at seroconversion and the severity of hemophilia. A piecewise exponential regression model for the calendar time at infection was used. If $\lambda_1(s; \mathbf{X}_1, \boldsymbol{\alpha})$ is the hazard function for infection at calendar time s for an individual with covariates $\mathbf{X}_1$, then

$$\log\{\lambda_1(s; \mathbf{X}_1, \boldsymbol{\alpha}\} = \alpha_0(s) + \alpha_1 \mathbf{X}_1,$$

where $\alpha_0(s) = \gamma_i$ for $w_{i-1} \leqslant s < w_i$. Calendar time s was measured from the origin, January 1, 1978, with changes in the hazard occurring at January 1, 1981, and January 1, 1983. A Weibull regression model was used for the incubation period. If $\lambda_2(t; \mathbf{X}_2, \boldsymbol{\beta})$ is the hazard of AIDS at time t units after seroconversion for an individual with covariate vector $\mathbf{X}_2$, then

$$\log\{\lambda_2(t; \mathbf{X}_2, \boldsymbol{\beta})] = \beta_0 + \beta_1 \mathbf{X}_2 + \log(pt^{p-1}).$$

Maximum likelihood estimates can be obtained by maximizing the log-likelihood by Newton–Raphson iteration. Good starting values are important to obtain rapid convergence. One simple approach for obtaining starting values is to augment the data with the midpoint estimate, $\hat{s}_i$, of the date of infection. Given $\hat{s}_i$, the likelihood for $\boldsymbol{\alpha}$ and $\boldsymbol{\beta}$ each have the usual form of likelihoods for right censored survival data, and the joint likelihood factors into two components, one involving only $\boldsymbol{\alpha}$ and the other involving only $\boldsymbol{\beta}$. Thus $\boldsymbol{\alpha}$ and $\boldsymbol{\beta}$ can be separately estimated using standard maximum likelihood algorithms for right censored data. Generalized linear interactive modeling (GLIM), for example, can be used to maximize likelihoods for right censored data under piecewise exponential and Weibull regression models (Aitkin and Clayton, 1980). Using these starting values for $\boldsymbol{\alpha}$ and $\boldsymbol{\beta}$, one can proceed to maximize the true likelihood function.

Maximum likelihood estimates along with the maximized log-likelihood are given in Table 5.2. Nested models can be compared by a likelihood ratio test. The broad conclusions from this model-building can be summarized as follows. Type A hemophiliacs with the highest severity of hemophilia (severity = 3) were at highest risk of infection This is consistent with the hypothesis that HIV preferentially precipitates out in Factor VIII concentrate, which is the replacement clotting factor for Type A hemophilia (Goedert, Sarngadharan, Eyster, et al., 1985). The importance of severity of hemophilia for risk of infection was also not unexpected, because more severe cases of hemophilia tend to receive more frequent and larger doses of replacement clotting factors. However severity does not appear to affect risk of progression to AIDS (compare models 1 and 2: $X^2(1) = 2(916.45 - 916.40) = .10$). If severity can be considered a surrogate measure of dose of innoculum, then the results suggest that innoculum does not affect the incubation period. Hemophiliacs who are older at

Table 5.2 Maximum Likelihood Estimates[a] Based on Piecewise Exponential/Weibull Two-Stage Model[b] for Infection and Disease (AIDS) Incidence

	Stage 1—Infection (X_1)				Stage 2—AIDS Incidence (X_2)				
Model	Type	N.Y.	Pittsburgh	Severity	Shape (p)	Intercept (β_0)	Age	Severity	Maximized loglikelihood
1	-1.286	.112	-.339	1.128	2.497	-22.447	1.432	.056	-916.40
2[c]	-1.287	.112	-.339	1.129	2.516	-22.444	1.432	—	-916.45
3	-1.307	.095	-.334	1.133	2.620	-22.298	—	.119	-924.69
4	-1.477	.627	-.043	—	2.346	-21.612	1.563	—	-978.06
5	—	.102	-.344	1.082	2.520	-22.443	1.432	—	-942.91
6	-1.472	.673	.021	—	2.423	-21.806	1.533	—	-978.10
7	-1.287	—	—	1.105	2.516	-22.444	1.432	—	-920.97
8	-1.286	—	-.339	1.141	2.517	-22.444	1.432	—	-916.74

Source: Brookmeyer and Goedert, 1989.

[a] Analyzed in time units of days.

[b] Covariates coded as follows: N.Y. and Pittsburgh were indicator variables; severity was coded 1, 2 and 3 for mild, moderate and severe, respectively; hemophilia type coded 0 for A and 1 for other; age coded 0 for <20 years and 1 for ⩾20 years.

[c] Intercept terms α_0 in piecewise exponential model for infection were -11.91 during 1978–80, -9.985 during 1981–83, and -10.01 during 1984–July 1985.

seroconversion ($\geq$ age 20) are at an increased risk of progression compared to younger hemophiliacs (compare models 2 and 3: $X^2(1) = 2(924.69 - 916.45) = 16.48$). Age has been found to be a cofactor in other studies as mentioned previously.

5.3 Cofactors and Prevalent Cohort Studies

The prevalent cohort study (Section 4.4) is a rapid and convenient approach to identify cofactors and markers of disease progression. However, because the time of viral infection is usually unknown in the cohort, there are several potential sources of bias. These biases arise from using follow-up time instead of time from infection in survival analyses of time to AIDS. We review two forms of bias in the analysis of cofactors in prevalent cohorts: onset confounding and differential length biased sampling. Our notation and setup is the same as in Section 4.4. A group of infected individuals are identified at calendar time Υ and followed for onset of AIDS.

5.3.1 Onset Confounding

Examples
The most important bias associated with identifying cofactors from prevalent cohorts is called onset confounding (Brookmeyer and Gail, 1987; Brookmeyer, Gail, and Polk, 1987). This occurs when the unknown calendar date of infection is associated both with the risk of AIDS and the cofactor under study. A subgroup may appear at higher risk of progression to AIDS simply because they were infected earlier than another subgroup. We give several examples of onset confounding:

1. Figure 5.1 shows estimates of the cumulative probabilities of progressing to AIDS within t years of follow-up, $F_p(t)$, based on prevalent cohorts of infected individuals in several cities. Because the hazard of AIDS increases with time since infection (Chapter 4), the higher estimate of $F_p(t)$ in the New York cohort of homosexual men suggests that the New York cohort was infected earlier than the other cohorts. However, these data are also consistent with the less plausible conclusion that geography is a cofactor, and, in particular, that the course of HIV infection is more rapid in New York than in the other cities.

2. Data from several prevalent cohorts have suggested that sexual exposure to an AIDS patient or to a person who subsequently develops AIDS accelerates progression to AIDS (Polk, Fox, Brookmeyer, et al.,

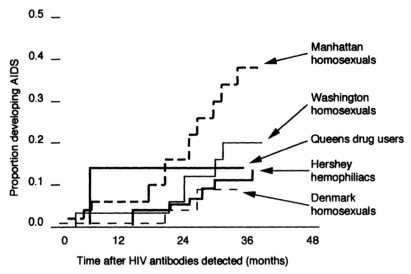

Figure 5.1 Cumulative proportions developing AIDS as a function of follow-up time in prevalent cohorts. (Source: Goedert, Biggar, Weiss, et al., 1986. Copyright 1986 by the American Association for the Advancement of Science.)

1987). This observation is consistent with the hypothesis that some strains of HIV are more virulent than others. However this observation may also be explained if the exposed group consisting of individuals who had sex with AIDS patients or with people who subsequently developed AIDS tended to be infected earlier than individuals who were not exposed (the unexposed group). Indeed, since partners of the exposed group had already developed AIDS while the partners of the unexposed group had not, it is very plausible that the exposed group had been infected for a longer time than the unexposed group. Because the hazard of AIDS increases with time since infection, the exposed group would tend to have higher rates of progression.

3.   The number of previous sex partners has been reported to be a predictor of progression to AIDS in a prevalent cohort (Schechter, Craib, Le, et al., 1989). This is consistent with the hypothesis that a large viral dose (for which number of partners could be a surrogate) accelerates progression. However, the data are also consistent with the very plausible hypothesis that individuals with higher numbers of partners were infected earlier in calendar time.

Mathematical Definition

The requirement to insure no onset confounding is that the probability densities of infection times among individuals infected before calendar time Υ is the same in the two subgroups that is, $g_0^*(s) \equiv g_1^*(s)$. A subtle point is that this requirement is weaker than the requirement that the rate of infection (Section 1.3) must be the same in both subgroups, that is $g_0(s) \equiv g_1(s)$. To clarify this distinction, suppose that the infection rate curve in group $X = 1$ has the same shape as the infection rate curve in group $X = 0$, but that the former is β times the latter, namely

$$g_1(s) = \beta g_0(s). \tag{5.4}$$

An example of a factor that obeys (5.4) is illustrated in Figure 5.2. Even though the *absolute* number of infected individuals is vastly different among those at levels $X = 1$ and $X = 0$, the probability densities of infection times among those infected before time Y are identical in the two subgroups. Whether or not the assumption $g_0^*(s) \equiv g_1^*(s)$ is reasonable for a covariate must be assessed from outside knowledge. For example, the calendar times at infection might not be expected to vary by HLA type, in which case condition $g_0^* = g_1^*$ is satisfied. However, if the virus was introduced earlier into one of two communities, then the probability densities in the two communities might differ by a translation rather than by a multiplicative constant, in which case $g_0^* \neq g_1^*$ (see Figure 5.3).

In the special case that the incubation distributions are exponential

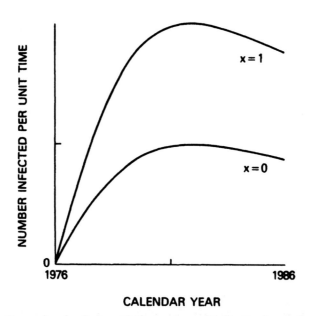

Figure 5.2 Example of a factor, X, that acts multiplicatively on the infection rate curve $g(s)$: X satisfies the condition for no onset confounding. (Source: Brookmeyer, Gail, and Polk, 1987.)

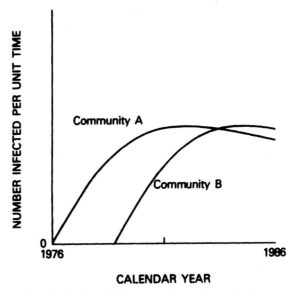

Figure 5.3 Examples of a factor, X, that translates the infection rate curve $g(s)$: X may induce onset confounding. (Source: Brookmeyer, Gail, and Polk 1987.)

in the subgroups $X = 1$ and $X = 0$, there will be no onset confounding even if $g_0^* \neq g_1^*$. This is because the hazard function for an exponential is constant; that is, the exponential distribution is "memoryless" regarding duration of infection.

Stratification to Control Onset Confounding

Onset confounding can be controlled by stratification on factors such as geographic region. Stratification on a covariate is useful provided we are not interested in determining whether the covariate itself is a cofactor of disease progression. In particular, if the analysis is stratified on a covariate that is thought to be related both to risk of infection and to risk of AIDS following infection, it cannot be evaluated as a cofactor of disease progression. For example, individuals with a high level of sexual activity may tend to be infected earlier in an epidemic. We cannot stratify on this variable and simultaneously examine it as a potential cofactor. Another approach that has been suggested to control onset confounding is to adjust for a baseline level of a marker, such as the number of CD4+ T cells at the beginning of follow-up. The appropriateness of this approach depends on how well the marker is correlated with duration of infection and on the mechanism by which the cofactor affects the risk of AIDS. These issues are discussed in Section 5.7.

5.3.2 Differential Length Biased Sampling

Unfortunately, even if X has no direct effect on the infection rate curve, so that there is no onset confounding, relative risk estimates obtained from prevalent cohorts may still be biased. Specifically, suppose a cofactor with two levels obeys the simple proportional hazards model (5.1),

$$\lambda_1(u) = \theta\lambda_o(u),$$

where u is time from infection and λ_1 and λ_o are hazards of developing AIDS. If a proportional hazards analysis is performed based on follow-up time and if there is no onset confounding, then tests of the null hypotheses $H_o : \theta = 1$ will be valid. However estimates of θ based on the incorrect assumption of proportional hazards on the observed follow-up time scale will usually be biased for θ. The term *differential length-biased sampling* is used to refer to this bias, which results from differences in the distributions of prior durations of infection (backward recurrence times) between the two prevalent subgroups. The magnitude and mathematical results concerning this bias have been described in Brookmeyer and Gail (1987).

The direction of the bias depends on whether the hazard function is increasing or decreasing. An intuitive explanation for this bias when the hazard function $\lambda_o(u)$ is increasing is as follows: Individuals in the group $X = 0$ with low hazard of AIDS will tend to have longer times since infection (backward recurrence times) than individuals in the group $X = 1$ with high hazard of AIDS, (see Figure 5.4). This is because people with $X = 1$ who were infected many years earlier are

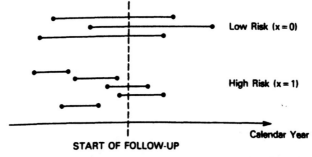

Figure 5.4 Illustration of differential length biased sampling in the prevalent cohort study: The low risk group ($X=0$) has been infected longer at the start of follow-up than the high risk group ($X=1$). (Source: Brookmeyer, Gail, and Polk 1987.)

more likely to have developed AIDS and thus be excluded from the prevalent cohort than people with $X = 0$ who were infected at the same calendar time. Because people with $X = 0$ in the prevalent cohort tend to have been infected for a longer time, and because $\lambda_o(u)$ increases with time since infection, the disparity in the risk of AIDS between the two groups is reduced, biasing the relative risk toward 1. For diseases with a decreasing hazard, the direction of the bias is reversed; the relative risk estimate will be biased away from 1.

Only in the special case when the hazard $\lambda_o(u)$ is constant over time (the exponential model) will the relative risk estimates be unbiased. The exponential model is "memoryless" and implies that individuals who have been infected for some time have the same risk of progression to AIDS as newly infected individuals.

5.4 COFACTORS AND RETROSPECTIVE STUDIES OF CASES

In this section we consider the analysis of cofactors from studies that involve only a sample of cases for whom the dates of infection are determined retrospectively (see Section 4.3). The best known example is the study of transfusion-associated AIDS (Lui, Lawrence, Morgan, et al., 1986). Analyses of data of this type suggested that age at infection is a cofactor of disease progression (Medley, Anderson, Cox, and Billard, 1987; Kalbfleisch and Lawless, 1989). Retrospective studies of this sort are useful for generating hypotheses about cofactors, but they are subject to two serious limitations: the effects of *truncation* and the effects of *competing causes of death*.

5.4.1 Effects of Truncation

The conditional incubation period distribution, $F^*(t) = F(t)/F(T^*)$, is the distribution of incubation periods given that the incubation period is less than T^*, the maximum truncation time.

Although the conditional incubation distribution F^* can be well estimated (Section 4.3.2), the unconditional incubation period distribution, F, cannot be estimated reliably from such studies. Inferences about cofactors based on estimates of a conditional incubation distribution F^* can be misleading. For example, subgroup 1 may appear to have shorter incubation periods than subgroup 0 because

$$F_1^*(t) > F_0^*(t).$$

However, the proportions of individuals with incubation periods less than T^* may in fact be much greater in subgroup 0 than subgroup 1, that is

$$F_1(T^*) < F_0(T^*).$$

Thus, subgroup 0 could in fact have a higher proportion of infected individuals progressing to AIDS within t time units of infection (that is, $F_1(t) < F_0(t)$ for all t). We would falsely conclude that subgroup 1 was at higher risk of disease progression if our inference was based solely on a comparison of the conditional distributions, F_1^* and F_0^*.

5.4.2 Effects of Competing Causes of Death

Differential risk of death from competing causes (i.e., causes of death other than AIDS) among subgroups can distort inferences on cofactors from these retrospective studies. The effect of mortality from competing causes is to exclude some individuals with long incubation periods from the retrospective sample, because such individuals may die before AIDS onset (Section 4.3.4). Thus, if the risk of death from competing causes is greater in subgroup 1 than subgroup 0, then subgroup 1 could artificially appear to have shorter incubation periods than subgroup 0. For example, suppose older individuals are at greater risk of death from a competing cause than younger individuals. Then, even if age at infection was not a true cofactor, it may falsely appear that individuals who were older at infection have shorter incubation periods.

To illustrate this phenomenon, suppose that the incubation distribution is exponential $F(t) = 1 - e^{-\lambda t}$. A binary covariate ($X = 1$ or 0) is under investigation. It is assumed that X has no effect on the incubation distribution but that the hazards of death from competing causes, δ_0 and δ_1, differ in the two subgroups. As pointed out in Section 4.3.4, the parametric methods of 4.3.3 estimate $F_s(t)$, which is the probability of developing AIDS within t time units given AIDS preceded death. The ratio of the median of the distribution F_s in subgroup 1 to the median of the distribution F_s in subgroup 0 is

$$\frac{\lambda + \delta_0}{\lambda + \delta_1}.$$

If $\delta_1 > \delta_0$, then the median incubation period in subgroup 1 will appear smaller than the median incubation period in subgroup 0, when in fact the covariate X has no effect on F.

5.5 MARKERS AS PROGNOSTIC FACTORS

Markers track the progression of HIV infection. Markers, unlike cofactors, are a consequence of infection and indicate the extent of disease progression. Markers are useful as prognostic factors for the risk of AIDS or death. For example, an HIV infected individual with fewer than 200 CD4+ T cells/μl but without AIDS could be expected to be at considerably higher risk of developing AIDS within the next 6 months than an HIV infected individual without AIDS who has more than 800 CD4+ T cells/μl. Knowledge of prognostic factors for progression to AIDS or death is important for the clinical management of patients and for the design and evaluation of clinical trials. Information on markers as prognostic factors has been obtained from *incident cohort studies,* in which the dates of infection of individuals in the cohort are known, and from *prevalent cohort studies,* in which individuals are known to be infected at baseline but the dates of infection are unknown.

Suppose that a set of markers are monitored from the date of infection to time t after infection. The measurements at time t since infection are denoted $\mathbf{Z}(t)$; the entire marker history is characterized by $H(t) = \{\mathbf{Z}(u): 0 \leqslant u \leqslant t\}$. The hazard, $\lambda(t)$, of developing AIDS at time t following infection can be modelled as a function of t and the marker history, $H(t)$. A special case of this hazard model is

$$\lambda(t) = \lambda_o(t) \exp\{\boldsymbol{\beta}'\mathbf{Z}(t)\}, \tag{5.5}$$

where $\mathbf{Z}(t)$ is some functional of the marker history, $H(t)$, and $\lambda_o(t)$ is the hazard of a patient with $\mathbf{Z}(t) = 0$. Gail (1981) applied this time-dependent covariate model (Cox, 1972) to the analysis of serial markers to predict recurrent colon cancer, and the same ideas have been used to model AIDS incidence (e.g., Eyster, Gail, Ballard, et al., 1987). Several introductory points are worth mentioning before more specific consideration of data from incident and prevalent cohorts.

1. Model (5.5) can only be used if the date of infection (or seroconversion) is known. Suppose model (5.5) is the true underlying model, where the time scale t is time since infection. Then if one applies model (5.5) using time since enrollment in a prevalent cohort instead of time since infection, the resulting estimates of $\boldsymbol{\beta}$ will usually be biased, and the direction of the bias is unpredictable (Brookmeyer and Gail, 1987; Brookmeyer, Gail and Polk, 1987).

2. The art of using time-dependent covariates to model the hazard of AIDS is to select a useful feature of the marker history, $H(t)$. For example, one

might choose for $\mathbf{Z}(t)$ the CD4+ T cell level at t, the CD4+ T cell level 12 months earlier (i.e., at time $t-12$), the slope of the least squares fit to a linear model for the CD4+ T cell count over the 6 month period preceeding t, or any other interesting and potentially useful feature of the marker history (Gail, 1981). More than one feature of the marker history can be accommodated in the vector $\mathbf{Z}(t)$.

3. Although equation (5.5) describes the evolving risk of AIDS, conditional on $\{\mathbf{Z}(u) : 0 \leqslant \mathbf{Z}(u) \leqslant t\}$, it does not provide a model for how $\mathbf{Z}(t)$ will evolve in the future. Thus, equation (5.5) can be used to compute the relative risk at t for a patient with $\mathbf{Z}^{(1)}(t)$ compared to another patient with $\mathbf{Z}^{(2)}(t)$; this relative risk is $\exp[\boldsymbol{\beta}'\{\mathbf{Z}^{(1}(t) - \mathbf{Z}^{(2)}(t)\}]$. However, equation (5.5) above cannot be used to compute the chance that the first patient will develop AIDS in the next year, without additional assumptions on how $\mathbf{Z}^{(1)}(t)$ will evolve over time.

4. Equation (5.5) can be used to ask the question: "Do the marker attributes $\mathbf{Z}(t)$ add prognostic information to time since infection for predicting AIDS risk?"

5. A nice feature of model (5.5) is that one need not study every member of an incident cohort to estimate the parameters $\boldsymbol{\beta}$. Efficient nested case-control designs and case-cohort designs can also be used (see section 3.2 in Gail, 1991a).

5.5.1 Prognostic Factor Studies of Markers from Incident Cohorts

Ideal data for studying the prognostic value of markers for predicting risk of AIDS could be derived from incident cohorts of newly infected individuals who are closely monitored for changes in markers levels and for onset of disease. Ideally, the timing and quantification of such marker measurements would be independent of disease status, and the assessment of disease status would be independent of marker measurements. The effects of the duration of infection can be controlled for in the statistical analysis of incident cohorts. Studies of incident cohorts can address the following question: "What prognostic information does a marker provide in addition to knowledge of time since infection?" This is in contrast to *prevalent cohort* studies in which the dates of infection are unknown and thus the effects of duration of infection cannot be controlled. Prevalent cohort studies of markers are discussed at the end of this section.

Suppose one wished to investigate whether the loss in CD4+ T cells in the year from $t-1$ to t provided additional prognostic information over and above the duration of infection, t, and the current CD4+ T cell level, $X(t)$. Using data from an incident cohort, we could apply model (5.5) with $\mathbf{Z}(t) = \{X(t) - X(t - 1), X(t)\}'$ and $\boldsymbol{\beta}' = (\beta_1, \beta_2)$. Suppose patient 1 had $X(t - 1) = 400$ cells/μl and $X(t) = 300$ cells/μl and suppose patient 2 had $X(t - 1) = 500$ cells/μl and $X(t) = 300$ cells/μl. Then, the relative risk comparing patient 1 to patient 2 would be $\exp[\beta_1\{-100 - (-200)\} + \beta_2(300 - 300)] = \exp(100\beta_1)$. A negative value of β_1 would imply that patient 1, who had the smaller CD4+ T cell decline, was at lower risk of AIDS, even though the current CD4+ T cell levels were the same in these two patients. The regression coefficients β_1 and β_2 reflect the *additional* prognostic information in CD4+ T cell levels over and above the prognostic information in duration of infection.

An example of an incident cohort study was the National Cancer Institute Multicenter Hemophilia Study (Goedert, Kessler, Aledort, et al., 1989; see Section 4.5.4). The dates of seroconversion were known to lie in an interval defined by the last stored serum sample that was negative and the most recent stored serum sample that was positive for HIV antibody. Seroconversion dates were estimated by the interval midpoint. A proportional hazards model was fit with CD4+ T cell level as a time dependent covariate. Different analyses were performed to determine how predictive current and past CD4+ T cell levels were of relative risk of AIDS. After controlling for infection duration, it was found that an individual who currently had <200 CD4+ T cells/μl had a relative risk of AIDS of 16 compared to an individual with $200-499$ CD4+ T cells/μl. It was also found that an individual's earlier CD4+ T cell level predicted current AIDS risk. For example, an individual with fewer than 200 CD4+ T cells/μl measured $12-36$ months previously had a relative risk of 3.0 compared to an individual with $200-499$ CD4+ T cells/μl measured $12-36$ months before. Other studies have shown that the risk of developing AIDS before the CD4+ T cell count declines below 200 is small (Phillips, Lee, Elford, et al., 1991).

5.5.2 Prognostic Factor Studies of Markers from Prevalent Cohorts

A prevalent cohort consists of infected AIDS-free patients whose earlier dates of infection are unknown. Thus, it is not possible to estimate the parameters $\boldsymbol{\beta}$ in equation (5.5) because it is not possible to control adequately for time since infection. These biases are particularly unpredictable when one attempts to study a time-varying marker by substituting time since enrollment in the cohort for time since infection in equation (5.5) (Brookmeyer and Gail, 1987; Brookmeyer, Gail, and

Polk, 1987). However, analyses of *baseline values* of markers, which are measured at the time of enrollment in a prevalent cohort, have proved useful for estimating relative risks and absolute risks of AIDS measured on the time scale of time since enrollment. Survival analyses and proportional hazards analyses on the scale of time since enrollment only answer the question: "What prognostic information does the baseline marker value provide in addition to time since *enrollment?*" The question "what prognostic information does the baseline marker value provide in addition to time since *infection?*" cannot be answered from such studies and analyses. Nonetheless, this information is useful, because the dates of infection are usually unknown in clinical practice. Thus, results from prevalent cohort studies provide important prognostic information for advising patients from similar prevalent cohorts about risk. Such studies may also identify important variables for stratification and adjustment in controlled clinical trials of individuals with prevalent infection (see Section 5.7, Example 2).

Fahey, Taylor, Detels, et al. (1990) assessed the prognostic value of a number of cellular and serological markers for progression to AIDS measured at baseline among prevalent seropositive homosexual men. They evaluated the absolute and relative risks for progression to AIDS associated with different levels of the number of CD4+ T cells at the beginning of follow-up. Individuals with fewer than 242 CD4+ T cells/μl had more than 8 times the risk of progression to AIDS of individuals with CD4+ T cell concentrations above 491 cells/μl. The cumulative proportions progressing to AIDS within 48 months was about 70% and 15% for those with less than 242, and those with more than 491 CD4+ T cells, respectively. Although many of the other markers were correlated with each other and with CD4+ T cell levels and did not contribute additional prognostic information to CD4+ T cell levels, the combination of CD4+ T cell levels and either serum neopterin concentration or serum beta-2 microglublin were especially predictive of AIDS. In a prevalent cohort study of gay men in San Francisco, Anderson, Lang, Shiboski, et al. (1990) also found that elevated levels of serum beta-2 microglobulin and low CD4+ T cell counts were especially predictive of AIDS. They found that 65.5% of HIV seropositive individuals with beta-2 microglobulin levels above 3.80 milligrams per liter and CD4+ T cell counts below 500 cells/μl developed AIDS in less than three years. Figure 5.5 from this study shows the cumulative probability of progression to AIDS as a function of follow-up time for different baseline combinations of beta-2 microglobulin and CD4+ T cell levels.

Combinations of baseline markers have been used to develop

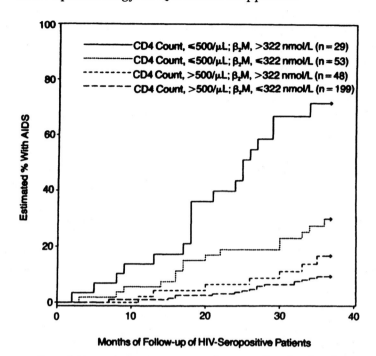

Figure 5.5 Cumulative proportion progressing to AIDS by baseline CD4 + T cell and serum beta-2 microglobulin levels among a prevalent cohort of 346 HIV-seropositive homosexual men in San Francisco. (Source: Anderson, Lang, Shiboski, et al. 1990. Copyright 1990, American Medical Association.)

simplified staging systems for HIV disease. An early example was the clinical classification called AIDS-related complex (ARC), which was based on a number of symptoms, such as those in Table 5.1. The Walter Reed staging system was based on combinations of both clinical and immunological markers (Redfield, Wright, and Tramont, 1986). Royce, Luckman, Fusaro, and Winkelstein (1991) compared various staging systems predictive of AIDS among individuals who were AIDS-free at baseline. Baseline clinical markers have also been used to develop a prognostic staging system for survival in AIDS patients. Justice, Feinstein, and Wells (1989) proposed three stages of AIDS based on nutritional, respiratory, serological and hematological parameters. The reported median survival from AIDS diagnosis in the three stages were 11.6, 5.1, and 2.1 months.

Baseline markers have also been used to predict particular AIDS-defining conditions. Phair, Muñoz, Detels, et al. (1990) evaluated the risk of *Pneumocystis carinii* pneumonia (PCP) in 1665 prevalent seropositive homosexual men. They found, for example, that 33% of infected individuals with fewer than 200 CD4 + T cells/μl developed PCP in less than 3 years. These data influenced public health officials to re-commend prophylaxis against PCP for patients with CD4+ T-lymphocyte levels below 200 cells/μl.

5.5.3 Prevalent Versus Incident Cohorts

The studies on prevalent cohorts are useful for identifying high risk persons and predicting risk among persons from similar prevalent cohorts. However risk estimates derived from prevalent cohorts may not be directly applicable to cohorts with different distributions of times since infection, and, in particular, to cohorts of newly infected individuals. Only if the markers are so informative that the current risk is conditionally independent of the duration of infection, given the current marker values, is it reasonable to suppose that estimates of risk from one prevalent cohort will be generally applicable. This assumption is implicit in stage models of HIV disease (Section 5.6).

Prevalent cohort studies cannot determine if markers carry information about risk of progression that is independent of duration of infection. The amount of information in a marker about disease risk over and above what it reflects about the duration of infection can be determined only from a study of newly infected individuals (an incident cohort). For example, persons with low numbers of CD4+ T cells at enrollment in a prevalent cohort have probably been infected much earlier and are thus at higher risk than patients with higher CD4+ T cell levels at enrollment. The excess risk associated with a longer duration of infection is incorporated into the relative risk associated with a low CD4+ T cell count from a prevalent cohort, but not into the relative risk estimates from an incident cohort that control for duration of infection. Thus, it is expected that relative risks associated with CD4+ T cell levels based on a prevalent cohort will tend to be greater than relative risks based on a cohort of newly infected individuals in which duration of infection is controlled.

5.6 THE MARKER TRAJECTORY

5.6.1 Introduction

In Section 5.5, we studied the risk of progression to AIDS as a function of current and past marker levels. In this section, our focus is on how marker values evolve over time. There are two methodological problems in studying the marker trajectory. First, the marker measurements can be extremely noisy because of considerable within individual and between individual variation. Second, marker information on an individual may not be available after onset of AIDS or shortly before death. Thus, individuals with the greatest rates of decline of CD4+ T cells may have the shortest follow-up. We call this *informative censoring*. A complete description of the disease process requires joint modelling of the marker trajectory and incidence of disease and death.

The depletion of CD4+ T lymphyocytes was one of the first immunological abnormalities found to be associated with AIDS, and there has been considerable research to characterize changes in the numbers of CD4+ T cells over time. Our focus in this section is on the CD4+ T cell trajectory.

Figure 5.6a shows the CD4+ T cell trajectory for 20 infected hemophiliacs from the National Cancer Institute Multicenter Hemophilia Cohort Study. The figure is a graph of peripheral blood CD4+ T cell concentrations as a function of time since seroconversion for each individual (dates of seroconversion were estimated by interval midpoints). This figure shows how variable CD4+ T cell measurements can be. Time trends are not readily discernible. There is considerable variation within and between individuals. As discussed in Section 5.8, laboratory measurement error and diurnal variation in

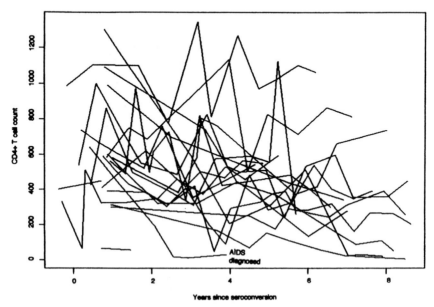

Figure 5.6a CD4+ T cell trajectories for 20 infected hemophiliacs. (Source: J. Goedert, National Cancer Institute, personal communication.)

CD4+ T cell levels obscure the general pattern of the marker trajectory for an individual. The interpretation of Figure 5.6a is further complicated by the fact that one of the 20 patients developed AIDS.

5.6.2 Approaches for Analyzing Trends in the CD4 + T Cell Trajectory Grouped Means

A simple, though possibly misleading, approach for summarizing data on the marker trajectories of a group of individuals is to take means at each point in time (i.e., average the CD4+ T cell values for all individuals at each time point). For example, Figure 5.6b is a graph of the means of CD4 + T cells and was obtained by grouping the time axis into 6 month intervals using the data in Figure 5.6a. A pattern of decreasing CD4+ T cell levels becomes apparent. However, the resulting (marginal or population average) marker trajectory may in fact not describe the trajectory for any individual patient. For example, consider a mixed cohort of newly infected individuals; half lose CD4 + T cells at a constant rate of 100 cells/year and the other half lose CD4 + T cells at a constant rate of 50 cells/year. If the CD4 + T cell count is averaged at each time point, the population average marker trajectory

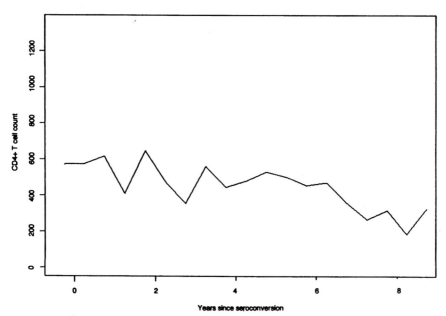

Figure 5.6b Mean CD4 + T cell trajectory for 20 infected hemophiliacs. Time axis grouped into 6-month intervals; means plotted at interval midpoint.

is linear with a slope of -75 cells/year, which does not correspond to any single patient's marker trajectory.

A number of selection biases may make it difficult to piece together the CD4+ T cell trajectory based on a graph of means at each time point. We shall discuss such biases in connection with data presented by Lang, Perkins, Anderson, et al. (1989), who describe changes in CD4+ and CD8+ T lymphocytes among subjects in the San Francisco Men's Health Study. They consider three groups of individuals: (1) individuals who seroconverted during follow-up; (2) individuals who were seropositive at study entry and remained AIDS free; and (3) individuals who were diagnosed with AIDS. Mean CD4+ T cell levels over time for the 3 groups are shown in Figure 5.7. The seroconverters had mean CD4+ T cell levels of $1119/\mu l$ at 18 months before seroconversion. Between the 6 months before seroconversion and 6 months after seroconversion, the CD4+ T cell levels dropped a mean of 360 cells/μl (34%). At 12 months after seroconversion, the seroconverters resembled the prevalent seropositives. The prevalent seropositives declined an average of 84 cells per year over the 3-year follow-up period. The data on AIDS cases in Figure 5.7 are aligned so that time 0 refers to AIDS diagnosis. The mean CD4+ T cell count at AIDS diagnosis was 190cells/μl. During the 18 months before diagnosis, the CD4+ T cell concentration declined an average of 160 cells/μl per year.

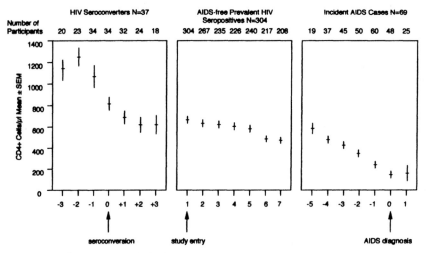

Figure 5.7 Illustration of declines in grouped means of numbers of CD4+ T cells based on three populations: HIV seroconverters, AIDS-free prevalent HIV seropositives, and incident AIDS cases. Unit changes in the abscissa represent 6 months. (Source: Lang, Perkins, Anderson, et al., 1989)

Possible selection biases should be considered when interpreting these trends. The sharp decline in CD4+ T cells among AIDS cases ($160/\mu l$ per year) may result from selection of those individuals (AIDS cases) with the greatest rates of CD4+ T cell decline. Both the prevalent seropositive and seroconverter trajectories suggest more modest rates of decline of CD4+ T cells. Further, Figure 5.7 indicates that the rate of loss of CD4+ T cells diminishes with time, both among the seroconverters and seropositive patients. This tendency could result in part from a selection bias whereby individuals with the greatest rates of CD4+ T cell decline are more likely to be lost to follow-up or be excluded because of an AIDS diagnosis. The prevalent seropositive trajectory also excludes individuals who developed AIDS before study entry. These excluded individuals may be the ones with the greatest rates of CD4+ T cell decline.

Statistical Models for the Marker Trajectory

An alternative to simply plotting grouped means is to use statistical models to describe the marker trajectory. For example, consider the linear regression model that relates the expected logarithm of the CD4+ T cell count to a linear function of the duration of infection; that is,

$$\log Z_i(t) = \beta_0 + \beta_1 t + \varepsilon_{it},$$

where $Z_i(t)$ is the CD4+ T cell measurement at time t following infection for individual i and ε_{it} are mutually independent random error terms with zero means. Note that each patient is assumed to have the same mean trajectory, defined by β_0 and β_1. Such simple regression models do not account for the correlation of measurements within an individual.

HIV disease, as measured by CD4+ T cell concentration, may progress more rapidly in some individuals than others. It is plausible that an individual with a large initial drop in the CD4+ T cells will "track," that is continue to lose CD4+ T cells at a relatively fast rate. An individual with a small initial drop in CD4+ T cells may continue to lose CD4+ cells at a slow rate. By tracking we mean that the slopes (rate of change of CD4+ T cells) for a particular individual over time are highly correlated.

Statistical models that incorporate tracking are based on random effects growth curve models (Laird and Ware, 1982; Ware, 1985). For example, consider the statistical model,

$$Z_{it} = \alpha_{0i} + \alpha_{1i}t + \varepsilon_{it} \tag{5.6}$$

where $\mathcal{Z}_{it}$ is the marker value for individual i at t time units following seroconversion. The quantities α_{0i} and α_{1i} are the random intercept and random slopes for the ith individual, respectively. Thus, the model allows for the intercept and slopes to vary among individuals. A simple model is to assume that the random effects $(\alpha_{0i}, \alpha_{1i})$ are drawn from a bivariate normal distribution, and that the errors, ε_{ij}, are also normal and independent of the random slope and intercept. This is one approach for introducing correlation among repeated marker measurements on the same individual. An important assumption of model (5.6) is that the ith individual's slope, α_{1i}, (i.e., change in the marker per unit time) remains constant over time although the model does allow for heterogeneity in slopes among individuals. Thus, the model implicitly assumes that individuals track.

De Gruttola, Lange, and Dafni (1991) applied model (5.6) to serial measurements of CD4+ T cell counts from individuals in the San Francisco Men's Health Study. Model estimation procedures were developed to account for the fact that the date of infection was unknown for some members of the cohort. This was done by incorporating prior information about the infection rate curve in San Francisco. A refinement of model (5.6) was considered that allowed an initial sharp drop in CD4+ cells at the time of seroconversion in addition to the long term decreasing trend. De Gruttola, Lange, and Dafni (1991) concluded that after a sharp drop in CD4+ T cell count at the time of seroconversion, the square root of CD4+ T cell count declines linearly. They also found considerable variation in the slopes and intercepts among individuals. Their results suggest that the approximate rate of loss of CD4+ T cells/μl per year for a "typical" individual at CD4+ T cell level $\mathcal{Z}$ is $4.26\sqrt{\mathcal{Z}}$. Thus, at CD4+ T cell levels $\mathcal{Z} = 800$, 600, and 100 cells/μl, an individual could expect to lose 120, 104, and 43 cells/μl per year, respectively.

Lange, Carlin, and Gelfand (1992) conducted a Bayesian analysis of the CD4+ T cell trajectory data from the San Francisco Men's Health Study. They allow for a nonlinear growth curve for $\sqrt{\mathcal{Z}}$, heterogeneous variances across individuals, covariate effects, unknown random infection times and varying numbers of observations per individual. The Gibbs sampler was used to obtain posterior distributions. They conclude there is considerable noise in the CD4+ T cell trajectory, and that one cannot reject a simple linear growth model for $\sqrt{\mathcal{Z}}$ in favor of more complicated models, based on these data.

A number of other statistical models have been proposed to describe the CD4+ T cell trajectory. For example, Berman (1990) assumed that the CD4+ T cell count at time t following seroconversion could be represented by

$$Z(t) = e^{X(t) - \delta t}$$

where $X(t)$ is a stationary Gaussian process. This model assumes that the effect of HIV infection is to decrease the expected log CD4+ T cell count by an amount $\delta \cdot t$ where t is the duration of infection. The model was applied to a cohort of intravenous drug users in detoxification and methadone maintenance programs in New York City. Taylor, Cumberland, and Sy (1992) considered a more general model which included random effects and measurement error as in model (5.6) as well as a stochastic process to account for additional within-subject covariance. The model was applied to a cohort of over 1600 homosexual and bisexual men in Los Angeles. It was found that the intra-individual correlations between two slopes (rate of change in CD4+ T cell count per microliter per unit time) 3 months apart was only 0.1. Thus, this analysis did not find that individuals track. In particular, individuals with large initial rates of decline in CD4+ T cell concentration do not necessarily continue to experience large rates of declines over the course of follow-up.

Joint Modeling of the Marker Trajectory and the Disease Process

An important complexity which the previous methods do not address concerns informative censoring. Specifically, individuals who are diagnosed with AIDS or other symptoms may be at greater risk of loss to follow-up or selective exclusion. Further, individuals who die may have the greatest rate of CD4+ T cell depletion. In order to account for these potential selection biases, it is necessary to jointly model the marker trajectory and the risk of progression to AIDS.

One approach for simultaneously modelling the marker trajectory and risk of AIDS progression or death is based on multistate survival models. The simplest such model assumes that individuals progress from one stage of HIV infection to the next. The stages are defined by marker levels, and the last stage is AIDS diagnosis or death.

Longini, Clark, Gardner, and Brundage (1991), for example, used a time homogeneous Markov chain to describe the transitions through seven states defined by CD4+ T cell numbers (>899, 700–899, 500–699, 350–499, 200–345, 0–199, AIDS diagnosis or death). The underlying assumptions were that individuals progress through a series of transient states, and the hazard of progression from stage i to stage $i + 1$ was a constant λ_i. Unlike the random effects growth models, the Markov model does not allow for tracking. The duration in a particular stage is independent of the durations in the other stages. These methods were applied to data from a cohort study of infected military personnel (Brundage, McNeil, Miller, et al., 1990). The results are given in Table 5.3. For an individual at 800, 600, and 100 CD4+ T cells/μl, the expected rate of decline is 160, 120, and 83 cells/μl per year, respectively. The expected time from first falling below 200 CD4+ T cells/μl to an AIDS diagnosis was 1.6 years. These investigators also identified an age effect. In particular, the waiting time in the last three states decreased with increasing age at first exam ($\leqslant 25$ years, 25–30 years, and >30 years). See also Longini (1990).

Although Markov models of this type have enough parameters to allow them to fit available data on rates of CD4+ T lymphocyte decline, and although such models yield estimates of the AIDS incubation distribution in good agreement with estimates derived from other methods (Chapter 4), the Markov assumption is a strong one and is probably not correct. Under the Markov stage model above, the time to death or AIDS is conditionally independent of time since infection, given a CD4+ T cell stage. Yet, using data from patients given AZT in the study reported by Fischl, Richman, Grieco, et al. (1987), Tsiastis, Dafni, De Gruttola, et al. (1992) have estimated that the hazard of death is more than three-fold greater 18 months after randomization than at 6 months after randomization when comparing patients with the same CD4+ T-lymphocyte levels at those two times. This is evidence that duration of illness has prognostic value above and beyond that provided by CD4+ T-lymphocyte levels and therefore that the Markov model cannot be strictly true. Moreover, that model

Table 5.3 Markov Model of CD4+ T Cell Decline among HIV Positive U.S. Army Personnel

State	CD4+ T Cell Range (per μl)	CD4+ T cell decline[a] (cells/μl/year)	Mean Waiting Time in State (years)	Cumulative Waiting Time (years)
1	>899	275	1.1	1.1
2	700–899	160	1.3	2.4
3	500–699	120	1.7	4.1
4	350–499	77	1.9	6.0
5	200–349	73	2.0	8.0
6	0–199	83	1.6	9.6
7	AIDS diagnosis[b]			

Source: Longini, Clark, Gardner, and Brundage, 1991.

[a]State 1 assumed to be 900–1200 CD4+ T cell range.

[b]Defined as Walter Reed Stage 6 case (see Redfield, Wright, and Tramont 1986).

does not allow for transitions from state $i + 1$ to state i, even though CD4+ T-lymphocyte trajectories from individual patients indicate that such transitions do occur.

Another approach for jointly modeling the marker trajectory and the progression of disease was proposed by Self and Pawitan (1992). Their basic idea was to use Cox proportional hazards regression models with time-dependent covariates to describe the relation between the marker and disease progression and a mixed linear model to describe the marker trajectory. Other approaches have also been proposed (De Gruttola and Tu, 1992; Jewell and Kalbfleisch, 1992).

5.7 OTHER USES OF MARKERS

A number of other uses for markers have been suggested. One suggestion has been to use markers to control for the effects of onset confounding in studies of prevalent cohorts. For example, to evaluate a cofactor (X_1), one might adjust for the baseline level (at beginning of follow-up) of a marker, X_2, (e.g. concentration of CD4+ T cells) that might be highly correlated with time since infection. The rationale for this approach is that since X_2 contains information about the duration of infection, adjustment on X_2 would control any onset confounding that might arise from the association of duration of infection with X_1. Adjustment could be accomplished either by stratifying on X_2 or by including X_2 in a regression model such as a proportional hazards model (model 5.1). The analysis is then performed using follow-up time as the time scale rather than time from infection. However, this approach is not always appropriate and its validity depends upon how well X_2 serves as a substitute for time since infection and on the mechanism by which X_1 affects the risk of AIDS. We illustrate with two examples:

Example 1.   Consider a cofactor X_1 whose value is fixed at the time of infection. Suppose its mode of action is to accelerate the decline in numbers of CD4+ cells, and thereby increase the hazard of AIDS, as indicated by the following schematic:

$$X_1 \rightarrow \text{Lowers CD4+ T Cells } (X_2) \rightarrow \text{AIDS}$$

The marker X_2 is part of the causal pathway. The effect of X_1 on the incubation period is revealed in part through depressed numbers of CD4+ T cells. Thus adjustment for X_2 may eliminate or obscure the very effects of X_1 we are trying to detect. Breslow and Day (1980) have described related phenomena, called overmatching, in the context of cancer case-control studies. Jewell and Kalbfleisch (1992) show under certain model assumptions that the relative risk of a cofactor will be biased toward 1 if one uses follow-up time and adjusts for the marker X_2 at entry.

Example 2.   Consider a time-dependent cofactor, X_1, which takes effect at the onset of follow-up. An example might be a treatment given to some members of a prevalent cohort at entry. In this second situation, unlike the first, the baseline marker X_2 contains no information about the effects of treatment X_1. Adjustment for the baseline marker X_2 helps to insure that the treated and untreated subgroups are comparable and to reduce the effects of onset confounding. In this example, even if the treatment is assigned randomly so that the condition for no onset confounding is satisfied ($g_0^* = g_1^*$), there is still good reason to adjust for baseline markers. This is because randomization does not guarantee that the distributions of prior infection times would be exactly the same in the two treatment groups. Brookmeyer and Gail (1987) show that failure to adequately adjust for duration of infection will under some conditions bias relative risk estimates toward 1.0. They call this potential bias "frailty selection."

Markers have been used to try to extract information on the incubation period distribution from prevalent cohorts. The basic idea is to try to use baseline markers measured at enrollment to estimate duration of infection. Muñoz, Wang, Bass, et al. (1989) analyzed data from 1628 prevalent homosexual men in the Multicenter AIDS Cohort Study (MACS) who were enrolled between April 1984 and March 1985. In 4 years of follow-up, 304 of those subjects developed AIDS, compared to only 12 of 233 men who were incident seroconverters in this period. In order to use the information from the prevalent cohort, these investigators imputed previous infection times by assuming that these times followed a Weibull distribution with parameters depending on the percentage of lymphocytes that were CD4+ T cells and on platelet levels. This model was fit to data from the seroconverters and then applied to the prevalent cohort. The resulting incubation distribution had a hazard (per person year) of approximately .004, .032, .064, .074, and .078 at years 1 through 5 respectively. Indications that the hazard might have been leveling off after only 3 years may be related to the use of zidovudine and other treatments beginning in 1987 or to the use of the Weibull model for imputing previous dates of infection. A theoretical concern with this methodology discussed by Jewell and Nielson (1993) is that it is not possible for the backward recurrence time (the time since infection) to follow a Weibull distribution for all times of enrollment, even if covariates in the Weibull model are allowed to vary with time since infection.

Taylor, Muñoz, Bass, et al. (1990) also tried to extend the range of the MACS data for estimating the incubation distribution by using markers. However, these authors imputed the residual time to AIDS among censored seroconverters. They estimated the residual time to AIDS distribution, conditional on each subject's percentage of CD4+ T cells. They assumed that this distribution was lognormal, and, importantly, that the residual time to AIDS was conditionally independent of duration of infection given the marker value. Having fit this model, they applied it to impute the missing residual times to AIDS among seroconverters. Standard survival methods were then used to estimate the incubation distribution from the "complete" data on seroconverters. Again, a theoretical concern discussed by Jewell and Nielson (1993) is that use of the lognormal model (or Weibull model) is "inconsistent" because it is impossible for the residual AIDS-free time for an individual infected t years to follow a lognormal distribution for all t.

Markov models have also been used to combine information from incident and prevalent cohorts. For example, the Markov model of Longini, Clark, Byers, et al. (1989) uses stages defined by CD4+ T cell count. An individual in stage i at entry contributes information only about transition rates beyond stage i. Thus data from prevalent cohorts can be used. Longini, Clark, Byers, et al. (1989) employed this model to combine information from incident and prevalent cohorts and to estimate the average duration in various stages of HIV infection as well as the distribution of the total incubation period.

5.8 VARIABILITY OF MARKERS

There can be considerable variability in repeat marker measurements from a given individual. The sources of variability include measurement errors in the assay, diurnal (i.e., time of day) variation and day-to-day variation in marker levels for a given individual. The effect of this variation is to bias relative risk estimates toward 1. Specifically suppose the underlying model for the hazard of progression is

$$\lambda(t) = \lambda_o(t)e^{\beta Z(t)},$$

where $Z(t)$ is a marker level at t time units after infection. We measure $\tilde{Z}(t)$ which is $Z(t)$ plus random measurement error ε,

$$\tilde{Z}(t) = Z(t) + \varepsilon.$$

If the measurement error ε has zero mean and variance σ^2, estimates $\hat{\beta}$ based on $\tilde{Z}$ will be biased toward 0. Measurement error attenuates the true marker disease risk association (Prentice, 1982; Pepe, Self, and

Prentice, 1989; Raboud, Reid, Coates, and Farewell, 1992). An adjusted or "deattenuated" estimate of β has been derived, and it depends on an estimate of σ^2 (Prentice, 1992; Raboud, Reid, Coates, and Farewell, 1992).

Smoothing techniques have been suggested to reduce the effects of marker measurement error. The basic idea is to adjust the marker value at a given time t by averaging the marker values in a neighborhood of t (Hastie and Tibshirani, 1990). Raboud, Reid, Coates, and Farewell (1992) compare a number of different smoothers, including a historical running mean which averages marker values from current and previous visits.

Malone, Simms, Gray, et al. (1990) considered the sources of variability in repeated CD4+ T cell counts among HIV infected individuals on three consecutive days. They reported a median coefficient of variation (standard deviation divided by the mean) of .145 when samples were drawn at a consistent time of day compared to a median coefficient of variation of .22 when samples were drawn throughout the day.

The CD4+ T cell count is calculated as the product of (1) the white blood cell count concentration (cells/μl), (2) the estimated fraction of white cells that are constituted by lymphocytes, and (3) the fraction of lymphocytes with CD4+ T cell receptors, as measured by flow cytometry. Error is introduced in the measurement of all three components. Another useful marker is simply the third component above, often called *percent CD4+ T cell* (CD4+%). An advantage of percent CD4+ T cell is that measurement error is introduced only through flow cytometry, because it is not necessary to measure the white blood cell count or the differential fraction of lymphocytes. Malone, Simms, Gray, et al. (1990) report a median coefficient of variation of only .075 for percent CD4+ T cell when drawn at a consistent time of day. Taylor, Fahey, Detels, et al. (1989) compared the prognostic value of percent CD4+ T cell with that of CD4+ T cell count and concluded that percent CD4+ T cell may be a better prognostic factor than the CD4+ T cell count.

5.9 SYNTHESIS OF KNOWLEDGE OF COFACTORS AND MARKERS

A large number of studies have investigated potential cofactors and markers of disease progression. This chapter highlighted a number of statistical issues in the interpretation and analysis of such studies.

The search for cofactors has been less fruitful than the search for markers (Table 5.1). Age at infection is the one cofactor that has been reported in a number of studies. Older hemophiliacs were at higher risk of progression to AIDS than younger hemophiliacs (Goedert, Kessler, Aledort, et al. 1989; Darby, Rizza, Doll, et al., 1989; Darby, Doll, Thakrar, et al., 1990; Phillips, Lee, Elford, et al., 1991). Darby, Doll, Thakrar, et al. (1990) report that the cumulative probabilities of developing AIDS within 5 years of seroconversion, $F(5)$, among hemophiliacs aged <25, 25–44 and >45 years at first seropositive test were .03, .07 and .20 respectively. This is illustrated in Figure 5.8. A prevalent cohort study (Moss, Bacchetti, Osmond, et al., 1988) among homosexual men also suggested a positive association between age and risk of AIDS progression, although onset confounding cannot be ruled out because older individuals may have been infected earlier in such a prevalent cohort. Retrospective studies of transfusion-associated AIDS cases (Medley, Anderson, Cox, and Billard et al., 1988) found a quadratic relation of age at infection with risk of AIDS progression. Children (0–4 years) and the elderly (⩽60 years) had shorter incubation periods than those 5–60 years at infection, although inferences about cofactors based on such studies are tenuous for the reasons outlined in section 5.4. Nevertheless, the cumulative evidence suggests age is a cofactor, at least among patients with hemophilia. No other cofactors have been consistently demonstrated.

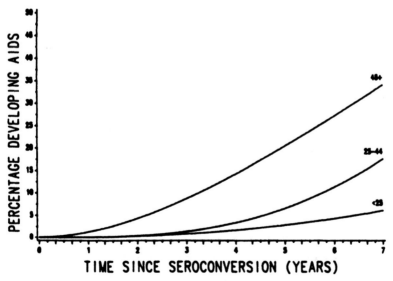

Figure 5.8 AIDS incubation distributions for hemophiliacs age <25 years, 25–44 years, and ⩾45 years at first seropositive test. (Source: Darby, Doll, Thakrar, et al., 1990.)

Numerous markers of progression of HIV disease have been identified and include CD4+ T cells, beta 2-microglobulin, serum neopterin, and various clinical and viral markers. The most intensively studied marker is the CD4+ T cell concentration. Both incident and prevalent cohort studies indicate that HIV infected individuals with depressed CD4+ T cells are at elevated risk of progression to AIDS. Thus, CD4+ T cells carry prognostic information over and above what it reflects about duration of infection.

The CD4+ T cell marker trajectory is difficult to study because of laboratory measurement error, day-to-day and diurnal variation, and informative censoring. Some estimates of the rates of CD4+ T cell decline based on different methodologies are summarized in Table 5.4. The rate of loss of CD4+ T cells declines as the CD4+ T cell level drops. In the range of 600 CD4+ T cells, the expected cell decline is approximately 100–200 cells per year. In the range of 300 CD4+ T cells, the expected cell decline is approximately 70–80 cells per year. More work is needed to determine the extent to which rates of change of CD4+ T cells "track" for a particular individual over time. The CD4+ T cell marker trajectory may also depend on covariates such as age at infection.

Table 5.4 Estimated Rates of CD4+T cell Decline

Current CD4+ T Cell Level (cells/μl)	Rate of CD4+ T Cell Decline (cells/μl/year)	
	Growth Curve Model[a]	Markov Model[b]
800	120	160
600	104	120
400	85	77
300	74	73
100	43	83

[a]Based on results reported in De Gruttola, Lange, and Dafni (1991) (see Section 5.6.2).
[b]Based on results reported in Longini, Clark, Gardner, and Brundage (1991).

6

Screening and Accuracy of Tests for HIV

6.1 INTRODUCTION

The isolation of the HIV virus from patients with AIDS led to the development of tests to detect viral antibodies in blood samples (Sarngadharan, Popovic, Bruch, et al., 1984). Such blood tests were used to demonstrate the frequent occurrence of HIV antibodies in persons with AIDS and their absence in healthy individuals and to monitor the development of HIV antibodies in persons who were inadvertently exposed to the virus through blood transfusions, hospital and laboratory accidents and other means. This evidence was decisive in supporting the hypothesis that HIV causes AIDS. The availability of such antibody tests also allowed epidemiologists to find risk factors for HIV infection, such as anal receptive intercourse with many homosexual partners (Chapter 2). Thus the availability of tests to detect the presence of HIV infection has been crucial in studying the etiology and epidemiology of AIDS.

Although accurate tests are important for studying AIDS etiology and epidemiology, high accuracy is even more important when such tests are applied to screening large populations to detect infected individuals and for advising patients. Even very good tests may needlessly alarm large numbers of healthy persons when used to screen large healthy populations (Meyer and Pauker, 1987). In this chapter we discuss measures of test accuracy, including sensitivity and specificity (Section 6.2); some of the more controversial proposals for screening populations using these tests in relationship to the likely proportions of false positive and false negative results to be obtained (Section 6.3); and the use of HIV tests to improve the safety of transfused blood products

(Section 6.4). Viral culture, the polymerase chain reaction to detect HIV genome, and assays for HIV antigen are described in Section 6.5. Sloand, Pitt, Chiarello, and Nemo (1991) review recent progress and procedures for HIV testing.

6.2 SENSITIVITY, SPECIFICITY AND RELATED MEASURES OF ACCURACY FOR DIAGNOSTIC TESTS

General principles and statistical methods for evaluating diagnostic tests are available in texts on clinical epidemiology (Fletcher, Fletcher, and Wagner, 1988) and expository articles (Begg, 1987; Gail, 1979 and 1991b). Schwartz, Dans, and Kinosian (1988) apply these ideas to tests for HIV, and Dodd (1986) gives a nice introduction to available HIV tests and concepts of specificity, sensitivity, and predictive value.

Often a diagnostic test is evaluated in a nondiseased population and in a population of individuals with the disease of interest, and test results are recorded as in Table 6.1. The *sensitivity* of the test is the probability that the test is positive among diseased individuals and is estimated by n_{11}/N_1 in Table 6.1. The *specificity* is the probability that the test will be negative in a nondiseased population; specificity is estimated by n_{22}/N_2.

6.2.1 The Effect of Changing the Definition of "Positive Test Result"

In applying these simple definitions, care must be taken to precisely define the criteria used to define a "positive" result, and one must precisely specify the nature of the non-diseased and diseased populations. Data in Table 6.2 are taken from a study by Weiss. Goedert, Sarngadharan, et al. (1985) of the performance of the enzyme-linked immunosorbent assay (ELISA assay). This assay detects antibodies in

Table 6.1 Cross-Classification by Disease Status and Test Status

		Disease	No Disease
Test	Positive	n_{11}	n_{12}
	Negative	n_{21}	n_{22}
		N_1	N_2

Table 6.2 Distribution of ELISA Absorbance Ratios in Healthy Blood Donors and AIDS Patients

	Absorbance Ratio Category							
	<2	2–2.99	3–3.99	4–4.99	5–5.99	6–11.99	≥12	Total
AIDS	0	2	7	7	15	36	21	88
Healthy blood donors	202	73	15	3	2	2	0	297

Source: From Weiss, Goedert, Sarngadharan, et al. (1985).

the blood specimen that bind to antigens from disrupted whole HIV virus. The bound HIV antibodies themselves become the binding sites for anti-human immunoglobulin antibodies that are attached to an enzyme, horseradish peroxidose, which catalyzes a color producing reaction. The optical absorbance of the color produced increases with increasing concentration of HIV antibodies in the original blood specimen. Sandler, Dodd, and Fang (1988) review ELISA assays and other types of enzyme immunoassays (EIA) that work on the same principles, as well as immunblot (Western blot) procedures used to obtain more specific tests. We use the term EIA to represent any type of enzyme immunoassay, including ELISA. The ELISA results in Table 6.2 are expressed as the ratio of the mean of duplicate absorbances in the test specimen to the mean of eight negative control absorbances.

It is evident that absorbance ratios tend to be higher among AIDS patients than among normal blood donors (Table 6.2). Formal tests for this trend may be based on the Wilcoxon two-sample test, adapted for ties (Lehmann, 1975; Gail, 1979) or, if one is willing to assign the scores $1, 2, 3, \ldots, 7$ to these categories, to standard tests for trend in $2 \times k$ contingency tables (Armitage, 1955; Mantel, 1963; Agresti, Mehta, and Patel, 1990). The two-sided Wilcoxon test yields significance level $p < 0.0001$ in this case.

Of greater interest than establishing that the ELISA absorbance is elevated among AIDS patients is estimating sensitivity and specificity. If the ELISA test is defined as positive whenever the ratio exceeds 4.99, the sensitivity is estimated from Table 2 as $72/88 = .818$ and the specificity is estimated as $293/297 = .987$. A higher sensitivity, $(72 + 7)/88 = .898$, is obtained by lowering the positivity cut-point to a ratio exceeding 3.99, but the corresponding specificity is reduced to $(293\text{-}3)/297 = .976$. This calculation illustrates the trade-off between sensitivity and specificity that occurs as one varies the cut-point used to define a "positive" result.

A much more complete description of the performance of the diagnostic test from Table 6.1 is obtained by plotting the sensitivity against one minus the specificity for all possible choices of cut-point. Such a plot of sensitivity versus one minus the specificity is called a *receiver operating curve* (ROC). A uniformly better assay than the ELISA assay would have a higher sensitivity for each fixed specificity and would lie above the ELISA locus on an ROC curve. Part of the difficulty in comparing various proposed tests for HIV is that data are often given corresponding only to a single point on the ROC curve, so that one cannot compare the sensitivities of various tests over a comparable range of specificities. Statistical methods are available for comparing ROC curves for two assays over the entire range of specificities (Hanley and McNeill, 1983) or only over the part of the specificity range of practical interest (Wieand, Gail, James, and James, 1989).

The estimated specificity $293/297 = 0.987$ for cut-point ratio 5.0 or higher is very promising, but it is subject to random error. The estimated standard deviation is $\{\hat{p}(1 - \hat{p})/N_2\}^{1/2} = \{(.987)(1 - .987)/297\}^{1/2} = .0066$, which leads to a 95% confidence interval $0.987 \pm 1.96 \times .0066 = (.974, 1.000)$. A more accurate lower 97.5% confidence limit is obtained by finding p such that

$$\sum_{X=293}^{297} C(X, 297) p^X (1 - p)^{297 - X} = .025, \qquad (6.1)$$

where $C(X, 297) = 297!/X!(297 - X)!$. This formula yields a lower 97.5% confidence limit of $p = .9659$ rather than .974 above. As we shall see, even small changes in specificity have implications for the usefulness of these tests. Similar formulas can be used for putting confidence limits on estimates of sensitivity.

The data in Table 6.2 were based on one of the first available EIA procedures. Current commercially available assays perform better (Reesink, Lelie, Huisman, et al., 1986).

6.2.2 Defining the "Infected" and "Uninfected" Populations Precisely

Another difficulty with the simple summary of test performance in Table 6.1 is in defining what is meant by the "nondiseased" and "diseased" categories. The specificity of a test may be reduced in persons who have never been exposed to the HIV virus (nondiseased) but who have other non-AIDS related disorders or other infections that give rise to antibodies and other products that may yield false positive tests for AIDS. Thus the type of nondiseased population must be carefully characterized in relation to the intended application of the diagnostic test. Failure to take such heterogeneity of nondiseased populations into account has been described as *spectrum bias* (Schwartz, Dans, and Kinosian, 1988; Ransohoff and Feinstein, 1978; Begg, 1987).

The spectrum of diseased populations is likewise very broad because different hosts react to the virus in different ways, and especially, because the interaction between the HIV virus and the host is a dynamic one that evolves over time. The state of health of the host and the biological and immunological evidences of infection vary over time. The word *sensitivity* thus has meaning only in relation to a well characterized stage of disease.

6.2.3 Time Course of Detectability of HIV by Various Assays

Some idea of the complex time course of the infection process is indicated in Figure 6.1, which depicts laboratory studies from a hypothetical person infected with HIV at time zero. The evolving patterns for various laboratory tests are based on the references in the legend to Figure 6.1. In this patient, antibody to HIV was not detectable by EIA until about month 2. Viral antigen (p24 protein) was detectable in the serum within one month of infection; it almost disappeared by 6 weeks however.

Whereas the EIA detects antibodies to a mixture of HIV proteins, the Western blot (WB) assay allows one to detect antibodies to specific HIV proteins and can be used to confirm an initial positive EIA, resulting in a combined test with enhanced specificity (Esteban, Shih, Tai, et al., 1985; Burke, Brundage, Redfield, et al., 1988). Western blot analyses can detect antibodies to proteins from the viral core ("gag" proteins) such as p17, p24, and p55, proteins produced by the polymerase ("pol") gene, such as p31, p51 and p66, and the envelope proteins gp41, gp120 and gp160. The manufacturer of the licensed Western blot (WB) procedure requires that antibody to proteins from each of these elements (core, polymerase, envelope) be present in order for the result to be positive—i.e., p24, p31 and either gp41 or gp160. In early studies, the U.S. Army (Burke, Brundage, Redfield, et al., 1988) considered the WB to be positive if either the gp41 band were present or if both the p24 and p55 bands were present. In the hypothetical example (Figure 6.1), the WB would be judged positive first at about

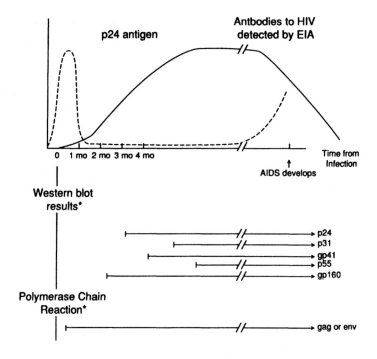

* arrows indicate the region over which the assay is positive

Figure 6.1. Time course of development of detectable viral antigens, antibodies and viral genome in a hypothetical patient. Modeled on data in Ranki, Valle, Krohn, et al. (1987); Bowen, Lobel, Caruana, et al. (1988); CDC (1988); Dodd and Fang (1990), and Haseltine (1989).

17 weeks under the U.S. Army criterion and about 5 weeks later under the manufacturer's criterion. Another widely used criterion (Association of State and Territorial Public Health Laboratory Directors, 1987; CDC, 1989b) is that the WB is positive if antibodies to any two of p24, gp41 and either gp120 or gp160 are present. This criterion has been adopted by the U.S. Army. Under this criterion, the hypothetical patient in Figure 6.1 would be judged positive at 13 weeks.

Of great concern is the "silent" interval or "window" following infection before sufficient antibody has developed to be detected by EIA. This window is thought to be on the order of a few months, with 95% of seroconversions occurring within 6 months (Horsburgh, Qu, Jason, et al., 1989). Nevertheless, some patients have expressed antibody to core proteins in the WB assay more than a year before seroconversion (Ranki, Valle, Krohn, et al., 1987), and segments of HIV DNA coding for core protein have been detected by the polymerase chain reaction method in peripheral-blood lymphocytes more than two years before EIA seroconversion (Imagawa, Lee, Wolinsky, et al., 1989; Wolinsky, Rinaldo, Kwok, et al., 1989). These very long silent periods are thought to be atypical, however, because the sample was selected to include only homosexuals with long EIA seronegative periods (Winkelstein, Royce, and Sheppard, 1990; Wolinsky, Rinaldo, and Phair, 1990).

The sensitivity of EIA thus depends on the stage of infection. In Section 6.5 we discuss the use of assays to detect p24 antigen, live virus, and HIV DNA. These assays have the potential to detect HIV early in the course of infection but have not proved practical for mass screening.

6.2.4 Detecting HIV-2

Another factor that can affect sensitivity is the evolution of new strains of HIV that can cause AIDS but are biologically distinct from HIV-1, the strain against which current assays are directed. In fact, a new strain, HIV-2, has been identified in Africa (De Cook and Brun-Vézinet, 1989). About 60–90% of people with HIV-2 test positive with currently used EIAs for HIV-1 (CDC, 1990b). Although HIV-2 is currently rare in the United States, the spectrum of current assays will need to be broadened, or routine testing for HIV-2 will need to be implemented, to retain high overall sensitivity in populations where the prevalence of HIV-2 is appreciable. Centers that collect blood donations began testing for HIV-2 in the United States in 1992.

6.2.5 Sensitivity and Specificity of EIA and WB Assays

The sensitivity of EIA assays is high in patients with AIDS or ARC. The data in Table 6.2 suggest a sensitivity of 82% with cut-off ratio 5.0 in patients with AIDS. Later studies of commercial assays in patients with AIDS or ARC yielded estimates of sensitivity ranging from 97.0% to 100.0% (Reesink, Lelie, Huisman, et al., 1986). The fact that sensitivity is less than 100% in patients with AIDS may reflect technical failures. A second factor is that antibodies can diminish in end-stage AIDS (Figure 6.1) and disappear, even in asymptomatic men with previously documented HIV antibody (Farzadegan, Polis, Wolinsky, et al., 1988). In very rare instances, a person may have clinical immunodeficiency and an AIDS-defining condition without HIV infection. If such a person were included in the panel of AIDS cases, the apparent sensitivity of the EIA would be reduced.

The sensitivity of the EIA is lower in recently infected individuals. von Sydow, Gaines, Sönnerborg, et al. (1988) found an EIA sensitivity of 0.0% (0/12) among homosexual men in the first week of their primary symptomatic illness. The sensitivity increased to 67% (8/12) in the second week (Table 6.3). Some of these patients are in the "silent" interval. Mayer, Stoddard, McCusker, et al. (1986) studied 26 EIA negative high risk homosexual men, 2 of whom had a partner with AIDS and 24 of whom had at least 100 lifetime partners. Among these patients, 2 were found to have HIV virus by direct viral cultures. Thus the negative predictive value (see Section 6.3.2) was 24/26, and, using formula (6.4) in Section 6.3.2, one can estimate the sensitivity of the EIA assay as about 91.8%. In this calculation we assumed that the prevalence of infection was 50% among the population of high risk homosexuals in Boston in 1984, when this study was conducted, and that the specificity of the test was 99%. This lower sensitivity among high risk homosexuals reflects the fact that new infections were occurring at a brisk rate, so that a substantial portion of these individuals were in the silent interval. In Section 6.4.2, we discuss the sensitivity of a test in relation to the length of the silent interval. Some positive viral cultures may result from viral contamination of cells used in the assay, and some positive viral cultures may represent "incomplete" infections that never progress to clinical HIV disease and are never transmitted (Imagawa and Detels, 1991). Suppose one of the two positive cultures mentioned above represented an "incomplete" infection or an artifact of the viral culture assay and should be ignored. Then the calculation above would yield an estimated EIA sensitivity of 96.0%, instead of 91.8%.

The specificity of the EIA assay has been calculated from samples of healthy blood donors by assuming that none of these persons were infected. Data in Table 6.2 would indicate a specificity of 198/202 = 98.0% for an absorbance cut-off above 4.99. Manufacturers recommend that an initially reactive EIA be repeated twice on the same sample and that only individuals whose sera are reactive on at least one of the two repeat assays be classified as positive. Reesink, Lelie, Huisman, et al. (1986) reported that specificities for initial EIA ranged from 98.7% to 99.9% for six commercial assays, whereas specificities increased to 99.6–100.0% when confirmation by a second positive EIA was required (Table 6.3). Specificity can be further enhanced by requiring that a repeatedly reactive EIA be confirmed by a positive Western blot. Such combined testing will enhance specificity but necessarily lower sensitivity somewhat. Cleary, Barry, Mayer, et al. (1987) estimated that the proportion of EIA true positive individuals

Table 6.3 Sensitivity and Specificity of Assays for HIV

	Specificity (%)		Sensitivity (%)		Sensitivity (%) Estimates During Primary Illness in Homosexual men	
	Population	Estimates	Population	Estimates		
EIA	Random blood donors	98.7–99.9[a]	AIDS/ARC	97.0–100.0[a]	First week / Second week	0.0(0/12)[f] / 67.0(8/12)[f]
EIA repeated[b] Western Blot	Random blood donors	99.6–100.0[a]	AIDS/ARC and EIA positive	96.8[g]		
EIA with Western Blot confirmation on two samples	17–18 year old applicants for military service from rural regions with prevalence <0.0015 in applicant pool	99.989[c]				
PCR	Repeat blood donors without risk factors	90.5–100.0[d] 94.7 (mean of 5 labs)	Homosexual/bisexual men who are EIA positive and viral culture positive	98.0–100.0[d] 99.0[d] (mean of 5 labs)		
p24 antigen			AIDS/ARC	34.0[e]	First week / Second week / Weeks 3–5	84.0(10/12)[f] / 75.0(6/8)[f] / 18.2(2/11)[f]
Viral culture from plasma			AIDS/ARC	65.6[e]		
Viral culture from peripheral blood mononuclear cells			AIDS/ARC	97.5[e]		

[a] Recsink, Lelie, Huismen, et al. (1986).
[b] EIA was repeated with a fresh set of reagents. Positive result required both EIA tests to be positive.
[c] Burke, Brundage, Redfield, et al. (1988). An estimate of 100.000% with lower two-sided 95% confidence limit 99.9987% has been given by MacDonald, Jackson, Bowman, et al. (1989) on the basis of viral culture confirmation of positive results.
[d] Sheppard, Ascher, Busch, et al. (1991).
[e] Coombs, Collier, Allain, et al. (1989).
[f] von Sydow, Gaines, Sönnerborg, et al. (1988).
[g] Association of State and Territorial Public Health Laboratory Directors (1987) and CDC (1989b). The criterion for positivity is any two of p24, gp41 and either gp120 or gp160.

6.3 SCREENING APPLICATIONS AND POSITIVE PREDICTIVE VALUE

6.3.1 Possible Screening Applications

By usual laboratory standards, the EIA assay with WB confirmation has very high sensitivity and specificity. It is therefore tempting to use this test: (1) To track the progress of the epidemic by estimating seroprevalence in various subgroups; (2) to prevent the spread of HIV infection by identifying infected individuals and counselling them on how to reduce the risks of transmission to others; and (3) to identify infected individuals so as to facilitate earlier and more effective treatment. Surveys to estimate seroprevalence (Chapter 3) are limited mainly by the willingness of persons to be screened for HIV rather than by the accuracy of these tests. Volberding (1989) has emphasized the importance of HIV testing for proper management of the HIV infected patient. Establishing the diagnosis of HIV infection allows the physician to advise the patient as to prognosis, plan further monitoring of the patient's immune status, and institute therapy in a timely manner rather than after serious complications have occurred. The most controversial proposals for using assays concern screening populations for prevention activities, though efforts to screen donated blood products (Section 6.4) are generally accepted.

The controversy about screening populations for prevention activities derives from two concerns. First, an appreciable number of false positive results may occur, especially when screening populations with low prevalence of HIV infection, resulting in needless anxiety and other possible adverse consequences in an uninfected individual. Second, whether or not the test positive individual is infected, he or she may be adversely affected by social ostracism or exclusion from insurance or employment opportunities if the test result is revealed.

6.3.2 Positive and Negative Predictive Value

The accuracy of a test in a given screening application is often quantified in terms of positive predictive value (PPV) and negative predictive value (NPV). The positive predictive value is the probability that a person with a positive test result (T) is truly diseased (D), and the negative predictive value is the probability that a person with a negative test value is truly negative. The PPV is of major importance for screening activities because (1-PPV) is the probability of a false positive test result. The PPV and NPV depend not only on the sensitivity and specificity of the test but also on the prevalence, $P(D)$ of disease in the population being screened. From Bayes theorem (Vecchio, 1966),

$$PPV = P(D) \times (\text{sens})/[P(D) \times (\text{sens}) + \{1 - P(D)\}(1 - \text{spec})] \qquad (6.3)$$

and

$$NPV = P(\bar{D}) \times (\text{spec})/[P(\bar{D}) \times (\text{spec}) + \{1 - P(\bar{D})\}(1 - \text{sens})], \qquad (6.4)$$

where $\bar{D}$ denotes absence of disease and $P(\bar{D}) = 1 - P(D)$.

To apply these ideas to the issue of false positives, consider a possible prevention program based on premarital HIV testing. Following Cleary, Barry, Mayer, et al. (1987), we assume that a combined EIA/WB test has sensitivity 0.92 and specificity 0.99990. From equation (6.4) we calculate (Table 6.4) that the negative predictive value remains very high over a broad range of population prevalences. For example, most general populations have prevalence rates well below 0.01, and for such populations, the NPV exceeds .999. Thus very few people with negative tests are infected. However, from equation (6.3), values of PPV are not as high, especially in populations with low disease prevalence (Table 6.4). For example, in a very low risk population with prevalence $P(D) = 0.0001$, more than half the positive results would be false positives, because PPV = 0.4792. Prevalences in the range 0.001 to 0.005 are found in candidates for the Army (Burke, Brundage, Herbold, et al., 1987). For $P(D) = 0.001$, PPV = 0.902 so that roughly 1 in 10 persons testing positive will be uninfected. The PPV increases with $P(D)$. In populations of intravenous drug users or homosexual men with prevalences above 0.10, the PPV exceeds 0.999, and very few false positive test results arise. As previously described, the data of Burke, Brundage, Redfield, et al. (1988) and of MacDonald, Jackson, Bowman, et al. (1989) suggest that specificity may approach 0.99999 in some programs with rigorous quality control. In this case, PPV = 0.902 for $P(D) = 0.0001$.

Table 6.4 Positive and Negative Predictive Values for Various Levels of Prevalence

	Prevalence $P(D)$						
	.0001	.0005	.001	.005	.01	.10	.30
PPV	.4792	.9788	.9020	.9788	.9894	.9990	.9997
NPV	1.0000	1.0000	.9999	.9996	.9992	.9912	.9668

Note: Based on an assumed sensitivity of 0.92 and specificity of 0.99990.

Formulas (6.3) and (6.4) are correct only if estimates of sensitivity, specificity and prevalence are correct. In Section 6.2 we described some of the systematic factors that can affect estimates of sensitivity and specificity as well as the random error associated with such estimates. Seroprevalence, $P(D)$, is even more difficult to estimate accurately and is subject to both systematic biases (Chapter 3) and random error. The reliability of estimates of PPV and NPV should therefore be studied by varying parameters over plausible ranges of systematic error and by calculating the statistical variance that arises from random error in estimates of sensitivity, specificity and prevalence (Gastwirth, 1987). Bayesian methods have been developed for determining the posterior distributions of PPV and NPV (Johnson and Gastwirth, 1991; Gastwirth, Johnson, and Reneau, 1991).

6.3.3 Benefits Versus Harm from Screening

Weiss and Thier (1988) stress the need to think carefully about how the results of a screening test might be used before adopting screening programs, because the benefits must outweigh the harm from false positive findings and from breeches of confidentiality. Cleary, Barry, Mayer, et al. (1987) conclude that premarital screening is not cost-effective and would yield an unacceptably large number of false-positive results, and Meyer and Pauker (1987) raise similar concerns for screening in the general population. Epidemic models suggest that voluntary confidential testing could retard the spread of the epidemic at modest cost for populations with prevalences of one percent or more (Gail, Preston, and Piantadosi, 1989). In populations with high prevalences, such as homosexual communities, voluntary confidential testing has been advocated (Institute of Medicine, 1988) in conjunction with a program of counselling to provide psychological support and to encourage measures to reduce the risk of transmission. Chapter 4 of *Confronting AIDS* (Institute of Medicine, 1988) reviews ethical, legal and social aspects of HIV screening and presents recommendations for selected applications. The U.S. Public Health Service has published guidelines for counseling and testing that emphasize prevention activities and high-risk exposure groups (CDC, 1987c).

6.3.4 Pooled Samples

It may be advantageous to pool samples and then determine whether the pooled sera contain evidence of HIV infection. This strategy of group testing may reduce the costs of screening (Cahoon-Young,

Chandler, Livermore, et al., 1989; Kline, Brothers, Brookmeyer, et al., 1989). Thus, group testing may be useful in countries where screening would otherwise be prohibitively expensive. Once a positive pool is detected, additional tests are required to identify infected individuals. Group testing may also be used to determine seroprevalence rates while helping to ensure that the serostatus of individuals who agree to participate in the survey remains confidential (Gastwirth and Hammick, 1989). In this application, no further testing is required once the status of the pooled sera is determined. Some experimental investigations require the use of group testing, such as a recent study to determine what proportion of blood donations screened negative by EIV were in fact infected with HIV (Busch, Eble, Khayam-Bashi, et al., 1991). By pooling 76,500 blood donations into 1530 groups and studying these groups with viral culture and DNA amplification methods, those investigators identified one infected donation. Gastwirth and Johnson (1991) calculate that group testing may be feasible as a quality control measure to monitor the sensitivity of screening programs.

6.4 SAFETY OF THE BLOOD SUPPLY

As of December 31, 1991, 4636 cases of AIDS reported to the Centers for Disease Control had been ascribed to receipt of infected transfusion products. An additional 1876 cases of AIDS reported to the Centers for Disease Control were ascribed to receipt of coagulation products. Patients with hemophilia were at very high risk because they required repeated doses of clotting factors that were obtained from the pooled sera from thousands of donors (Peterman and Allen, 1989). This route of exposure has been largely eliminated by encouraging donors with risk factors not to donate blood, by screening the blood for HIV, and by taking measures to inactivate HIV in coagulation products (Goedert, Kessler, Aledort, et al., 1989). Therefore, we shall confine the present discussion to risks of HIV transmission from transfusion of whole blood and closely related products like packed red cells, platelets and white cells. Ward, Bush, Perkins, et al. (1989) found that 119 (59%) of 203 living recipients of infected blood were infected, indicating a high rate of transmission by this route.

6.4.1 Prevention Efforts

In order to prevent infection from contaminated blood, efforts have been made to reduce HIV prevalence in the population of donors and to screen donated blood for HIV. To increase the sensitivity of the screening procedure, blood is ejected if the first EIA is positive, even if that result is not later confirmed by a second EIA or by WB. Nonetheless, because of the "silent" interval, there remain rare instances of infection from blood products. Risks of failing to detect blood from infections in the silent interval are greater in populations with a preponderance of recent infections. Thus a donor population that contains 0.01% of infected people, most of whom are infected in the recent past, poses a greater risk than a donor population that contains 0.01% of infected people, most of whom were infected years before.

Several steps have been taken to prevent HIV transmission through the blood supply. In 1983, the U.S. Public Health Service first recommended that members of high risk groups be urged not to give blood. In the spring of 1985, compulsory ELISA screening of donated blood and blood products for HIV began. If the initial test was positive, the blood was not to be transfused or manufactured into other products capable of transmitting infectious agents (CDC, 1985a). This procedure maximizes sensitivity for detecting contaminated blood. To improve specificity for counselling donors, the test is only regarded as positive if the ELISA assay is repeatedly positive and if a subsequent positive WB result is obtained. Persons found to be positive are urged not to donate again. It is common practice for a blood bank to retain a confidential list of persons previously tested positive at that facility, and to use that list to prevent subsequent donations by such persons. Since the spring of 1985, the information given to potential donors on who should defer from donating blood has become more explicit (e.g., "males who have had sex with another male at any time since 1977"), and donors have been given the option to confidentially indicate that their blood should not be used for transfusion. The establishment of HIV testing facilities apart from transfusion centers has also been promoted to discourage the use of blood donation as a means of checking HIV status. These measures have reduced the risk of infection from blood transfusion dramatically.

There has been an important decline in HIV prevalence among donors and in the proportion of blood donations that are confirmed WB positive (Table 6.5). In every time period, repeat female donors have much lower seroprevalence than other classes of donors, and new male donors have much higher HIV antibody prevalence rates (Table 6.5). The effects of voluntary deferral are seen among new male donors and new female donors. There has been a 44% drop in seroprevalence among new male donors from 1985 to 1987, and a 10% drop among

Table 6.5 Rates of Positive Western Blot Results per Million Donations to the American Red Cross

	New Male Donors	Repeat Male Donors	New Female Donors	Repeat Female Donors
April–December,				
1985	898	402	171	51
1986	717	187	148	34
1987	589	123	154	36

Source: From Cumming, Wallace, Schorr, and Dodd (1989).

new female donors. Possibly there is less awareness among females of what constitutes risk of exposure. The largest percentage drops in seropositivity are seen in repeat donors, where the combined effects of voluntary deferral and blood bank imposed deferral operate. There has been a 69% drop in seropositivity among repeat male donors from 1985 to 1987 and a 29% among repeat female donors.

6.4.2 Effect of the "Silent" Window on the Sensitivity of the EIA Assay

If the EIA test had 100% sensitivity, all infected donors would be screened out. However, as we discussed in Section 6.2, the EIA assay will be negative in the silent time window between infection and the evolution of antibody to HIV. Consider a population of potential blood donors for whom the infection rate is $g(s)$ (see Section 1.3) and for whom the probability of surviving greater than u years after infection is $\mathcal{J}(u)$. Let $\psi(u)$ be the sensitivity of the ELISA assay as a function of time, u, from infection. Define the normalized density of previous infection times among infected donors alive at calendar time T as

$$g^*(s|T) = g(s)\mathcal{J}(T-s)/\int_{-\infty}^{T} g(s)\mathcal{J}(T-s)ds. \qquad (6.5)$$

The density $g^*(s|T)$ describes the distribution of previous infection times among the infected members of the donor pool at time T. Then the effective sensitivity of the test at calendar time T for this group of infected donors is

$$\text{sens} = \int_{-\infty}^{T} g^*(s|T)\psi(T-s)ds. \qquad (6.6)$$

To simplify, suppose $\psi(u) = 0$ for $0 \leqslant u \leqslant w$ and 1 for $u > w$. The sensitivity is thus zero within a window of length w. Under this model, equation (6.6) reduces to

$$\int_{-\infty}^{T-w} g^*(s|T)\,ds,$$

namely the probability that infection occurred before $T - w$. For repeat donors it is reasonable to suppose that new infections occur uniformly in the interval between screens, which we take to be 54 weeks, following Cumming, Wallace, Schorr, and Dodd (1989). Since the chance of death is nearly zero within this time period, the sensitivity of the EIA assay is about $(54-w)/54$ for persons infected since their last donation, where the window width, w, is measured in weeks.

The situation is more complicated for first time donors because we have less knowledge about $g^*(s|T)$. To be concrete, suppose $T = $ January 1, 1988. We make a rough estimate of $g^*(s|T)$ by assuming it is proportional to the infection curve, $g(s)$, in the United States. This assumption would not be true if a substantial fraction of those infected early in the epidemic had died, or if programs to discourage donations by high risk donors had been more effective for people infected early in the epidemic than for those infected later. Both these effects would produce distributions of times of infection more weighted toward recent infections. Back-calculated estimates of the infection curve in the United States (see Figure 8.11) suggest that $g^*(s|T)$ can be approximated by the following piecewise linear model: $g^*(s|T) = 0$ for $s < 1979$, $0.0342 \times (s - 1979)$ for $1979 \leqslant s < 1984$, 0.1711 for $1984 \leqslant s < 1985$, and $0.1711 - 0.0250 \times (s - 1985)$ for $1985 \leqslant s < 1988$. Thus 59.9% of the infections among potential first time donors in January 1988, occurred before January 1, 1985. Assuming the window, w, is less than 3 years, the sensitivity of EIA is, from equation (6.6) $0.599 + 0.1711 \times (3 - w/52) - 0.025 \times (3 - w/52)^2/2$, where w is expressed in weeks. For $w = 8$ weeks, the sensitivity among first time donors is thus .9847, whereas for repeat donors, the sensitivity is only $(54 - 8)/54 = 0.8519$.

We can estimate the number of units of contaminated blood that get through the HIV screen, per million donated units, by considering the proportion of blood donated by various types of donors and the corresponding estimated EIA sensitivity (Table 6.6). The prevalences for each of these six donor groups in 1987 are taken from the Red Cross study by Cumming, Wallace, Schorr, and Dodd (1989), as are the proportions of donors constituted by these groups. We treat new and untested repeat donors as having the same high sensitivity, 0.9847, as calculated above, whereas tested repeat donors have the lower sensitivity 0.8519.

Table 6.6 Estimated Number of HIV-positive Units Entering the Blood Supply in 1987, per Million Donated Units

	Prevalence (per million)	Proportion of Donors	EIA Sensitivity	Undetected Units[a]
New male	589	.080	.9847	0.72
Untested repeat Male	319	.140	.9847	0.68
Tested repeat male	46	.358	.8519	2.44
New female	154	.076	.9847	0.18
Untested repeat female	94	.097	.9847	0.14
Tested repeat female	13	.249	.8519	0.48
		1.000		4.64

Source: Adapted from table 5 in Cumming, Wallace, Schorr, and Dodd (1989).

Note: Prevalence is based on repeatedly EIA reactive Western blot confirmed units.

[a]Calculated as prevalence times the proportion of donors times 1 minus the sensitivity.

These calculations lead to an estimate of 4.64 contaminated units per million donated units (Table 6.6). Ward, Holmberg, Allen, et al. (1988) outlined the window calculation and obtained a rate of 2.6 contaminated samples per million by simply dichotomizing the donor pool into first time donors and repeat donors and by assuming a sensitivity of 0.99 for first-time donors. Cumming, Wallace, Schorr, and Dodd (1989) obtained a somewhat higher rate of 6.5 contaminated units per million donations from the data in Table 6.6 because they assumed $g^*(s)$ was uniform over the 5 years preceding donation for first time donors and uninfected repeat donors, yielding an EIA sensitivity of $(5 \times 52 - w)/5 \times 52 = 0.9692$ for a window of 8 weeks, instead of the value 0.9847 in Table 6.6.

One can compare estimates of the chance of false negative screening results based on the window calculation with the scant available empirical data. Cohen, Muñoz, Reitz, et al. (1989) found one sero-conversion among cardiac surgery patients who received 36,282 units, for a rate of 28 per million units. Based on Poisson sampling, the corresponding 95% confidence interval is 6.7 to 154 per million units. Busch, Eble, Khayam-Bashi, et al. (1991) found one positive unit confirmed by culture and DNA amplication among 76,500 donations in San Francisco. Based on Poisson variation, the corresponding estimated rate of false negative results would be 13 per million units, with 95% confidence interval 3.2 to 73 per million units. The empirical data thus yield estimates of false negativity rates in reasonable concordance with the window calculation, especially in view of the considerable random uncertainty associated with empirical estimates.

Based on window calculations, one can assert that the risk of contracting HIV from a blood transfusion is small. A patient requiring 20 units of blood might have a risk on the order of $1-(1 - 4.6 \times 10^{-6})^{20} = .00009$. If the recent estimate (Petersen, Satten, and Dodd, 1992) that the average window width is only 45 days is correct, the risk would be even smaller. To get an idea of the maximum plausible risk, we assume a window of width $w = 16$ weeks. Then the sensitivity for first-time donors decreases to 0.9690, and the sensitivity for repeat donors decreases to 0.7037. The expected number of contaminated units per million donations increases to 9.33, and the chance of infection from receiving 20 randomly selected units increases to 0.00019. If we further assume that the HIV prevalences in Table 6.6 are too small because the testing procedure with Western blot confirmation used to estimate these prevalences has sensitivity 0.90, the chance of a false negative result is increased further to $9.33/0.90 = 10.37$ per million, and the chance of infection from 20 units increases to 0.00021. If, based on empirical data, we assume the rate of false negative results is 20 per million units, then the chance of infection from 20 units increases further to 0.00040. Such risks are small compared to the risks of not receiving needed blood products.

The window calculations can be refined to take into account the fact that some persons who tested negative at year $T - 1$ and donated again at year T were, in fact, already infected at or before $T - 1$. The screening assay at T would have 100% sensitivity to detect such persons for window widths less than one year. Hence the sensitivity would be somewhat higher than the value $(54 - w)/54 = (54 - 8)/54 = .8519$ calculated previously. The improvement is small, however, as illustrated by the following calculations. We assume that mortality is negligible and consider the population of individuals infected before T whose first donation is at $T - 1$, and who subsequently donated at T. We assume that the chance, π, of donating at $T - 1$ and T is the same for persons who were infected before $T - 1$ and tested negative at $T - 1$ as for persons who were first infected between $T - 1$ and T. Then, of the infected persons at T who tested negative at $T - 1$, a proportion $\gamma = A/(A + B)$ were already infected by $T - 1$, where A and B are approximately

$$A \doteq \pi \times \{1 - \text{sensitivity at } T - 1 \text{ for a first time}$$
$$\text{donor who is infected}\} \times \int_{-\infty}^{T-1} g(s)\,ds$$

and

$$B \doteq \pi \times \{\text{specificity for a first time donor at } T - 1$$

$$\text{who is uninfected}\} \times \int_{T-1}^{T} g(s)\,ds.$$

Supposing $g(s)$ was proportional to $g^*(s|T = 1988)$, which was defined previously, and setting $T - 1 = 1987$, we obtain $A = \pi c(1 - 0.9847) \times (.8912)$ by assuming the sensitivity for first time donors is 0.9847 as before, and $B = \pi c(0.98) \times (.1088)$, by assuming the specificity for a single unconfirmed EIA is 0.98. Here c is a proportionality constant that cancels out when calculating $\gamma = 0.113$. Based on this calculation, the window model with $w = 8$ weeks predicts a sensitivity of $0.113 + (1 - 0.113) \times (52 - 8)/52 = 0.864$ for persons screened negative one year before. This value is 1.4% greater than the value .852 obtained by ignoring the possibility of false negative screens at $T - 1$. Such calculations suggest that the previous simple window calculations are sufficiently accurate given other uncertainties, but that they slightly underestimate the sensitivity of the screening procedure. A simulation study by Le Pont, Costagliola, Massari, and Valleron (1989) yields results similar to calculations based on the window model.

6.4.3 Screening Blood in Developing Countries

In a developing country with high seroprevalence rates, screening can reduce numbers of transfusion-related infections drastically. Even in a rapidly growing epidemic in which there are many recent infections so that the dates of infection among infected donors are uniformly distributed over the previous 5 years, a window calculation with $w = 2$ months suggests an effective sensitivity of about $\{(60 - 2)/60\} = 0.967$. If the prevalence of infection among donors were 5%, screening could thus reduce the chance that a transfused unit was infected from 5% to $5\% \times (1 - .967) = .17\%$. The chance that a person receiving three units would become infected would thereby be reduced from $1 - (1 - .05)^3 = .142$ to $1 - (1 - .0017)^3 = .005$, a dramatic improvement. To achieve such gains, developing countries must be able to find economic and logistical support for screening facilities, and the tests must be simple and reliable enough to use without the need for elaborate laboratory facilities and quality control systems. Quinn and Mann (1989) discuss the role of transfusion of blood products and other factors that promoted the spread of HIV in Africa.

6.5 ASSAYS FOR LIVE VIRUS, FOR HIV ANTIGEN, AND FOR HIV GENOME

Partly in an effort to reduce or eliminate the "silent" interval and thereby increase the sensitivity of tests for HIV, researchers have investigated assays based on viral culture, on detection of HIV p24 antigen, and on detection of viral DNA through the polymerase chain reaction (PCR). Studies of patients in the acute primary phase of illness indicate that p24 antigen, live virus and viral DNA may be found within one month of infection and before antibody is detectable by EIA (Bowen, Lobel, Caruana, et al., 1988; Clark, Saag, Don Decker, et al., 1991; Daar, Moudgil, Meyer, and Ho, 1991). Earlier studies on high risk seronegative homosexual men and on men who had recently seroconverted had indicated that HIV genome might be detectable through PCR or hybridization assays months or years before sero-conversion (Ranki, Valle, Krohn, et al., 1987; Wolinsky, Rinaldo, Kwok, et al., 1989; Imagawa, Lee, Wolinsky, et al., 1989).

Antigen to p24 has been extensively studied as a means to shorten the silent interval. In a prospective study, 515,494 blood donations from thirteen centers in the United States were tested, and 5 samples were positive for p24 antigen (Alter, Epstein, Swenson, et al., 1990). However, these same 5 samples were EIA positive. A similar study of 595,000 donations in Austria and Germany between March 1987 and April 1988 also failed to reveal a single p24 positive, EIA negative case (Baecker, Weinauer, Cathof, et al., 1988). These data demonstrate that p24 antigen adds very little to the sensitivity of available EIA tests for contaminated blood, despite its appearance in the acute phase of primary infection (Table 6.3). The p24 assay has low sensitivity in patients with AIDS or ARC (Table 6.3).

A similar large-scale investigation of viral culture for screening blood has not been undertaken, perhaps because viral culture is expensive and poses risks to laboratory workers. These practical considerations make it unlikely that viral culture assays will be widely used for screening blood (Sloand, Pitt, Chiarello, and Nemo, 1991).

Viral culture is an important research tool and is usually regarded as the "gold standard" indicator of infection. However, occasionally, it may be difficult to determine the biological significance of a positive viral culture. For example, Imagawa, Lee, Wolinsky, et al. (1989) isolated HIV-1 from 31 (23%) of 133 seronegative homosexual men who continued to engage in high risk behaviors such as unprotected anal-receptive intercourse with more than one partner in the previous 6 months. Four men later seroconverted. Subsequent testing of the 27 men who did not seroconvert yielded only one instance of viral isolation in 151 samples (Imagawa and Detels, 1991). These investigators concluded that these 27 cases probably represented "incomplete infections" that would not progress to clinical HIV disease or infect other partners. Positive viral assays may also result from contamination and other laboratory errors.

The PCR assay amplifies HIV DNA present in a sample and can detect even a single DNA molecule. As a consequence, any contamination of laboratory facilities or specimens can result in low specificity and false positive results. Sheppard, Ascher, Busch, et al. (1991) used coded samples to test the performance of five laboratories with extensive experience in handling PCR. Ninety-four specimens were from seropositive, culture-positive homosexual or bisexual men. One hundred five specimens were from seronegative regular blood donors without known risk factors. The sensitivities for the five laboratories ranged from 98.0% to 100.0%. The specificities ranged from 90.5% to 100.0%. The average sensitivity was 99.0%, and the average specificity was 94.7%.

Such specificities are too low for mass screening. Assuming an average prevalence of HIV of 0.0001 among donors (Table 6.5) and a sensitivity of 99%, a PCR specificity of 96% would yield a positive predictive value of 0.0025 (see equation (6.3)). Of each 10,000 bloods screened positive by PCR, 25 would be infected and 9,975 would be uninfected. Put another way, one must throw away $9,975/25 = 399$ units of good blood to prevent one infection. Thus, at present, PCR does not have high enough specificity for screening blood. By comparison, a single EIA test might have a sensitivity of 0.98 and specificity of 0.995 or greater. With this procedure one throws away about 51 units of good blood to prevent one infection.

7

Statistical Issues in Surveillance of AIDS Incidence

7.1 INTRODUCTION

AIDS incidence refers to the numbers of newly diagnosed cases per unit time. Before the development of the HIV antibody screening test (Chapter 6), AIDS incidence data were the only available data for tracking the course of the epidemic. However, trends in AIDS incidence do not reflect current trends in the spread of HIV infection because incubation times are long and variable. Nevertheless, because of the difficulty in conducting representative HIV seroprevalence surveys (Chapter 3), AIDS surveillance remains one of the more reliable tools for monitoring the epidemic. Since 1981, sophisticated registries have been developed for tracking and counting AIDS cases. The objective of this chapter is to address a number of statistical and epidemiological issues that arise in the interpretation of AIDS surveillance data. These issues include delays in reporting, incomplete reporting, changing surveillance definitions and empirical extrapolation of AIDS incidence curves.

7.2 AIDS INCIDENCE DATA

Registries of AIDS cases have been established for tracking the epidemic in many countries. The Global Programme on AIDS at the World Health Organization (WHO) is responsible for worldwide AIDS surveillance. Countries are requested to report AIDS cases to WHO at least once per year even if there were no AIDS cases to report.

The Centers for Disease Control in the United States developed the first national AIDS surveillance system. All states, the District of

Columbia, U.S. dependencies and possessions report cases using a standardized case definition and report form. Cases are classified by risk group. A hierarchical scheme is used whereby individuals with two or more risk factors are classified in the category listed first, with the exception that homosexual men who are intravenous drug users are placed in a separate category (see, e.g., CDC, 1990d, and Table 1.1). Individuals without an identified risk factor are listed as "no identified risk" (see Section 7.4) and further investigations are conducted. The reports include information on age, race, sex, geographic region, and date of diagnosis.

Graphical displays of AIDS incidence data are invaluable for monitoring the epidemic. The number of newly diagnosed AIDS cases are grouped into calendar intervals, typically either 6-month, 3-month or monthly intervals. Before trends can be interpreted, AIDS incidence data must be adjusted for reporting delays as described in Section (7.3). Because the reporting delay adjustments are highly uncertain for AIDS cases diagnosed in the most recent 6 months, analyses are often based on "delay-corrected" AIDS incidence data up to 6 months before the analysis.

Green, Karon, and Nwanyanwu (1991) interpreted trends by a graphical analysis of U.S. AIDS incidence data. Their analyses emphasized the heterogeneity in trends and the importance of stratifying by risk group and demographic factors. Quarterly AIDS incidence data were adjusted for reporting delays and smoothed using a locally weighted moving average (the weights were taken from a normal distribution with a standard deviation of one year). Their general conclusions were that the rate of growth of AIDS cases diagnosed per quarter in the United States increased until 1987. After that time, the rate of growth declined. However there is considerable geographic and demographic variation. For example, outside New York City, San Francisco, and Los Angeles, the slowing in growth in AIDS incidence is seen only in non-Hispanic whites. Further, Green, Karon, and Nwanyanwu (1991) conclude there was no evidence for slowing through mid-1990 among heterosexual cases.

7.3 STATISTICAL ANALYSIS OF REPORTING DELAYS

There can be considerable delays before newly diagnosed AIDS cases are reported to central registries. For example, AIDS cases diagnosed in the United States are first reported to the staff of state health departments, who, in turn, report the cases to the national AIDS surveillance system at the Centers for Disease Control. Reporting

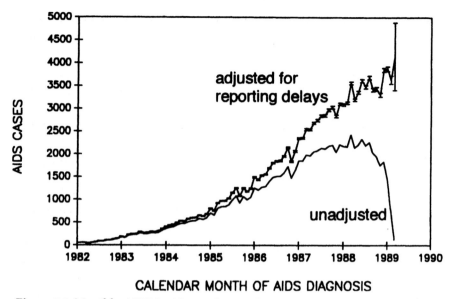

Figure 7.1 Monthly AIDS incidence data in the U.S., adjusted and unadjusted for reporting delays. Error bars represent 95% confidence intervals. (Source: Harris, 1990a.)

delays may falsely give the appearance of a recent decline in disease incidence when, in fact, the apparent decline in incidence is due to incomplete reporting of the most recently diagnosed cases. In order to accurately monitor disease incidence trends it is necessary to adjust for delays in disease reporting. Figure 7.1 is a graph of numbers of cases in the United States by date of diagnosis for cases reported by March 31, 1989 (Harris, 1990a). The lower curve is unadjusted for reporting delays and suggests a decline in recent AIDS incidence. When the curve is appropriately adjusted for reporting delays, a different picture of rising disease incidence emerges.

The statistical analysis of reporting delays is complicated by the fact that the data are right truncated. This truncation refers to the exclusion from a data set of individuals with long reporting delays. Very similar statistical problems arise in the analysis of incubation periods of transfusion-associated AIDS cases (Chapter 4). Generally, failure to account for such right truncation will lead to biased results that underestimate reporting delays. The following discussion is adapted from Brookmeyer and Liao (1990b).

The data available for analysis consist of all cases reported to a registry as of the current calendar time, say C. The calendar time of diagnosis, U_i, and the calendar time of report to the registry, R_i, are recorded on each case (i indexes the case). The reporting delay for the ith case is $d_i = R_i - U_i$. We also record covariate values for each case, such as geographic region of diagnosis, risk group, or calendar time of diagnosis. Such covariates may explain heterogeneity in reporting delays. Again, the main complexity with the analysis of reporting delays is that the data are right truncated; that is, a case is included in the registry only if the reporting delay d_i is less than or equal to $T_i = C - U_i$. We call T_i the truncation time for the ith individual.

The cumulative probability that the reporting delay is less than or equal to t is called the reporting delay distribution, and we use the notation $F(t) = P(d \leqslant t)$. The most important limitation of our data for estimating $F(t)$, is that we cannot observe reporting delays larger than the maximum truncation time. For example, suppose a disease registry is examined on January 1, 1989, and it is found that the earliest diagnosis time of a reported case is January 1, 1983. The maximum truncation time is 6 years. The best we can do is estimate the reporting delay distribution conditional on the delay being less than or equal to 6 years. We call this the conditional reporting delay distribution, $F^*(t)$, and it is related to $F(t)$ according to $F^*(t) = F(t)/F(6)$.

Our subsequent discussion refers to methods for estimating the conditional reporting delay distribution $F^*(t) = F(t)/F(t_m)$ for some value t_m which is not greater than the maximum truncation time. If t_m is sufficiently large, then F^* may be a good approximation to F. In our analysis of AIDS reporting delays (Section 7.3.3), we will estimate the reporting delay distribution conditionally on the delay being less than 4 years. An important point is that there is no information in the data about the proportion of AIDS cases with long reporting delays that exceed the maximum truncation time or the proportion of AIDS cases who are never reported (Lagakos, Barraj, and DeGruttola, 1988; Kalbfleisch and Lawless, 1989; Brookmeyer and Liao, 1990b). Additional epidemiological studies, such as death certificate reviews, are needed to address these important issues, and we return to this point in Section 7.4. An important caveat associated with an analysis based on the conditional distribution F^* is that it could indicate delays are longer in subgroup A than subgroup B, but nevertheless, the proportion of cases that are never reported or have very long delays (greater than t_m) could be larger in subgroup B than subgroup A.

We note that a simple linear regression analysis of observed delays d_i on calendar time of diagnosis u_i can be highly misleading, because we only get to observe AIDS cases if d_i is smaller than $T_i = C - u_i$. Thus, a naive regression analysis of this type will show a trend of reporting delays becoming shorter over time, even if, in fact, there were no trends in the reporting delay distribution or possibly even if there were a trend toward larger delays.

7.3.1 Nonparametric Estimation

The method for finding the nonparametric estimate of the conditional reporting delay distribution adapts survival analysis and life table techniques for use with right truncated data. This approach involves expressing the conditional reporting delay distribution, $F^*(t)$, as the product of conditional probabilities. We define the conditional probability p_j to be the probability that the reporting delay is equal to t_j given it is less than or equal to t_j; that is, $p_j = P(d = t_j | d \leqslant t_j)$. Then,

$$F^*(t_s) = \prod_{j=s+1}^{m} (1 - p_j) \qquad s = 1, \ldots, m-1,$$

where $(1 - p_j) = P(d < t_j | d \leqslant t_j)$ and $F(t_m) = 1.0$. The estimate of the reporting delay distribution is obtained by substituting estimates of the conditional probabilities into the above expression. The only cases who can contribute information about p_j are those cases whose truncation times are greater than or equal to t_j and whose reporting delays are less than or equal to t_j. We call these individuals the "risk set at t_j" to emphasize the analogy with life table analysis. The number of individuals in the risk set at t_j is called n_j, and the number of cases with reporting delays of duration t_j is called Y_j. Thus, an estimate of p_j is Y_j/n_j. Then substituting this into the expression for F^*, the nonparametric estimate of F^* is

$$\hat{F}^*(t_s) = \prod_{j=s+1}^{m} \left(1 - \frac{Y_j}{n_j} \right) \qquad s = 1, \ldots, m-1. \tag{7.1}$$

The variance is given by

$$\operatorname{var}(\hat{F}^*(t_s)) = [\hat{F}^*(t_s)]^2 \sum_{j=s+1}^{m} \frac{Y_j}{n_j(n_j - Y_j)}$$

$$s = 1, \ldots, m-1, \tag{7.2}$$

which is analogous to Greenwood's formula.

These methods for nonparametrically estimating the reporting delay distribution are illustrated with hypothetical reporting delay data given in Table 7.1. Table 7.1 is hypothetical data of cases cross classified by the month of diagnosis and the reporting delay (in months). Since the maximum reporting delay which could possibly be observed was 5 months, the best that can be done (nonparametrically)

Table 7.1 Hypothetical Data of Cases Reported by April 30, 1991:
Illustration of Reporting Delay Calculations

Month of Diagnosis	Reporting Delay (months)					
	1	2	3	4	5	6
Dec. '90	50	20	10	6	2	—
Jan. '91	100	55	20	12	— (273)	(88)
Feb. '91	171	115	45	— (586)	—	—
Mar. '91	207	118	— (836)	—		
April '91	220	—	—	—	—	—

Note: Numbers in parentheses are total cases in rectangular boxes.

is to estimate the conditional reporting delay distribution given that the reporting delay is not greater than 5 months. The conditional probabilities p_j are

$$p_2 = P(d = 2 | d \leqslant 2) = \frac{308}{836} = .368$$

$$p_3 = P(d = 3 | d \leqslant 3) = \frac{75}{586} = .128$$

$$p_4 = P(d = 4 | d \leqslant 4) = \frac{18}{273} = .066$$

$$p_5 = P(d = 5 | d \leqslant 5) = \frac{2}{88} = .023$$

Then the reporting delay distribution given that the delay is less than or equal to 5 months is calculated from equation (7.1) as follows:

$$\hat{F}^*(5) = 1.0$$
$$\hat{F}^*(4) = 1 - .023 = .977$$
$$\hat{F}^*(3) = .977(1 - .066) = .913$$
$$\hat{F}^*(2) = .913(1 - .128) = .796$$
$$\hat{F}^*(1) = .796(1 - .368) = .503$$

The incidence data adjusted for reporting delays is obtained by appropriately dividing the observed cases by the reporting delay distribution. If Z is the number of reported cases who were diagnosed u time units ago, then the adjusted incidence is $Z^* = Z/F^*(u)$. Again, this adjusted number does not account for cases with reporting delays longer than t_m (in the hypothetical example, $t_m = 5$ months). The calculations are illustrated in Table 7.2. There are two sources of uncertainty associated with the adjusted incidence data Z^*: uncertainty in the estimated reporting delay distribution; and uncertainty due to binomial variation. The variance of $Z^* = Z/\hat{F}^*$ is approximately (for large Z)

$$\frac{Z^*(1 - \hat{F}^*)}{\hat{F}^*} + \frac{(Z^*)^2 \hat{\sigma}^2}{\hat{F}^{*2}}. \tag{7.3}$$

where $\hat{\sigma}^2$, the estimated variance of $\hat{F}^*$, is obtained from equation (7.2) (see Brookmeyer and Liao, 1990). This formula is obtained by applying the delta method (Fienberg, 1980) to the ratio $Z/\hat{F}^*$ with the binomial variance for Z and the variance of $\hat{F}^*$.

There are alternative approaches for estimating the reporting delay distribution. An alternative computational approach which produces the same estimate given by equation (7.1) is based on Poisson regression methods for the analysis of triangular incomplete contingency tables. Rosenberg (1990) gives a noniterative computational approach. These approaches are maximizing a conditional likelihood that is conditional on the numbers of cases that were reported to be diagnosed at each calendar time (Brookmeyer and Daminao, 1989; Harris, 1990a; Kalbfleisch and Lawless, 1989; Lagakos, Barraj, and De Gruttola, 1988). Another approach assumes a parametric model for the AIDS incidence curve and maximizes an unconditional likelihood. This approach is considered in Section 7.5.

7.3.2 Regression Analysis

In this section, statistical techniques for the regression analysis of reporting delays are briefly outlined. Regression techniques are important for assessing calendar time (secular) trends in reporting delay and

Table 7.2 Illustration of Adjustment of Hypothetical Incidence Data for Reporting Delays

	Observed Incidence	Adjusted Incidence
Dec. 90	88	88
Jan. 91	187	187/.977 = 191
Feb. 91	331	331/.913 = 363
Mar. 91	325	325/.796 = 408
April 91	220	220/.503 = 437

identifying covariates, such as geographic region or risk group, that affect the reporting delay distribution. The main statistical problem is that the data are right truncated. We assume that there are r covariates $(X_1, \ldots, X_r)$ and that each covariate can take a finite number of values. Thus, each individual can be grouped into one of K strata defined by the values of the covariates. We label these strata by the covariate vector $\mathbf{X}_k$, $k = 1, \ldots, K$. The approach is to model the conditional probabilities p_j as a function of covariates.

We extend the notation in the preceeding section by adding an additional subscript k to index the covariate strata. Thus, in the kth stratum, the conditional probability at t_j is called p_{jk}; the numbers of cases with reporting delay equal to t_j is called Y_{jk}; and the size of the risk set at t_j is called n_{jk}. Our model is that, conditional on n_{jk}, the Y_{jk} have independent binomial distributions, that is,

$$Y_{jk} = \text{binomial } (n_{jk}, p_{jk}) \qquad j = 1, \ldots, m-1 \qquad k = 1, \ldots, K. \qquad (7.4)$$

Although the independence assumption is not strictly correct, it can be shown that the maximum likelihood estimates and their estimated variances are not affected by this assumption (Efron, 1988). In order to allow reporting delays to depend on covariates, we model the binomial probabilities as follows:

$$g(p_{jk}) = \alpha_j + \boldsymbol{\beta} \mathbf{X}_k \qquad (7.5)$$

where α_j and $\boldsymbol{\beta} = (\beta_1, \beta_2, \ldots, \beta_r)$ are parameters to be estimated. The function g is called the *link function* in the theory of generalized linear models (McCullagh and Nelder, 1989).

Two leading choices for the link function are the logistic link, $g(p_{jk}) = \log\{p_{jk}/(1 - p_{jk})\}$ and the complementary log-log link, $g(p_{jk}) = \log\{-\log(1 - p_{jk})\}$. The model given by equations (7.4) and (7.5) with a logistic link has been termed a continuation ratio model in the contingency table literature (Fienberg, 1980; McCullagh and Nelder, 1989). The complementary log-log link is especially attractive because it induces a simple relation among the distribution functions of reporting delays:

$$F_k^*(t_s) = \{F^*(t_s)\}^{\theta_k} \qquad \theta_k = \exp(\boldsymbol{\beta} \mathbf{X}_k) \qquad s = 1, \ldots, m-1, \qquad (7.6)$$

where

$$F^*(t_s) = \prod_{i=s+1}^{m} \exp(-e^{\alpha_i})$$

is the reporting delay distribution function when all the covariates are 0. The interpretation of a regression coefficient β_l associated with one of the covariates X_i is as follows: a positive β_i indicates delays are longer with increasing values of X_i after controlling for the other covariates; a negative β_i indicates delays are shorter with increasing values of X_i; and a β_i equal to zero suggests no association between delays and the covariate X_i.

7.3.3 Reporting Delays in the United States

The methods described in Sections 7.3.1 and 7.3.2 were used to analyze reporting delays of AIDS in the United States (Brookmeyer and Liao, 1990b). The analyses were based on the October 1989 AIDS Public Information Data Set. This data set included 109,168 AIDS cases diagnosed in the United States and reported to CDC before October 1, 1989. The analysis included only cases who met the pre-1987 AIDS surveillance definition. This restriction is important because some cases who met only the expanded 1987 surveillance definition were reported to have been diagnosed months, and in some cases years, before the new definition went into effect, which could artificially give the appearance of long reporting delays.

Table 7.3 presents the nonparametric estimates of the reporting delay distribution for the entire United States and for each of the six geographic regions (using equation (7.1)). Overall, 51% of cases are reported within 3 months of diagnosis, and 84% within 12 months. The fastest reporting occurred in the Northeast and the slowest in the South. For example, the proportion of cases diagnosed within three months ranged from 0.56 in the Northeast to only 0.39 in the South.

An important question is whether the distribution of reporting delays has changed over calendar times. The regression methods of Section 7.3.2 were used to evaluate the separate effects of calendar time, risk group, and geography on the reporting delay distribution. These analyses suggested significant geographic variation. The influences of risk groups and calendar year of diagnosis were not consistent across each of the geographic regions. Variation among risk groups was attributed primarily to slower reporting of transfusion-associated and pediatric AIDS cases. An overall trend toward longer delays with calendar time of diagnosis was attributed primarily to a trend toward longer delays in the Northeast.

Adjusted AIDS incidence in the most recent month is very uncertain. For example, suppose the reporting delay distribution were known precisely, so that $\hat{\sigma} = 0$ in equation (7.3). Then, even with a true monthly incidence as large as 200 cases/month, the coefficient of variation of the adjusted incidence in the most recent month, $\mathcal{Z}^*$,

Table 7.3 Conditional Reporting Delay Distribution[a] by Geographic Region of Diagnosis Among Cases Meeting the Pre-1987 Surveillance Definition

Reporting Delay in Months (number of cases)[b]	U.S. (88,037)[c]	Northeast (22,738)	Central (6,375)	West (18,471)	South (11,342)	Mid-Atlantic (5,585)	Other (22,249)
1	0.05	0.07	0.05	0.05	0.02	0.07	0.04
2	0.31	0.35	0.32	0.35	0.19	0.32	0.28
3	0.51	0.56	0.53	0.54	0.39	0.51	0.49
4	0.62	0.67	0.63	0.64	0.52	0.62	0.59
5	0.68	0.73	0.69	0.70	0.61	0.69	0.65
6	0.72	0.76	0.73	0.74	0.67	0.73	0.69
7	0.75	0.79	0.76	0.77	0.70	0.76	0.72
8	0.78	0.82	0.78	0.79	0.74	0.78	0.75
9	0.80	0.83	0.80	0.81	0.76	0.80	0.77
10	0.82	0.85	0.82	0.83	0.78	0.82	0.79
11	0.83	0.86	0.83	0.84	0.81	0.83	0.80
12	0.84	0.87	0.84	0.85	0.83	0.85	0.82
18	0.90	0.92	0.90	0.90	0.90	0.90	0.88
24	0.93	0.95	0.93	0.93	0.94	0.93	0.92
36	0.97	0.98	0.97	0.97	0.98	0.98	0.97
48	1.00	1.00	1.00	1.00	1.00	1.00	1.00

Source: Brookmeyer and Liao, 1990b.

[a]Cumulative probability $F^*(t)$, of a reporting delay less than or equal to t months given the delay is less than or equal to 48 months. Cases reported within same month of diagnosis coded 1; cases reported in month following diagnosis coded 2, etc.

[b]Number of cases reported to the CDC before October 1, 1989, that met the pre-1987 surveillance definition.

[c]Includes an additional 1277 pediatric AIDS cases with missing geographic region information.

would be over 30% (from equation (7.3)). For this reason, adjusted AIDS incidence for the most recent month should be typically ignored when assessing trends. Many analysts recommend ignoring the most recent 3 or even 6 months of adjusted incidence data.

7.4 UNDERREPORTING OF AIDS CASES

Some AIDS cases may never be reported, and these cases are not accounted for by the reporting delay adjustments described in Section 7.3. Cases may not be reported either because they were never properly diagnosed, or, if diagnosed, may not have been reported to the surveillance system (General Accounting Office, 1989).

One method for assessing underreporting of cases is to identify individuals who died from AIDS by reviewing death certificates and to match these individuals to the AIDS surveillance registry. A measure of the completeness of reporting, f, is the fraction of cases identified by the death certificate review who are found in the AIDS surveillance registry:

$$f = \frac{\text{Number of death certificate cases also in registry}}{\text{Number of AIDS cases found from death certificates}}.$$

Hardy, Starcher, and Morgan (1987) used this methodology and searched death certificates from 1985 in four U.S. cities. They report $f = 487/548 = .89$. A source of uncertainty with this methodology is error in identification of all AIDS-related deaths from death certificates. AIDS cases that are not reported to the surveillance system may also be less likely to be correctly classified as an AIDS-related death on the death certificate.

A disadvantage of the above methodology is that it requires an identifier (record linkage) to match cases from death certificates with cases in the registry. An alternate methodology that does not require identifiers was proposed by Remis and Palmer (1991). Remis and Palmer assessed the completeness of reporting in the Quebec AIDS surveillance program by comparing deaths modelled from reported AIDS cases to AIDS mortality based on death certificates. They predicted AIDS deaths by propagating forward reported AIDS cases to obtain predicted dates of death, according to a survival distribution for AIDS patients. Based on a comparison of predicted and observed AIDS deaths in 1987–88, they estimated that the completeness of reporting was 92%.

A separate issue from the underreporting of cases concerns individuals with severe HIV disease who do not meet the AIDS surveillance definition. Stoneburner, Des Jarlais, Benezra (1988) studied the increased mortality in the 1980s among New York intravenous drug users. The death certificates among the IV drug users for whom the causes of death were AIDS-related were matched to the New York City Department of Health AIDS Surveillance Registry. They concluded that there was a large spectrum of severe HIV disease that does not qualify as AIDS.

An additional problem with tracking trends in individual risk groups is that the risk group for some cases may be unknown. The practice in the United States is to temporarily assign these individuals to a category with undetermined risk ("no identified risk"). Some of these individuals may then be reclassified to other risk groups, following the results of more intensive investigation and interviewing. As a result, trends in the undetermined group typically show pronounced growth in the most recent past. This "growth" must be interpreted very cautiously since it is likely due to using the undetermined classification as a temporary holding category. For example, as of November 1990, 9920 AIDS cases in United States were initially reported as no identified risk. Additional interviews and follow-up information were collected from 4863 of these cases, of which 4416 were eventually reclassified. Only 447 remained classified as no identified risk/other (Centers for Disease Control, 1990d).

In order to monitor risk group specific trends in AIDS incidence, it is necessary to redistribute cases with undetermined risk. Green, Karon, and Nwanyanwu (1992) have performed an analysis to examine past trends in these redistribution fractions among cases initially with undetermined risk for whom additional follow-up information and interviews were obtained. For example, among adult white males with initially undetermined risk, Green, Karon, Nwanyanwu (1992) report that eventually 72% are reclassified as gay, 7% as IVDU, 3% as gay/IVDU, 6% as heterosexual, 4% as transfusion-related, and 8% as no identified risk/other.

7.5 CHANGES IN THE SURVEILLANCE DEFINITION

The AIDS surveillance definition in the U.S. has been revised several times. These revisions reflect increasing knowledge of the pathogenesis of HIV infection and a desire to make sure that the surveillance definition reflects current diagnostic practice. Before 1985, the surveillance definition was not based on a positive HIV antibody test but required pathological evidence of AIDS-defining conditions. In 1985, the definition was expanded to include individuals who also had diseases such as disseminated histoplasmosis, chronic isosporiasis, and high grade or B-cell non-Hodgkins lymphoma (Centers for Disease Control, 1985b). A more significant revision occurred in 1987 (Centers for Disease Control, 1987d) when the definition was expanded to include HIV positive persons with diseases such as extrapulmonary tuberculosis, HIV dementia, and HIV wasting syndrome. The 1987 definition also included individuals who were HIV antibody positive and who were diagnosed with certain diseases, such as *Pneunocystis carinii* pneumonia and cerebral toxoplasmosis on a presumptive clinical basis rather than by histological proof. In 1993, the CDC revised the surveillance definition of AIDS. The case definition was expanded to include all HIV-infected persons who have <200 CD4$+$ T cells or a CD4$+$ T-lymphocyte percentage of total lymphocytes of less than 14. The expansion includes 3 clinical conditions—pulmonary tuberculosis, recurrent pneumonia, and invasive cervical cancer—as well as 23 specific clinical conditions in the 1987 AIDS surveillance definition (Centers for Disease Control, 1992b).

The impact of the definitional changes on reported AIDS incidence is illustrated graphically in Figure 7.2. Selik, Buehler, Karon, et al. (1990) report that about 28% of cases diagnosed and reported from September 1, 1987, to December 31, 1988, met only the new criteria of the 1987 revision. This proportion was highest among heterosexual intravenous drug users (43%) and lowest among male homosexuals (21%).

In general, the effect of broadening the surveillance definition is to

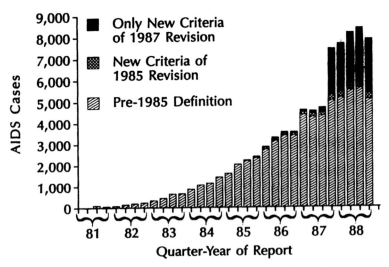

Figure 7.2 U.S. AIDS cases by quarter year of report by category of case surveillance definition. (Source: Selik, Buehler, Karon, et al., 1990.)

cause an abrupt increase in AIDS incidence (Figure 7.2). An important objective of the broadened definition is to capture a wider spectrum of HIV-related disease. Unfortunately, sudden changes in the surveillance definition make it difficult to interpret trends in AIDS incidence. There have been several attempts to reconstruct the AIDS incidence curve that would have been observed if there had been no definitional changes. Karon, Dondero, and Curran (1988) suggested the concept of a "consistent" AIDS case series. These cases include individuals who were diagnosed, either presumptively or definitively, with any one of the 1985 AIDS defining conditions. The consistent case series excluded AIDS cases who were diagnosed on the basis of the new 1987 AIDS defining conditions such as wasting syndrome or HIV encephalopathy.

A limitation of the consistent series is that it does not account for individuals who are diagnosed with AIDS by one of the new criteria and then subsequently develop a disease included in the old criteria. To address this concern, Gail, Rosenberg, and Goedert (1990a) introduced the concept of an "augmented consistent" case series. The idea is based on a three-state competing-risk model. The model is illustrated in Figure 7.3 where λ_1 is the hazard of death for individuals diagnosed under the new definition and λ_2 is the hazard of progression to the old definition for individuals diagnosed under the new definition. Then, the probability that an individual diagnosed by the new definitional criteria would subsequently qualify for diagnosis with the old criteria in the tth month following the first diagnosis is

$$p_t = \frac{\lambda_2}{\lambda_1 + \lambda_2}[e^{-(\lambda_1+\lambda_2)(t-1)} - e^{-(\lambda_1+\lambda_2)(t)}]. \tag{7.7}$$

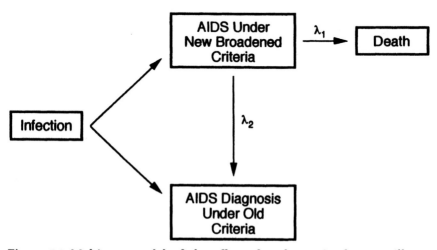

Figure 7.3 Multistate model of the effect of a change in the surveillance definition.

Equation (7.7) is used to obtain an augmented case series as follows: Suppose n_i individuals are diagnosed under the new criteria in calendar month i. Then the diagnosis times of these n_i individuals are reallocated forward in time so that $n_i p_t$ individuals are considered to have been diagnosed under the old definition at calendar month $(i + t)$. Figure 7.4 shows trends in both overall AIDS incidence and the augmented consistent case series among gay men in the United States.

7.6 EMPIRICAL EXTRAPOLATION OF AIDS INCIDENCE

7.6.1 General Considerations

The simplest spproach for obtaining projections of AIDS incidence is extrapolation of the AIDS incidence curve. The first Public Health Service projection made in 1986 estimated 270,000 cumulative AIDS cases in the United States by the end of 1991 (Public Health Service, 1986; Morgan and Curran, 1986). This projection was based on the extrapolation of a quadratic polynomial model for transformed monthly AIDS incidence. AIDS incidence was transformed using a Box–Cox transformation before fitting the polynomial model. The projections of annual U.S. AIDS incidence were 45,000, 58,000, and 74,000 in 1989, 1990, and 1991, respectively (Morgan and Curran, 1986).

The most serious limitation with extrapolation is that the projections depend crucially on the mathematical function used as the basis for the extrapolation. Furthermore, as discussed in the preceeding sections, AIDS incidence data are subject to a number of sources of uncertainty including reporting delays, underreporting, and changes in the surveillance definition. In this section, we discuss approaches for extrapolating the AIDS incidence curve and situations when extrapolation can produce useful short term projections of AIDS incidence.

The first step is to adjust AIDS incidence data for reporting delays as described in Section 7.3. Figure 1.1 displays the delay-adjusted AIDS incidence data by calendar quarter of diagnosis separately by risk group. This figure was based on all cases reported to the CDC by March 31, 1990. A simple log-linear model for extrapolation implies exponential growth in AIDS incidence. If $E(Y_t)$ is the expected AIDS incidence at calendar time t, then

$$\log E(Y_t) = b_0 + b_1 t. \tag{7.8}$$

The regression parameters b_0 and b_1 can be estimated from statistical computing algorithms for Poisson regression (GLIM, for example,

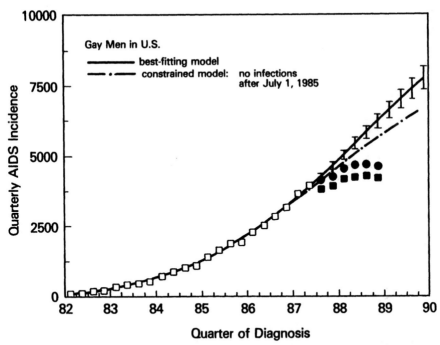

Figure 7.4 Projected and observed quarterly AIDS incidence among homosexual and bisexual men in the United States. Projections were based on consistently defined AIDS incidence counts through June 30, 1987 (open squares) without constraints (solid line) and under the constraints that no infections occurred after July 1, 1985 (dot-dash line), as described by Gail, Rosenberg, and Goedert (1990a). Vertical lines indicate 95% confidence intervals, and solid squares depict augmented consistently defined quarterly AIDS incidence beginning in July, 1987. Solid circles depict all AIDS incidence beginning in July 1, 1987. (Source: figure 1 in Gail, Rosenberg, and Goedert, 1990a.)

Payne, 1986) under the assumption that AIDS incidence approximates a nonhomogeneous Poisson process. Equation (7.8) forces the expected AIDS incidence to keep growing exponentially, which is not consistent with epidemic theory. Indeed Figure 1.1 exhibits subexponential growth beginning in the early 1980s. Accordingly, it is necessary to add quadratic time terms to equation (7.8) to obtain

$$\log E(Y_t) = b_0 + b_1 t + b_2 t^2.$$

The Public Health Service (PHS) projection in 1986 that there would be 270,000 cumulative AIDS cases by the end of 1991 was based on an extrapolation of a model of the form

$$E(Y_t^*) = b_0 + b_1 t + b_2 t^2, \tag{7.9}$$

where α is a power transformation. This model was applied to reporting-delay-corrected AIDS incidence data. The projection agreed with observed AIDS incidence until 1989, when the projections began to exceed AIDS incidence. By April 1, 1992, 215,263 cumulative AIDS cases with diagnoses through December 31, 1991, had been reported to the CDC, and the delay-corrected cumulative projection of AIDS cases through 1991 was 240,000.

The addition to equation (7.9) of higher order terms in time (e.g., t^3 or t^4) is not usually recommended. The most recent data points can have high influence on these regression coefficients and could result in AIDS incidence curves that predict dramatic changes in incidence in the short-term.

Even if the mathematical function used for the extrapolation agrees perfectly with observed counts of AIDS cases, the assumption that the mathematical function will agree with future AIDS incidence cannot be verified. Furthermore, any one of a number of statistical models may fit the observed AIDS incidence data equally well but give radically different long-term projections. Indeed, extrapolation of some models may yield anomalous and misleading results. For example, extrapolation of U.S. AIDS incidence data through 1987 using a normal density curve predicted sharp decreases in AIDS incidence and a cumulative final number of AIDS cases of about 200,000 (Bregman and Langmuir, 1990). The basis for this anomalous results was that although AIDS incidence was still increasing, it was increasing more slowly than previously (Gail and Brookmeyer, 1990a).

Conventional confidence intervals for the expected AIDS incidence at a future time, based on extrapolation methods, reflect the statistical uncertainty in the estimated regression parameters, but do not reflect the uncertainty in selecting the assumed parametric regression model. For example, the confidence bounds reported for the 1986 PHS projections are correct provided the assumed parametric model is correct. Conventional confidence intervals also do not reflect the random variation in future AIDS incidence.

Although these problems with extrapolation limit its usefulness for obtaining reliable long-term projections, extrapolation may still be useful for short-term projections. Observed trends in AIDS incidence may persist over the short term because even abrupt changes in the underlying transmission of HIV infection would not be seen in counts of AIDS cases for many years and then only gradually. This is because the AIDS incidence curve is smoothed when changes in the infection rate are convolved with the incubation period distribution (Chapter 8). Smooth curves may lend themselves to simple extrapolation. However in some circumstances, even short-term extrapolation can be in error. For example, some events may have an immediate impact on AIDS incidence, such as the advent of a new therapy to prevent or delay AIDS, a sudden increase in reporting delays, or a major change in the surveillance definitions. In these situations, historical trends in incidence cannot be reliably extrapolated.

7.6.2 Joint Modeling of Reporting Delays and AIDS Incidence

An alternative to, first, estimating the reporting delay distribution and then empirically modelling the delay-adjusted incidence data is to jointly model reporting delays and AIDS incidence (Harris, 1990a; Zeger, See, and Diggle, 1989). The basic idea is to model, Y_{tu}, the number of AIDS cases diagnosed in calendar time (month) t and reported u time units (months) later. Zeger, See, and Diggle (1989) proposed a Poisson model for Y_{tu} with expectation given by

$$\log E(Y_{tu}) = f(t; \beta) + d(u; \alpha)$$

where $f(t; \beta)$ is a function of calendar time (t) with unknown parameters β, which describes the calendar time trends in AIDS incidence, and $d(u; \alpha)$ is a function of the reporting delay (u) with unknown parameters α, which describes the reporting delay distribution. Specifically,

$$\frac{e^{d(u; \alpha)}}{\sum_j e^{d(j; \alpha)}}$$

is the probability of a reporting delay equal to u months (actually, it is the conditional probability given that the delay is less than or equal to the maximum observed reporting delay; see Section 7.3). A simple choice for $f(t)$ is a quadratic function $f(t; \beta) = \beta_0 + \beta_1 t + \beta_2 t^2$. Zeger, See, and Diggle (1989) suggest a cubic spline. A very flexible model for the delay function is the step function model $d(u, \alpha) = \alpha_u$. Models such as these can be fit using Poisson regression methods (e.g., GLIM in Payne [1986].

There are several advantages to joint modeling of reporting delays and AIDS incidence. First, a correctly specified parametric model for AIDS incidence can increase the precision of delay-adjusted AIDS incidence considerably for the most recent time periods. Second, joint modeling accounts for two sources of uncertainty: uncertainty in the reporting delay adjustments and uncertainty in the estimated regression coefficients.

Fitted models of AIDS incidence will be unreliable in small subgroups with few numbers of AIDS cases (for example, subgroups defined by small geographic areas and risk groups). Zeger, See, and Diggle (1989) propose an empirical Bayes approach to predict AIDS incidence in small subgroups. The basic idea is to *borrow strength* from other similar subgroups to improve the trend estimates for a given subgroup. The empirical Bayes estimate for a given subgroup is a weighted average of a trend estimate obtained from modelling geographic and risk group effects from data from many subgroups and the trend estimate obtained only from the given subgroup.

8

Back-Calculation

8.1 INTRODUCTION

Back-calculation is a method for estimating past infection rates from AIDS incidence data. The method has been useful for obtaining short-term projections of AIDS incidence and estimating HIV prevalence. Back-calculation requires reliable counts of the numbers of AIDS cases diagnosed over time and a reliable estimate of the incubation period distribution. Early references on back-calculation are Brookmeyer and Gail (1986; 1988).

The basic idea is to use AIDS incidence data together with an estimate of the incubation period distribution to reconstruct the numbers of individuals who must have been previously infected in order to give rise to the observed pattern of AIDS incidence. Then, the incubation distribution is applied to these estimated numbers of previously infected individuals to project AIDS incidence. The fundamental relation between the expected cumulative number of AIDS cases diagnosed by calendar time t, $A(t)$, the infection rate $g(s)$ at calendar time s, and the incubation period distribution $F(t)$, is given by the convolution equation

$$A(t) = \int_0^t g(s) \cdot F(t - s)ds. \qquad (8.1)$$

The convolution equation (8.1) is justified by noting that in order for an individual to be diagnosed by calendar time t, he or she must have been infected at some prior time s and then have an incubation period less than $t - s$. Essentially, the back-calculation methodology uses equation (8.1) together with knowledge of $A(t)$ (obtained from registries of AIDS cases as described in Chapter 7) and $F(t)$ (obtained from epidemiological studies as described in Chapter 4) to glean information about previous infection rates $g(s)$. Differentiation of equation (8.1) yields the relationship between AIDS incidence rates and the infection rate, equation (1.3). Integral equations such as equation (8.1) arise in many different scientific applications (O'Sullivan, 1986; Mendelsohn and Rice, 1982; McMahan, Maxwell, and Shephard, 1986) and have been called Volterra equations of the first kind and are a special case of Fredholm integral equations (Wahba, 1990; Press, Teukolsky, Vetterling, and Flannery, 1992).

The relationship between AIDS cases, the infection rate and the incubation period distribution can be illustrated empirically with data from San Francisco (Figure 1.5). Estimates of the infection rates were obtained from epidemiological HIV seroprevalence surveys (Bacchetti, 1990). The figure illustrates how AIDS cases lag behind the infections. This lag is determined by the incubation period distribution. The figure also shows that the AIDS incidence curve increases steadily and is considerably smoother than the underlying infection curve, which rises and falls sharply. Indeed, the effect of the long and variable incubation period is to smear out the infection curve so that sudden changes in the infection curve are not clearly reflected in the AIDS incidence series.

Back-calculation allows us to reconstruct the gross behavior of the underlying infection curve; however, the finer structure is often lost. Additional modeling and empirical data are necessary to reconstruct finer aspects of the shape of the infection curve. Furthermore, because the incubation period is long there is little statistical information in AIDS incidence data about the numbers of individuals most recently infected. As such, two infection curves that are similar early on, but differ dramatically later on, can produce very similar observed AIDS incidence curves. However, they have very different long term implications about the scope of the epidemic. For example, De Gruttola and Lagakos (1989b) fit four different parametric models for the infection curve to AIDS incidence in the United States in the period 1981–87. Figure 8.1a shows that the four fitted infection curves differ dramatically in the most recent years but nevertheless yield similar AIDS incidence curves in the period 1981–87 (Figure 8.1b).

Back-calculation is one of the most useful methods for obtaining quantitative estimates of HIV prevalence and future AIDS incidence. Nevertheless, before proceeding with the technical development of the back-calculation methodology, it is important to emphasize a number of limitations and underlying assumptions of the methodology.

given functions, and an attempt is made to find the infection curve $g(s)$, that fits $A(t)$ exactly or that minimizes

$$\int \left\{ A(t) - \int_0^t g(s) F(t-s)\, ds \right\}^2 dt.$$

If the model for $g(s)$ involves too many parameters, the estimate of $g(s)$ may be very irregular or even negative in places. Such phenomena also arises in statistical deconvolution (Section 8.3). The major drawback of deterministic deconvolution is that it provides no framework for estimating the uncertainty in estimates of $g(s)$. Nevertheless, deterministic deconvolution provides a useful introduction to the method of back-calculation that is easy to understand and that provides insight into the effects of systematic perturbations in the AIDS incidence data and the incubation distribution (Hyman and Stanley, 1988).

8.2.1 Discrete Time

Deterministic deconvolution has an especially simple solution if we assume that infections occur at discrete points in calendar time, such as the beginning of each calendar year. The unknown numbers of individuals infected at the beginning of the jth year of the epidemic is called g_j. The known number of AIDS cases diagnosed in the jth year, namely in the interval $[j-1, j)$, is called Y_j. Below is a schematic illustration:

Y_j = Number of new AIDS cases

g_j = Number of new infections

AIDS incidence data, the Y's, are used to estimate the unknown numbers infected, the g's, by solving a system of linear equations that involve the incubation distribution, F, which is assumed known. Let $f_i = F(i) - F(i-1)$ be the probability that an individual develops AIDS during the ith year following infection. If equation (8.1) is obeyed exactly, then Y_1 must be equal to the number infected in year 1 who have incubation periods less than 1 year: $Y_1 = g_1 f_1$. The number of AIDS cases diagnosed during year 2 of the epidemic is the sum of two components: individuals infected in year 2 with incubation periods less than one year and individuals infected in year 1 with incubation periods between 1 and 2 years duration, as in $Y_2 = g_1 f_2 + g_2 f_1$. Similarly,

$Y_3 = g_1 f_3 + g_2 f_2 + g_3 f_1$. In general, the number of AIDS cases diagnosed during the jth year of the epidemic satisfies

$$Y_j = g_1 f_j + g_2 f_{j-1} + \cdots + g_j f_1. \tag{8.2}$$

AIDS incidence data that span n years generate a system of n linear equations (one for each of the Y's) in n unknowns (one for each of the g's), for which there is a simple solution. The number infected in year 1 is $g_1 = Y_1 / f_1$. Note that this estimate g_1 is very sensitive to small changes in the AIDS incidence counts or small errors in specifying the incubation curve $F(t)$, because f_1 is very small. For this reason, equation (8.1) defines an "ill-posed inverse" problem (O'Sullivan, 1986; Hyman and Stanley, 1988). The other g's can be obtained recursively from the equation

$$g_j = \frac{Y_j - (g_1 f_j + g_2 f_{j-1} + \cdots + g_{j-1} f_2)}{f_1}. \tag{8.3}$$

There are two limitations with this procedure for estimating the infection rates. First, the estimated infections rates $\{g_j\}$ can exhibit saw-toothed, irregular behavior and can even be negative. More plausible estimates for the infection rates would be smoother and nonnegative. One could try to alleviate these problems by smoothing the g's in some manner. Second, estimates of the precision of the estimated infection rates are not readily available. Statistical deconvolution considered in Section 8.3 addresses some of these problems.

8.2.2 Continuous Time

Several approaches have been proposed for deterministic deconvolution of AIDS incidence data in continuous time. Hyman and Stanley (1988) fit a smooth function, namely a polynomial, to the cumulative AIDS incidence function $A(t)$. The infection rate curve, $g(s)$, was approximated by a spline (piecewise cubic Hermite polynomial). Then, the infection rate curve $g(s)$ was estimated by minimizing $\int [A(t) - \hat{A}(t)]^2 dt$ where $\hat{A}(t)$ are the fitted values of the cumulative AIDS incidence at calendar time t. Hyman and Stanley (1988) point out that if there are too many knots in the spline, the solution for $g(s)$ will exhibit irregular behavior and high frequency oscillations.

Freund and Book (1990) use Laplace transforms to perform the deterministic deconvolution. They first fit a smooth function, $a(u)$, to AIDS incidence. They show that

$$g(t) = \int_o^t a(u) f^*(t - u) du,$$

where f^* is the inverse Laplace transform of $1/f_L(u)$ and where

$$f_L(u) = \int_0^\infty e^{-u(s)} f(s)\,ds$$

is the Laplace transform of the incubation density. If the incubation distribution is assumed to be gamma with integer shape parameter k and scale parameter λ (Section 4.2), then $f^*(u) = [1 + (u/\lambda)]^k$. Thus, the problem of solving for $g(t)$ is reduced to integration. Freund and Book use a cubic polynomial for $a(t)$ and show that this produces a cubic polynomial solution for $g(s)$. An alternative approach is given in Isham (1989).

8.3 STATISTICAL DECONVOLUTION

8.3.1 Analysis in Discrete Time

Statistical deconvolution with a discrete time infection curve is relatively simple. The *expected* AIDS incidence is required to follow an equation analogous to (8.2):

$$\mu_j = E(Y_j) = g_1 f_j + g_2 f_{j-1} + \cdots + g_j f_1 \tag{8.4}$$

where, as in Section 8.2, g_j is the number infected in the beginning of the jth year of the epidemic, and Y_j are the number of AIDS cases diagnosed in the jth year, namely in the interval $[j-1, j)$. It is often appropriate with count data, such as AIDS incidence, to assume that the variance of Y_j is equal to the mean $E(Y_j)$. This assumption would be justified for example, if the Y's have a Poisson distribution. Model (8.4) can be fit to AIDS incidence data using Poisson regression analyses. Poisson regression relates the expected values of Y to a function of covariates, and assumes Y has a Poisson distribution (McCullagh and Nelder, 1989). In our application, the f's in equation (8.4) play the role of the covariates (the design matrix) and the g's play the role of the regression coefficients. The regression model would be fit without an intercept term. A difficulty with model (8.4) is that it is not parsimonious. There are n data points and n parameters. The estimated g's can exhibit saw-toothed or irregular and unstable behavior and have very large variances, especially for the most recent infection rates. O'Sullivan (1986) calls this problem "ill-posed." One approach is to introduce certain smoothness assumptions on the infection rates (Bacchetti, Segal, and Jewell, 1993; Becker, Watson, and Carlin, 1991; Brookmeyer, 1991; Brookmeyer and Liao, 1992). The smoothness assumptions will reduce variances and problems of instability, but biased estimates of infection rates could result if the smoothness assumptions are incorrect. One faces the usual tradeoff between bias and variance in making such assumptions.

A simple smoothness assumption is to require that the numbers of individuals infected, g_j, be constant over specified intervals. For example, suppose $g_j = g_{j+1} = \beta_j$ in successive pairs of intervals as illustrated in Figure 8.2. In this figure, β_i is the annual infection rate at calendar time i. As before, we assume for simplicity that infections occur only at discrete points in calendar time, for example, on January 1 of each calendar year. Then it follows from equation (8.4), for example, that the expected AIDS incidences in the first three years are:

$$E(Y_1) = \beta_1 f_1$$
$$E(Y_2) = \beta_1 f_1 + \beta_1 f_2 = \beta_1 (f_1 + f_2)$$
$$E(Y_3) = \beta_1 (f_3 + f_2) + \beta_2 f_1.$$

In general, the expression for $E(Y_j)$ is linear in the unknown parameters, the β's. Estimates of β_i can be obtained using Poisson regression analysis.

The statistical methods for discrete deconvolutions are illustrated in Table 8.1 with hypothetical AIDS incidence data and an incubation distribution. It was assumed that infection rates were constant over two-year intervals. A Poisson regression analysis was performed using the generalized linear interactive modelling computing software (GLIM, see Payne, 1986) by declaring the "error" as Poisson and the "link" as the identity, and by fitting the model with four independent

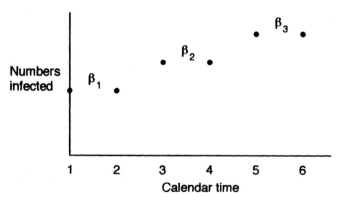

Figure 8.2 Illustration of discrete time infection curve.

Table 8.1 Illustration of Statistical Deconvolution in Discrete Time

Input Data

AIDS Incidence Data		Incubation		
$Y_1 = 20$	$Y_5 = 330$	$f_1 = .01$	$f_5 = .10$	$f_9 = .08$
$Y_2 = 39$	$Y_6 = 500$	$f_2 = .06$	$f_6 = .17$	$f_{10} = .07$
$Y_3 = 80$	$Y_7 = 700$	$f_3 = .08$	$f_7 = .14$	$f_{11} = .04$
$Y_4 = 200$	$Y_8 = 930$	$f_4 = .10$	$f_8 = .10$	$f_{12} = .05$

Model $E(Y) = X\beta$ (Matrix notation)

$$\begin{bmatrix} E(Y_1) \\ E(Y_2) \\ E(Y_3) \\ E(Y_4) \\ E(Y_5) \\ E(Y_6) \\ E(Y_7) \\ E(Y_8) \end{bmatrix} = \begin{bmatrix} .01 & 0 & 0 & 0 \\ .07 & 0 & 0 & 0 \\ .14 & .01 & 0 & 0 \\ .18 & .07 & 0 & 0 \\ .20 & .14 & .01 & 0 \\ .27 & .18 & .07 & 0 \\ .31 & .20 & .14 & .01 \\ .24 & .27 & .18 & .07 \end{bmatrix} \begin{bmatrix} \beta_1 \\ \beta_2 \\ \beta_3 \\ \beta_4 \end{bmatrix}$$

Results

	Poisson	Normal Unweighted	Normal Weights $= 1/Y$
$\hat{\beta}_1$ (SE)	587 (56)	516 (72)	525 (95)
$\hat{\beta}_2$ (SE)	1348 (155)	1466 (139)	1463 (272)
$\hat{\beta}_3$ (SE)	1556 (290)	1559 (158)	1521 (513)
$\hat{\beta}_4$ (SE)	2378 (722)	2153 (358)	2240 (1265)

variables without an intercept term. The estimated regression coefficients (the β's) along with standard errors are shown under the results column of Table 8.1 labeled "Poisson." We have also computed the results using normal unweighted linear regression and using normal weighted linear regression with weight equal to $1/Y_j$. The estimates are quite similar, although the standard errors (SE) are considerably different. The normal linear regression with weights equal to $1/Y_j$ is a rough approximation to the Poisson regression analysis.

The standard errors reported in Table 8.1 do not account for a number of important sources of uncertainty. These include: (1) uncertainty in the incubation distribution; (2) uncertainty in the AIDS incidence data due to reporting delay adjustments and underreporting; and (3) uncertainty in the parametric model used for the infection rate (in this example, it was assumed that infections occur at discrete points in time (January 1) and that annual rates were constant over 2-year intervals). Uncertainty in the incubation distribution is often the main source of uncertainty.

The results in Table 8.1 can be used to estimate cumulative

infections and forecast AIDS incidence. For example, the estimated cumulative number infected by the end of year 8 is (using the Poisson estimates) $2(587 + 1348 + 1556 + 2378) = 11{,}738$. The predicted AIDS incidence in year 9 is obtained by projecting forward the estimated infection rates:

$$\hat{Y}_9 = \hat{\beta}_1 \cdot f_9 + \hat{\beta}_1 f_8 + \hat{\beta}_2 f_7 + \hat{\beta}_3 f_6 + \cdots + \hat{\beta}_4 f_2 = 1167.$$

This projection does not account for any AIDS cases that occur among individuals infected in year 9. Various adjustments have been suggested to account for future infections in AIDS projections. One approach assumes the infection rate in year 8, $\hat{\beta}_4$, can be extrapolated through year 9. Under this assumption the term $\hat{\beta}_4 f_1 = 24$ would be added to the projection. Then, the adjusted projection is $1167 + 24 = 1191$. Other adjustments have also been suggested (see Section 8.3.2), but because the incubation period tends to be long and f_1 is small, these adjustments are minor and have little effect on short term projections of AIDS incidence.

8.3.2 General Statistical Framework and Maximum Likelihood Estimation

We outline a general statistical framework for back-calculation in which we no longer require the infection curve to be discrete. The data consist of the number of AIDS cases diagnosed over calendar time. Let $\mathbf{Y} = (Y_1, Y_2, \ldots, Y_n)$ where Y_i represents the number of AIDS cases diagnosed in the calendar time interval $[T_{i-1}, T_i)$, $i = 1, \ldots, n$. It is assumed that individuals become infected according to a nonhomogeneous Poisson process, although, as indicated in Section 8.8.2, the results hold more generally. The intensity function of the Poisson process, $g(s; \boldsymbol{\beta})$, is assumed to come from a parametric family with p unknown parameters $\boldsymbol{\beta}$. The objective is to estimate the parameters $\boldsymbol{\beta}$. If infections follow a Poisson process then Y_i has a Poisson distribution (Cox, 1963) with mean

$$E(Y_i) = \mu_i = \int_{T_0}^{T_i} g(s; \boldsymbol{\beta}) \cdot (F(T_i - s) - F(T_{i-1} - s)) ds, \tag{8.5}$$

where $F(t)$ is defined to be 0 for $t \leqslant 0$. The variance of Y_i is $\mathrm{Var}(Y_i) = \mu_i$. By convention, we shall define calendar time 0 to be the start of the epidemic (that is $g(s) = 0$ prior to that time) and thus $T_0 = 0$. The log-likelihood function for the parameters $\boldsymbol{\beta}$, $\mathrm{LL}(\boldsymbol{\beta}; \mathbf{Y})$ is

$$\mathrm{LL}(\boldsymbol{\beta}; \mathbf{Y}) = \sum_{i=1}^{n} Y_i \log \mu_i - \mu_i - \log(Y_i!).$$

The log-likelihood function can be maximized to obtain the maximum likelihood estimates $\hat{\boldsymbol{\beta}}$. The variance-covariance matrix of $\hat{\boldsymbol{\beta}}$, $\mathrm{Var}(\hat{\boldsymbol{\beta}})$, is given by the negative inverse of second derivatives of the log-likelihood function,

$$\mathrm{Var}(\hat{\boldsymbol{\beta}}) = \left[-\frac{\partial^2 \mathrm{LL}(\boldsymbol{\beta}; \mathbf{Y})}{\partial \beta_i \partial \beta_j} \right]_{\boldsymbol{\beta} = \hat{\boldsymbol{\beta}}}^{-1},$$

provided $\hat{\boldsymbol{\beta}}$ lies in the interior of the parameter space. If the parameters $\boldsymbol{\beta}$ are constrained so that the infection rates are nonnegative, the maximization must be done over the restricted parameter space where $g(s; \boldsymbol{\beta}) \geqslant 0$. When constraints such as these are placed on the parameters, it often occurs that $\hat{\boldsymbol{\beta}}$ lies on a boundary of the restricted parameter space. In this event, standard variance estimates such as those based on the second derivatives of the log-likelihood are not correct (Chernoff, 1954). In this situation, the parametric bootstrap has been used to estimate variances (Gail, Rosenberg, and Goedert, 1990a). In the present context, one would generate a large number, B, of bootstrap samples of AIDS incidence data $\{Y_i^*\}$ by sampling Y_i^* as independent Poisson variates with mean $\hat{\mu}_i$. Then parameter estimates $\hat{\boldsymbol{\beta}}^*$ and estimated infection rates $g(s, \hat{\boldsymbol{\beta}}^*)$ are obtained for each bootstrap sample. The sample variance of the B bootstrap estimates is used to approximate the variance $\hat{\boldsymbol{\beta}}$ (Efron, 1982).

In practice, the AIDS incidence data exhibit extra-Poisson variation. The overdispersion could be due to a number of sources of including heterogeneity in reporting delays and incubation distributions. A more realistic model for the variance of AIDS incidence is to assume $\mathrm{Var}(Y_j) = \sigma^2 E(Y_j)$ where σ^2 is the overdispersion parameter (Brookmeyer and Liao, 1990a). The overdispersion parameter is estimated by

$$\hat{\sigma}^2 = \frac{1}{n-p} \sum_{i=1}^{n} (Y_i - \hat{Y}_i)^2 / \hat{Y}_i,$$

where $\hat{Y}_i$ is the predicted AIDS incidence obtained by substituting $\hat{\boldsymbol{\beta}}$ into (8.5). Rosenberg, Gail, and Carroll (1992) account for overdispersion by generating bootstrap samples of AIDS incidence data from a normal approximation to a negative binomial distribution that has mean $\hat{\mu}_i$ and variance $\hat{\sigma}^2 \hat{\mu}_i$.

Cumulative Number of HIV Infections
The maximum likelihood estimate of the expected cumulative number of HIV infections that occurred prior to calendar time T (where $T \leqslant T_n$) is

$$\hat{G}(T) = \int_0^T g(s; \hat{\boldsymbol{\beta}}) ds. \tag{8.6}$$

The standard error of this estimate can be obtained by an application of the delta method provided $g(s; \hat{\beta}) > 0$ or by bootstrapping if constrained optimization is required. Estimates of cumulative infections are statistically imprecise and are sensitive to model assumptions when $T = T_n$ because then $\hat{G}(T)$ depends on estimates of recent infection rates. HIV prevalence is defined to be the number of HIV infected individuals who are alive. An estimate of current HIV prevalence is obtained by subtracting the cumulative number of deaths among HIV infected individuals from $\hat{G}(T_n)$.

Projections of AIDS Incidence

A lower bound estimate of the expected number of AIDS cases diagnosed in a future calendar interval $[T_{l-1}, T_l)$ is obtained by projecting forward the number of individuals previously infected according to the incubation period distribution. This estimate is given by

$$\int_0^{T_n} g(s; \hat{\beta}) \cdot \{F(T_l - s) - F(T_{l-1} - s)\} ds, \qquad (8.7)$$

where $F(t)$ is defined to be 0 for $t \leq 0$. This is a lower bound since it projects cases only from among individuals infected prior to calendar time T_n.

Effect of Future Infections on Projections of AIDS Incidence

An important question concerns the effect of future infections on projections of AIDS incidence. In the long term, future infections will be the main determinant of AIDS incidence. However, in the short term, future infections have only a minor impact on AIDS incidence because the incubation periods tend to be long. In principle, one approach to account for future infections is to hypothesize a future infection rate curve and project these rates forward using the incubation period distribution (Brookmeyer and Damiano, 1989). For example, if future infections occurring after T_n arrive according to a non-homogeneous Poisson process with intensity $g(s; \beta)$, then the expected number of new AIDS cases to be diagnosed on the interval $[T_{l-1}, T_l)$ who will be infected after T_n is given by

$$\int_{T_n}^{T_l} g(s; \beta) \{F(T_l - s) - F(T_{l-1} - s)\} ds. \qquad (8.8)$$

Expression (8.8) is added to (8.7) to obtain an estimate of AIDS incidence that accounts for future infections.

The problem, of course, is that the future infection rate $g(s; \boldsymbol{\beta})$ is unknown. One approach to the problem is to assume different values for $g(s; \boldsymbol{\beta})$ and perform sensitivity analyses. However, since a very small proportion of individuals progress within three years of infection, even extremely high assumptions about the future infection rate have a relatively small effect on three-year projections of AIDS incidence. A range of values for $g(s; \boldsymbol{\beta})$ for the sensitivity analyses could be suggested from seroprevalence survey data (Chapter 3). For example, monitoring selected cohorts has yielded estimates of current infection rates (Section 3.5.1).

Another approach is to extrapolate the current infection rate, estimated from back-calculation, into the future. The assumption is that the current infection rate remains unchanged in the short-term. For example, suppose that $g(s; \boldsymbol{\beta})$ has been parameterized as a piecewise constant step function with p steps and that the estimated infection rate in the last step is $\hat{\beta}_p$. Then, equation (8.8) becomes

$$\hat{\beta}_p \int_o^{T_l - T_n} [F(T_l - T_n - s) - F(T_{l-1} - T_n - s)]ds.$$

More generally, one could use the average value $g(s; \hat{\boldsymbol{\beta}})$ over the previous few years instead of $\hat{\beta}_p$ (Rosenberg and Gail, 1991). There are two limitations with this approach. First, the estimate of $\hat{\beta}_p$ obtained from back-calculation is highly uncertain. Second, even if β_p was known exactly, there is no a priori reason why the current infection rate should persist into the future. Nevertheless, it is important to reemphasize that adjustments of this sort typically have a small effect on projections of AIDS incidence over three years.

Use of the Conditional Incubation Period Distribution in Back-Calculation

In some situations, the method of back-calculation can be used with an estimate of a "conditional incubation distribution" rather than $F(t)$.

For example, suppose infected individuals are a mixture of a proportion, α, of infected individuals who develop AIDS according to the incubation period distribution, F_1 and a proportion $(1 - \alpha)$ of infected individuals who never develop AIDS. Then $F(t) = \alpha F_1(t)$. If one had only an estimate of F_1, it would still be possible to forecast AIDS incidence. The idea is to back-calculate using F_1 in place of F. However, the resulting estimates of infection rates, $\hat{g}$, refer to the numbers of infected individuals who would eventually develop AIDS rather than to the total numbers of infected individuals. In order to estimate the total infection rate, an estimate of α is required and $\hat{g}$ would be inflated by the factor $1/\alpha$. Similarly, estimates of the cumulative number of infections refer only to those individuals who would eventually develop AIDS. The projections of AIDS incidence obtained by back-calculating with F_1 would be correct because in order to forecast AIDS incidence it is only necessary to estimate infection rates among individuals destined to develop AIDS. Of course, AIDS case projections alone do not reveal the entire scope of the epidemic. Nevertheless, the ability to project cases based only on F_1 could be important, especially early in the epidemic. This is because, early in the epidemic, retrospective data on the dates of infection and diagnosis among AIDS cases may yield an estimate of F_1, but not F (see Section 4.3.3). Only later may prospective follow-up data become available to yield an estimate of F.

Suppose one is unwilling to assume the mixture model $(F = \alpha F_1)$. Under some conditions it is still possible to back-calculate using an estimate of the conditional distribution given that the incubation period is less than T years, $F^*(t) = F(t)/F(T)$. However the estimable quantities using F^* have peculiar interpretations and are of limited interest. For example, suppose the AIDS incidence series spans a period that is less than T years (i.e., the epidemic is less than T years old). If one back-calculates using F^* instead of F, $g(s)$ refers to the infection rate among individuals who would have incubation periods less than T years. Estimates of the cumulative number of infected individuals refer to the cumulative number of infected individuals with incubation periods less than T years.

8.3.3 Models for the Infection Curve

The statistical framework for back-calculation outlined in Section 8.3.2 can be used with any parametric model for the infection curve, $g(s)$. Models for the infection curve that have been used in back-calculation have ranged from strongly to weakly parametric. We give several examples below in terms of parameters β_1, β_2, and K.

Strongly Parametric Models
(Damped) Exponential Model
$$g(s) = K^{\beta_1 s^{\beta_2}}$$

The model allows for exponential growth if $\beta_2 = 1$ and subexponential growth if $\beta_2 < 1$. It has been used by Taylor (1989), De Gruttola and

Lagakos (1989) and in Morbidity and Mortality Weekly Report (Centers for Disease Control, 1987b).

Log-Logistic Model

$$g(s) = K \frac{\beta_1 \beta_2 (\beta_1 s)^{\beta_2 - 1}}{[1 + (\beta_1 s)^{\beta_2}]^2}$$

Under this model, if $\beta_2 > 1$, infection rates increase monotonically until they peak at $s = \{(\beta_2 - 1)/(\beta_2 + 1)\}^{1/\beta_2}/\beta_1$. If $\beta_2 \leqslant 1$, infection rates decrease monotonically. This model has been considered by Brookmeyer and Damiano (1989).

Logistic (Prevalence) Model

$$g(s) = \frac{K e^{\beta_1 + \beta_3 s}}{1 - e^{\beta_2 + \beta_3 s^2}}$$

This model allows for initial exponential growth followed by subexponential growth and possibly decreasing infection rates in later years. The model has been considered by Taylor (1989) and by Rosenberg, Gail, and Pee (1991).

The three models mentioned above are strongly parametric. Once the infection rates in the early years of the epidemic are fixed, the model assumption forces infection rates in later years to follow the shape of the assumed curve. Thus, estimated infection rates in the recent past are very sensitive to the model assumptions. If the assumptions are incorrect, estimates of infection rates, especially in the recent past, can be very biased. Furthermore, usual estimates of standard errors of infection rate are unrealistically small as a result of the strong parametric assumptions.

Weakly Parametric Models

An alternative to strongly parametric models are weakly parametric models, such as a piecewise constant step function model. The piecewise constant step function is

$$g(s) - \beta_1, \qquad c_{i-1} \leqslant s < c_i.$$

This model assumes the infection rate is constant at level β_i in the interval $[c_{i-1}, c_i)$. The calendar times at which the step function jumps, the c's, are called the knots. It is a flexible parametric model because the behavior of the early part of the curve does not pin down the later behavior.

The main issue with flexible models such as the piecewise constant step function is how to choose the number and spacings of the knots. Because there is little information about infection rates in the recent past, the standard error of the estimated infection rate in the last step, $\hat{\beta}_p$, becomes very large as the width of this step is decreased. On the other hand, if the width of the last step is too large, this infection rate could be very biased if in fact infection rates are rapidly rising or falling in this interval. Rosenberg, Gail, and Pee (1991) suggest that a width of about four years in the last step yields a good compromise between bias and variance.

Splines and Smoothing Approaches

A disadvantage of the piecewise constant step function model is that $g(s; \boldsymbol{\beta})$ has discontinuities at the knots. Splines have the advantage of yielding smoothed estimates of the infection curve without invoking strong assumptions about the shape of the infection curve. Rosenberg and Gail (1991) considered continuous spline function models, which are polynomial functions between prespecified knots, $c_0, c_1, c_2, \ldots, c_p$. For example, the continuous linear spline is

$$g(s) = \beta_0 + \sum_{j=1}^{p} \beta_j (s - c_{j-1})_+,$$

where $(s - c_{j-1})_+$ is defined to be 0 if $s < c_{j-1}$ and $(s - c_{j-1})$ otherwise. A spline that is smoother than the continuous linear spline is the quadratic spline with a continuous first derivative:

$$g(s) = \beta_0 + \beta_1 s + \sum_{j=1}^{p} \beta_{j+1} \{(s - c_{j-1})_+\}^2.$$

Rosenberg and Gail (1991) showed how back-calculation could be performed using regression methods for very general models of the infection curve,

$$g(s) = \sum_{i=1}^{p} g_i(s),$$

where $g_i(\cdot)$ are known functions. This general class includes spline models. Constrained optimization is required to insure that the estimated infection rates are nonnegative.

An alternative to the spline approach outlined above is based on Phillips–Tikhonov regularization (Phillips, 1962; Tikhonov, 1963). This approach was used by Brookmeyer (1991) and Brookmeyer and Liao (1992). Bacchetti (1990) and Taylor, Kuo, and Detels (1991) used a similar approach to estimate the incubation distribution (see

Section 4.6). The basic idea is to approximate the infection curve by a step function with a large number of short steps,

$$g(s) = \beta_j, \qquad c_{j-1} \leqslant s < c_j,$$

and then to impose smoothness requirements on the estimated infection rates to avoid wild oscillations. This is accomplished by maximizing a penalized log-likelihood function

$$\text{Log L} - \frac{\lambda}{2} \mathcal{J}$$

where Log L is the log likelihood function, $\mathcal{J}$ measures the roughness of the infection curve and λ is the smoothing parameter that determines the degree of smoothness of the infection curve. Constrained optimization is required to ensure that estimated infection rates are nonnegative. For a Poisson likelihood, this is equivalent to minimizing (O'Sullivan, Yandell, and Raynor, 1986)

$$\sum_{i=1}^{n} \frac{(y_i - \mu_i)^2}{\mu_i} + \lambda \mathcal{J},$$

where the first term measures the closeness of the observed AIDS incidence data to the expected values and the second term is the roughness penalty. One measure of roughness is a discrete approximation to the integrated squared second derivative of the infection curve, and when the knots are equally spaced, this is given by

$$\mathcal{J} = \frac{1}{w^3} \sum_{k=1}^{p-2} (\beta_{k+2} - 2\beta_{k+1} + \beta_k)^2,$$

where $w = c_j - c_{j-1}$ is the spacing between the knots.

A major issue with this approach is how to choose the smoothing parameter λ. Various automatic smoothing procedures have been suggested to guide the degree of smoothing, such as generalized cross-validation. Generalized cross-validation was proposed by Craven and Wahba (see Wahba, 1983, 1990) and extended to the case of generalized linear models by O'Sullivan, Yandell, and Raynor (1986). Some theoretical work and simulation work suggest that the λ that minimizes the generalized cross validation score will minimize a weighted mean squared error criterion for the AIDS incidence curve (O'Sullivan, Yandell, and Raynor, 1987). For our purpose, a more relevant criterion might be a mean square error criterion for the infection curve rather than the AIDS incidence curve. An alternative to automatic smoothing is to perform sensitivity analyses to different choices of the smoothing parameter λ. Brookmeyer and Liao (1992) show that estimated infection rates in the recent past are much more sensitive to the choice of smoothing parameter than are estimated infection rates in the distant past. They also quantify the tradeoff between bias and variance. In general, less smoothing yields smaller bias but greater variance in the estimated infection rates.

Another smoothing approach, called EMS, was investigated by Becker, Watson, and Carlin (1991). This approach also approximates the infection curve by a large number of narrow step functions but uses an EM algorithm to estimate the infection rates. At the end of each cycle of the EM algorithm, the step height parameters are smoothed by taking running averages. An advantage of this approach is that it automatically produces positive estimates of infection rates. However, special methods are needed to assess random variability.

8.4 UNCERTAINTY IN BACK-CALCULATION

8.4.1 Sources of Uncertainty

The Incubation Distribution

Lack of information about the incubation distribution is perhaps the most important source of uncertainty in back-calculation. A shorter assumed incubation distribution leads to a lower estimated cumulative number of infections. Standard errors based on Fisher information and an assumed incubation distribution do not account for uncertainty in the incubation period distribution. Sensitivity analyses to different assumptions about the incubation distribution are important. Estimates of cumulative infections are much more sensitive to the incubation distribution than are short term projections of AIDS incidence.

Rosenberg and Gail (1990) performed a detailed sensitivity analysis of the choice of incubation distribution on back-calculated estimates of cumulative infections based on U.S. AIDS incidence data through July 1, 1987. They considered five different incubation distributions (Figure 8.3) and back-calculated the infection rate using a piecewise constant step function model. Figure 8.4 shows joint confidence regions for the cumulative numbers infected by January 1, 1985, and July 1, 1987. These confidence ellipsoids were based on a parametric bootstrap and account for variability in choosing the placement of the knots in the step function model as well as for random variation in the AIDS incidence data. Figure 8.4 shows that systematic uncertainty in the choice of incubation distribution can overwhelm random uncertainty in knot selection and model fitting.

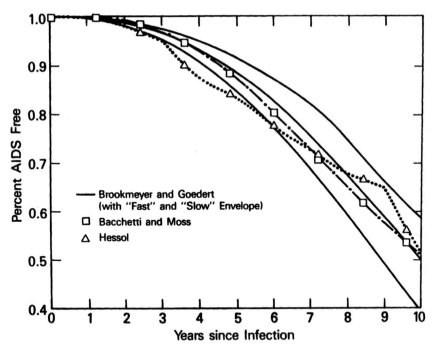

Figure 8.3 Incubation period distributions used in sensitivity analysis of back-calculation estimates. (Source: Rosenberg and Gail, 1990. Reprinted by permission of Elsevier Science Publishing Co.)

The Infection Curve Model

The infection curve model, $g(s)$, needs to be chosen with care. There is a great deal of information in AIDS incidence data about $g(s)$ in the distant past but little information about $g(s)$ in the recent past. If strong parametric models, such as an exponential growth model, are used for $g(s)$ and if the model chosen is not correct, estimates of the infection rate in the recent past can be severely biased. Furthermore, the resulting confidence intervals can be very narrow as a result of the strong parametric assumptions, making it appear that the estimates are more accurate than they really are. On the other hand, if the model for $g(s)$ is too flexible, especially within the most recent 2 or 3 years, the standard errors of estimated recent infection rates will be quite large. The choice between weakly and strongly parametric models for the infection curve represents the usual statistical tradeoff between bias and variance. In the absence of epidemiological data to suggest the parametric family, we prefer the use of flexible models, such as splines or step functions. The resulting estimates of infection rates will have wide confidence intervals, which we believe is preferable to potentially biased estimates with narrow confidence intervals.

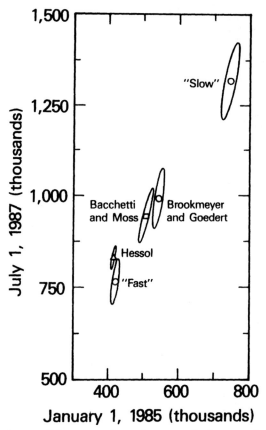

Figure 8.4 Joint confidence regions for cumulative numbers infected by January 1, 1985, and July 1, 1987: Sensitivity to the incubation period distribution. (Source: Rosenberg and Gail, 1990. Reprinted by permission of Elsevier Science Publishing Co.)

Rosenberg, Gail, and Pee (1991) performed a simulation study to examine the performance of piecewise constant step functions for a range of epidemics. Figure 8.5 shows nine different hypothesized infection curves where time 0 corresponds to January 1, 1977. They considered different step function models, varying the number and placement of knots. The simulation study was based on simulating quarterly AIDS incidence data (counts of AIDS cases in three month intervals) during the period January 1, 1977, through July 1, 1987. They considered four families of models with 3, 4 or 5 steps and used a Pearson chi-square statistic to choose the best fitting model within each

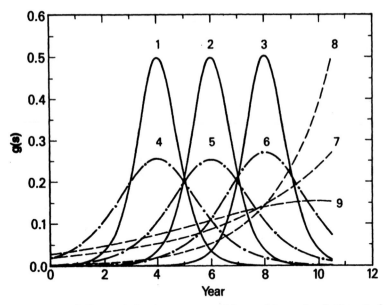

Figure 8.5 Nine different infection curves, $g(s)$, used in a simulation study of back-calculation procedures. (Source: Rosenberg, Gail, and Pee, 1991. Reprinted by permission of John Wiley & Sons, Ltd.)

family. The performance of an estimator $\hat{\theta}$ of θ was measured by the percent root mean square error (PRMSE) defined as

$$\text{PRMSE} = \frac{100}{\theta} \cdot \left\{ \sum_{i=1}^{N} (\hat{\theta}_i - \theta)^2 / N \right\}^{1/2},$$

where $\hat{\theta}_i$ is the estimate from the ith simulation. The percent bias was defined as $100 \cdot (\bar{\hat{\theta}} - \theta)/\theta$, and the percent standard deviation was defined as

$$\frac{100}{\theta} \cdot \{ \Sigma (\hat{\theta}_i - \bar{\hat{\theta}})^2 / N \}^{1/2},$$

where $\bar{\hat{\theta}}$ is the mean value of $\hat{\theta}_i$ over the N simulations.

Figure 8.6 gives the percent root mean square error for cumulative numbers of infected individuals and projections of AIDS incidence. The estimated cumulative HIV infections through January 1, 1985, yielded percent root mean square error (PRMSE) of less than 14% for each of the nine infection curves. However, the PRMSE for estimated cumulative infections through July 1, 1987, ranged as high as 33%. Short-term projection of AIDS incidence (2–3 years ahead) always

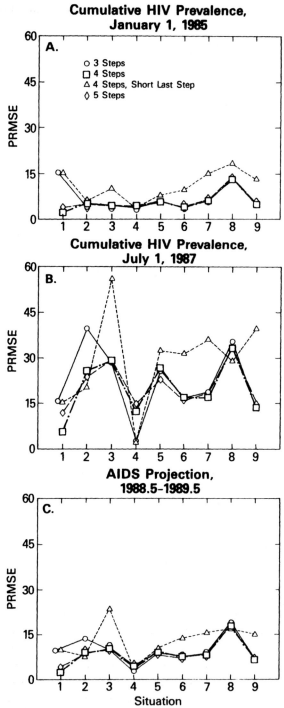

Figure 8.6 Simulation study of percent root mean square error for different step function models for the nine infection curves in Figure 8.5. (Source: Rosenberg, Gail, and Pee, 1991. Reprinted by permission of John Wiley & Sons, Ltd.)

had a PRMSE less than 18%. The simulation studies suggested that step function models with a long last step of about 4 years yielded a favorable tradeoff between bias and variance.

A "bull's-eye plot" shows the percent standard deviation and percent bias for fitting step function models with four steps and a last step of 4 years, for each of the nine epidemics (Figure 8.7). The circular contours in these plots correspond to constant values of the PRMSE. The fitting procedure produces small PRMSE for projecting AIDS incidence and for estimating cumulative numbers infected through January, 1985, for all nine epidemics. However, biased estimates of cumulative numbers infected through July 1, 1987, are obtained when the infection curve is either rapidly rising or decreasing in the period shortly before mid-1987. For example, if the epidemic is decreasing rapidly (epidemic 3 in Figure 8.5), step function models with a long last step can overestimate cumulative numbers infected through July 1, 1987, by about 30% (Figure 8.7b). It would be interesting to carry out similar studies of the performance of spline models and other smoothing approaches and to examine the tradeoff between bias and variance for various choices of smoothing parameters and procedures.

AIDS Incidence Data: Reporting Delay Adjustments and Underreporting

Back-calculation relies on accurate AIDS incidence data. One source of error in the data arises because of uncertainty in the reporting delay adjustments (Chapter 7). Reporting delay adjustments have the most impact on the recent AIDS incidence data, and recent AIDS incidence data can have high leverage (Weisberg, 1985) on back-calculation estimates. One approach is to not use the most recent AIDS incidence data in back-calculation, because delay adjustments and other uncertainties are greatest in the most recent AIDS incidence counts (Section 7.3). Many analysts exclude the most recent six months of reporting-delay adjusted AIDS incidence data from back-calculation analyses. Another approach is to formally account for these uncertainties in the analysis (Harris, 1990a). The approach involves modeling Y_{ij}, the number of cases diagnosed in the ith interval with delay j, rather than modeling Y_i, the number of cases diagnosed in the ith interval. The model contains reporting delay "effects" as well as effects that depend on infection rates and incubation periods. Lawless and Sun (1992) have also provided a general framework to account for errors in reporting delay adjustments in back-calculation.

A certain proportion of cases may never be reported. Suppose γ is the probability that a case will be reported, and we assume that γ is constant over time. The back-calculation methodology could still be

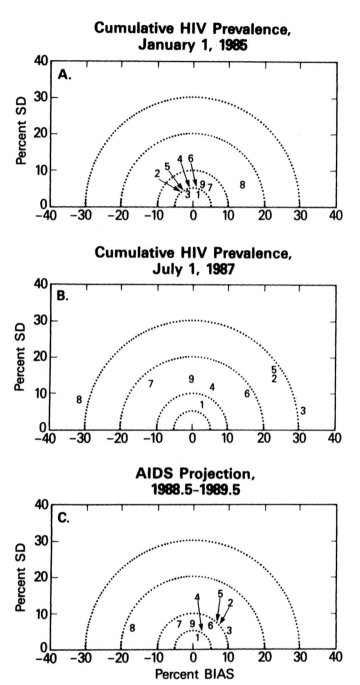

Figure 8.7 Bulls-eye plot (relative percent SD vs. relative percent bias) for a step function model for $g(s)$ with four steps for the nine infection curves in Figure 8.5. (Source: Rosenberg, Gail, and Pee, 1991. Reprinted by permission of John Wiley & Sons, Ltd.)

used, but in this case the infection rate, $g(s)$, refers only to infected individuals who would be reported if diagnosed with AIDS. In order to obtain an estimate of the total infection rate, it is necessary to inflate estimated infection rates by the factor $1/\gamma$. Similarly the projections of the total numbers of AIDS cases, both reported and unreported, are obtained by inflating by the factor $1/\gamma$. For example, if 90% of cases are eventually reported, it would be necessary to inflate infection rates and AIDS incidence projections by the factor $1/.90 = 1.11$. The crucial assumption that justifies this simple adjustment is that the proportion of cases that are reported, γ, has remained constant over calendar time.

Rosenberg and Gail (1990) performed a sensitivity analysis to evaluate the effect of differential underreporting over calendar time (i.e., γ changes over time). Of particular concern was the possibility of more underreporting early in the epidemic due to lack of recognition of AIDS. Also of interest was the effect of increased reporting in later years due to increased awareness of AIDS and to changes in the surveillance definition. Table 8.2 shows the sensitivity of the estimated cumulative numbers infected to perturbations in the AIDS incidence data. Perturbations of AIDS cases in more recent years have a greater effect than perturbations in the early years (see also Brookmeyer and Gail, 1986). However, these perturbations do not change estimated cumulative infections by more than 15%.

Effects of Immigration and Emigration
Individuals may become infected in one community but immigrate into another community before or after the diagnosis of AIDS. We consider the situation in which some individuals born in community A become infected when living abroad and then return home to community A to receive health care after AIDS diagnosis. The effects of this

Table 8.2 Sensitivity of Estimate of Cumulative Number Infected in the United States by July 1, 1987, to Perturbations in AIDS Incidence Data

Multiplier of AIDS Incidence Data			Cumulative infections by July 1, 1987
1977–82	1983–84	1987	
1.0	1.0	1.0	992,000
1.5	1.15	0.95	916,000
1.5	1.0	1.0	1,048,000
1.0	1.0	0.95	903,000
1.0	1.15	1.0	930,000

Source: Adapted from Rosenberg and Gail (1990).

type of immigration on back-calculation are similar to the effects of underreporting. Suppose we wish to back-calculate AIDS incidence data based on cases reported in community A. Let ϕ be the probability that an infected individual who was born in community A is in fact diagnosed and reported in community A. This individual may have been infected in community A or perhaps another community. Back-calculation of AIDS incidence data from community A yields an estimate $g(s)$, which refers to the infection rate among individuals who would be reported in community A if diagnosed with AIDS. Forecasts of AIDS incidence based on $g(s)$ refer to cases reported in community A. In fact, this is precisely what is of interest for forecasting future health care needs in community A. The crucial assumption is that ϕ is constant over calendar time. However, $g(s)$ does not refer to the infection rate occurring in community A, but rather to the infection rate among individuals who would be diagnosed and reported in community A. This latter rate includes some infections that occur outside community A and excludes some infections that occur in community A among individuals who later emigrate from that community. Although we are unaware of studies of the importance of migration on back-calculation, the effects of immigration and emigration are probably less important for analyzing national AIDS incidence data than for analyzing local AIDS incidence data.

8.4.2 Plausible Ranges and Quantifying Uncertainty

It is important to indicate the substantial uncertainty in back-calculated estimates by presenting plausible ranges for parameter values rather than simple point estimates.

It also is important to perform sensitivity analyses to investigate the impact of different underlying assumptions. An ad hoc approach for obtaining a plausible range on a parameter (such as the cumulative numbers infected) is to compute confidence limits on the parameter under each set of postulated assumptions. The plausible range is determined by the smallest of the lower confidence limits and the largest of the upper confidence limits. Some investigators have used this approach to establish plausible ranges on cumulative infections by considering different assumptions about the incubation distributions with weakly parametric models for the infection curve (Rosenberg, Biggar, Goedert, and Gail, 1991; Brookmeyer, 1991; Rosenberg, Gail, and Carroll, 1992). If strongly parametric models are used instead of weakly parametric models, it is also important to consider a number of different parametric families for the infection curve, $g(s)$.

More formal Bayesian approaches have been suggested for incorporating uncertainty in model assumptions. For example, Taylor (1989) considered 105 different sets of model assumptions determined by different combinations of the incubation distribution and infection curve model. Taylor assumed a uniform discrete prior on the various models and used Bayes' theorem to obtain posterior distributions for various parameters.

In order to obtain a plausible range on projected AIDS incidence it is also important to account for uncertainty in the future infection rate. Brookmeyer (1991) accounted for this uncertainty by performing calculations under different assumptions about the future infection rate.

8.5 BACK-CALCULATION FOR INVESTIGATING HYPOTHESES ABOUT THE INFECTION RATE

Back-calculation is useful for investigating hypotheses about the infection rate. The basic idea is to use the incubation period distribution to test if a hypothesis about the infection rate is consistent with the observed pattern of AIDS cases.

For example, Gail, Rosenberg, and Goedert (1990a) observed a decrease in the rate of increase in AIDS incidence in the United States, especially among homosexual men in Los Angeles, New York, and San Francisco beginning in the middle of 1987. One possible explanation for the improvement in AIDS incidence trends was that there had been a marked drop in the infection rate years earlier. Back-calculation methods were used to test the hypothesis that the fall off in AIDS incidence was due completely to a drop in the infection rate. This was done by considering the extreme hypothesis that infections actually stopped after a certain point in calendar time and constraining the model for the infection rate accordingly.

Figure 8.8 shows AIDS incidence for homosexual men in Los Angeles, New York, and San Francisco. A step-function model for the infection rate that was constrained was used so that the infection rate was 0 after December 31, 1982. The predicted AIDS incidence based on back-calculation still overestimated the observed AIDS incidence after 1987 even under this extreme assumption of no infections after 1982. Thus, even a sharp decline in the infection rate beginning in 1983 cannot fully explain the observed AIDS incidence, and other explanations must be entertained. Other possible explanations include misspecification of the incubation distribution, increased reporting delays, changes in the definition of AIDS, and secular changes in the

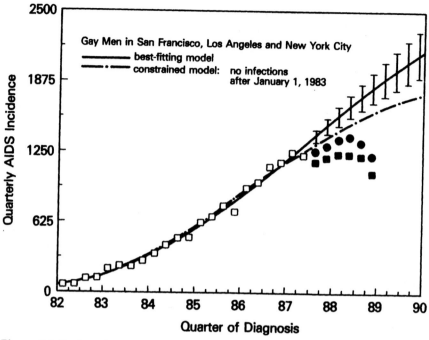

Figure 8.8 Projected and observed quarterly AIDS incidence among homosexual and bisexual men in San Francisco, Los Angeles, and New York City. Projections were based on consistently defined AIDS incidence counts through June 30, 1987 (open squares) without constraints (solid line) and under the constraints that no infections occurred after January 1, 1983 (dot-dash line), as described by Gail, Rosenberg, and Goedert (1990a). Vertical lines indicate 95% confidence intervals, and solid squares depict augmented consistently defined quarterly AIDS incidence beginning in July 1987. Solid circles depict all AIDS incidence beginning in July 1, 1987. (Source: figure 2 in Gail, Rosenberg, and Goedert, 1990a.)

incubation period distribution. Gail, Rosenberg, and Goedert (1990a) concluded that the most likely explanation was a secular change in the incubation period distribution due to the introduction of effective treatments, such as zidovudine and prophylactic inhaled pentamidine (see Section 11.4), for AIDS-free patients with advanced HIV disease.

Back-calculation thus led to new hypotheses and focused attention on the need to consider treatment when forecasting AIDS incidence and interpreting trends in AIDS incidence. We now discuss how to adapt back-calculation to account for treatment and other factors that affect the incubation distribution.

8.6 GENERALIZED BACK-CALCULATION: EXTENSION TO ACCOUNT FOR NONSTATIONARY INCUBATION DISTRIBUTIONS

A fundamental assumption of the back-calculation methods considered in the preceeding sections is that the incubation period distribution is stable over calendar time. However, a number of factors, including treatment of HIV infected individuals who have not progressed to AIDS could alter the incubation period distribution. For example, the drug zidovudine was approved by the U.S. Food and Drug Administration in March of 1987 for the treatment of AIDS patients as well as for AIDS-free HIV infected individuals with CD4+ T cell counts below 200 cells/μl. Inhaled pentamidine was approved in 1988 for use with HIV infected patients to prevent *Pneumocystis carinii* pneumonia. These treatments can delay the onset of AIDS and thus lengthen the incubation period.

In this section, we extend the method of back-calculation to account for a nonstationary incubation distribution. The basic approach is to consider not a single incubation distribution but rather a family of distributions indexed by the calendar year of infection. The fundamental equation underlying the back-calculation method can be generalized to account for changes in the incubation period distribution (Brookmeyer and Liao, 1990a). The generalization of equation (8.1) is

$$A(t) = \int_0^t g(s) \cdot F(t - s|s)ds,$$

where $F(t|s)$ is the incubation period distribution for an individual infected at calendar time s; that is $F(t|s)$ is the probability of developing AIDS within t years of infection for an individual who was infected at calendar time s. Thus, instead of a single incubation distribution we have a family of distributions indexed by the calendar time of infection. The equation for the expected AIDS incidence and the methods described in Section 8.3 generalize simply by substituting $F(t|s)$ for $F(t)$.

In order to proceed with this methodology, information about $F(t|s)$ is required. Ideally, separate Kaplan–Meier estimates of the incubation period distribution could be computed from separate cohorts defined by calendar year of infection. There are two difficulties with this empirical approach. First, most cohorts contain relatively few individuals with known calendar dates of infection, and thus there is insufficient information for estimating separate incubation distributions, corresponding to different calendar years of infection. Second, changes in the incubation period distribution observed in one population may not be applicable to another population because such changes depend both on the efficacy of treatment and on the proportions of infected individuals in treatment. The proportions of infected individuals in treatment may vary widely across populations. The efficacy of treatment might be expected to be more nearly constant across populations, though differences in efficacy could arise if compliance to treatment varies across populations of if the effectiveness of treatment depends on factors like age, race, sex, or general health status.

Even though available empirical data are insufficient to specify the family of distribution functions $F(t|s)$ with confidence, there is solid empirical evidence that treatment has affected the incubation distribution. Clinical trials have shown that zidovudine can delay the onset of AIDS (Chapter 11), and data on the extent of zidovudine in AIDS-free patients with advanced HIV disease suggest that sufficient zidovudine and other treatments have been used to alter the incubation distribution significantly (Gail, Rosenberg, and Goedert, 1990a; Rosenberg, Gail, Schrager, et al., 1991; Graham, Zeger, Kuo, et al., 1991). Moreover, there is evidence for a secular trend in the incubation distribution that is temporally related to the introduction of effective treatments in 1987 in a cohort of homosexual men in Vancouver (Schechter, Craib, Le, et al., 1989b) and in a cohort of homosexual men in Los Angeles (Taylor, Kuo, and Detels, 1991).

An alternative to the completely empirical approach for estimating $F(t|s)$ outlined above is to introduce additional modelling assumptions. Below we consider some specific models for accounting for secular trends in the incubation distribution due to the introduction of treatment.

8.6.1 Models for the Effect of Treatment on the Incubation Period

Several issues must be addressed in order to model the effect of treatment on the incubation period. First, antiretroviral treatments for HIV infection, such as zidovudine, were not available, except in clinical trials, before March of 1987. Likewise, although some forms of prophylaxis against *Pneumocystis carnii* pneumonia were being used earlier, it was not until 1988 that inhaled pentamidine was widely recommended for this purpose. Second, some treatments were only prescribed for individuals in late stages of HIV disease. For example, zidovudine was first approved only for HIV infected individuals with fewer than 200 CD4+ T cells/μl.

One model to account for secular trends in the incubation period is called a *staging model* (Brookmeyer, 1991; Longini, 1990; Brookmeyer and Liao, 1990a, 1992). It is assumed individuals progress from infection (stage 1) to an advanced stage of HIV disease without an AIDS diagnosis (stage 2) to AIDS (stage 3). Advanced stage HIV disease (stage 2) could be defined in terms of CD4+ T cell levels or clinical signs and symptoms. The main assumptions of this staging model are as follows: Individuals in advanced stage HIV disease (stage 2) may be treated but individuals with early stage HIV disease are not treated. An individual who entered stage 2 at calendar time s has a hazard, $h(u|s)$ of beginning treatment u time units after entry into stage 2. The effect of treatment is to reduce the hazard of progression to AIDS by the factor θ (the treatment relative risk). A schematic illustration of this four-state model is shown in Figure 8.9. In the absence of treatment, the hazard of progressing from stage i to stage $i+1$ after u time units in stage i is called $\lambda_i(u)$. These assumptions induce changes in the incubation period distribution. Analytic expressions for the resulting nonstationary family of incubation period distributions have been developed (Brookmeyer and Liao, 1990a).

An example of the nonstationary incubation distribution is illustrated in Figure 8.10. Figure 8.10 was based on assuming $\lambda_1(u)$ was Weibull $(\lambda_1(u) = .029u^{2.08}$, median $= 6.5$ years) and $\lambda_2(u)$ was exponential $(\lambda_2 = .277$, median $= 2.5$ years). Treatment was assumed to be phased in at a constant rate of .20 per year beginning July 1, 1987. To be precise, $h(u|s) = 0$ for $u + s \leqslant 1987.5$ and $h(u|s) = .20$ for

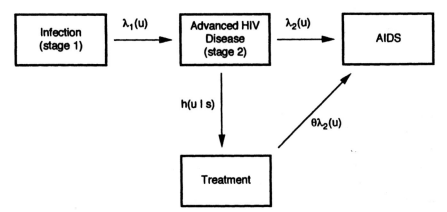

Figure 8.9 Four state (staging) model of Brookmeyer (1991) to incorporate secular changes in the incubation period due to treatment.

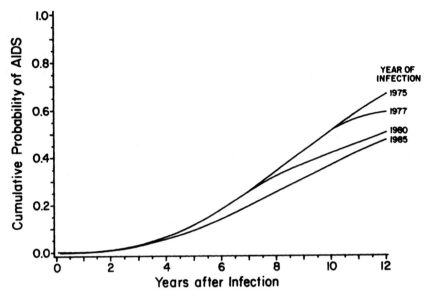

Figure 8.10 Nonstationary family of incubation period distributions resulting from phase-in of treatment. (Source: Brookmeyer, 1991.)

$u + s > 1987.5$. However, studies have shown considerable variation across both transmission and demographic groups in access to treatment (Rosenberg, Gail, Schrager, et al., 1991; Moore, Hidalgo, Sugland, and Chaisson, 1991; Graham, Zeger, Kuo, et al., 1991). The curve labeled 1975 in Figure 8.10 refers to individuals infected in 1975 and essentially represents the natural history of HIV disease, because treatment was unavailable during the period 1975–87. The incubation distribution for cohorts infected in 1980 overlaps the 1975 curve for the first 7.5 years because treatment was introduced in mid-1987 according to this model. The longer incubation periods associated with cohorts infected later in calendar time are attributable to the increasing availability of treatment as soon as patients enter stage 2.

The staging model makes a number of important assumptions. First it assumes that treatment reduces the hazard of AIDS by a constant factor, θ (i.e., a proportional hazards model). However studies have suggested that the efficacy of zidovudine may diminish in time, perhaps due to viral drug resistance (Larder, Darby, and Richman, 1989). The model could be generalized to allow θ to depend on time in treatment. Second, the model does not account for any future therapeutic advances that could effect the incubation period.

Third, the model assumes individuals must successively pass through each stage. In fact, individuals may regress from an advanced stage of disease back to an earlier stage, for example, if CD4+ T cells rise sharply. Fourth, the model assumes that durations spent in each stage are independent within an individual. However, it is plausible that some infected individuals are *fast progressors* and some are *slow progressors*. If so, sojourn times in successive stages would be correlated and individual rates of progression would "track" (Section 5.6).

An alternative to the staging model described above is a "time since infection" model (Rosenberg, Gail, and Carroll, 1992). In this model, the hazard of AIDS at t years after infection for a person infected at calendar time s and given access to treatment at calendar time τ is

$$h(t|s, \tau) = \begin{array}{ll} h_o(t) & t + s < \tau \\ h_o(t) \cdot \theta(t) & t + s \geq \tau \end{array}$$

where $h_o(t)$ is the "natural history" hazard function for an untreated patient and $\theta(t)$ is an efficacy function that accounts for treatment effects. Just because a patient has access to effective treatments at time τ does not imply that powerful drugs will be used immediately. In fact, Rosenberg, Gail, and Carroll assume that the use of drugs that can alter the natural history hazard will be phased in as the disease progresses. The efficacy function thus depends on time since infection. It is assumed that $\theta(t)$ is near 1 when t is near 0 because individuals are typically not treated shortly after infection. After about 5 years, $\theta(t)$ decreases to a plateau value θ_{min}, which resembles θ in the stage model above. Rosenberg, Gail, and Carroll (1992) also multiplied the natural history hazard by a factor to account for changes in the incubation period that resulted from broadening the AIDS surveillance definition of AIDS to include dementia, wasting syndrome, extrapulmonary tuberculosis and a few other conditions in the fall of 1987. The effect of broadening the AIDS surveillance definition on the incubation period is to increase the hazard, which partially offsets the favorable changes induced by treatment.

Both the staging model and the time-since-treatment model allow for a gradual increase in access to effective treatments beginning in 1987, resulting in a family of gradually decreasing incubation distributions. An earlier back-calculation model to accommodate treatment assumed that the incubation distribution changed suddenly at a single point in calendar time (Solomon and Wilson, 1990).

An advantage of the staging model is that it permits estimation of the numbers of individuals in different stages of HIV infection (Brookmeyer and Liao, 1990). This is important for forecasting health care needs because it is established that individuals in advanced stages of HIV infection can benefit from treatment. Estimates of the numbers of individuals in different stages of HIV infection are obtained by taking the back-calculated infection rates and forward calculating using the stage specific incubation period distributions. Brookmeyer (1991) used this methodology to estimate the numbers of HIV infected individuals with fewer than 200 CD4+ T cell/μl (Section 8.7). Longini, Byers, Hessol, and Tan (1992) extended the staging model to allow for seven stages of HIV infection that were defined by symptoms and markers (Chapter 5). They assumed a Markov model where the hazards of progression from one stage to the next were constant (i.e., the distribution of durations in each stage were assumed to be exponential). They applied the model to estimate numbers of individuals in different stages of HIV infection in the San Francisco City Clinic Cohort.

8.6.2 Qualitative Effects of a Nonstationary Incubation Distribution

Failure to account for secular changes in the incubation distribution can lead to severely biased estimates by back-calculations. If the effect of a treatment is to lengthen the incubation period, a model that incorporates a treatment effect would estimate a much higher cumulative number of HIV infections than a model based on a stationary incubation distribution. The reason is that back-calculation based on a stationary incubation distribution attributes any fall off in AIDS incidence to an earlier drop in the infection rate, while back-calculation based on a nonstationary incubation distribution attributes some of the fall off to a lengthening of the incubation period. The larger estimates of HIV prevalence eventually lead to larger numbers of projected AIDS cases. Thus, paradoxically, back-calculation models that account for treatment can produce higher AIDS incidence projections than a model that assumes a stationary incubation distribution (Gail and Brookmeyer, 1990b).

8.7 APPLICATION TO THE U.S. AIDS EPIDEMIC

The back-calculation methods described in the previous sections were applied to the AIDS epidemic in the United States (Brookmeyer, 1991). The methods were based on the smoothing splines using Phillips Tikhonov regularization (Section 8.3.3) and the nonstationary incubation distribution illustrated in Figure 8.10.

This analysis was based on AIDS cases diagnosed before April 1, 1990, and reported by September 1990. The AIDS incidence data were grouped into 3-month (quarterly) intervals, adjusted for reporting delays, and inflated 10% for underreporting. The infection curve was parameterized as a step function with 12 steps spanning the period January 1977 to April 1990. The lengths of the first and last intervals were 2 and 1.25 years, respectively; all other intervals were yearly. Generalized crossvalidation was used to guide the degree of smoothing (see comments in Section 8.3.3). Figure 8.11 shows the reconstruction of the infection curve in the United States. Infection rates grew rapidly during the period 1978–81. The estimated doubling time (time for the cumulative number of infections to double) increased from 7.8 months in the beginning of 1981 to 12.7 months in the beginning of 1982 to 19.2 months in the beginning of 1983. The infection rate appears to have peaked in 1984 at about 160,000 infections per year. There were marked declines in the infection rate between 1985 and 1987.

Figure 8.11 shows plausible ranges on the estimated infection rates. The ranges are based on 95% confidence limits (conditional on the degree of smoothness, that is, the smoothing parameter) using three different incubation distributions. The ranges are the maximum of the three upper and minimum of the three lower confidence limits computed from the three incubation distributions. The hazards of AIDS for these three distributions rise rapidly with time from infection and eventually level off. The three distributions account for some

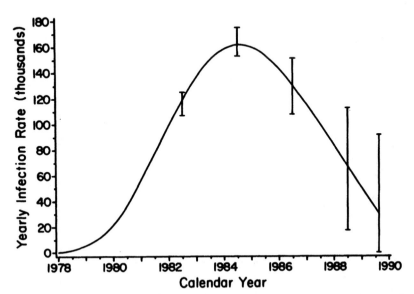

Figure 8.11 Reconstruction of HIV infection rates in the United States. Estimates based on nonstationary distributions illustrated in Figure 8.10. (Source: Brookmeyer, 1991.)

uncertainty in how quickly the hazard levels. The median of each distribution was about 10 years. The estimated cumulative number of infections by April 1, 1990, was 1,050,000 with a plausible range of 850,000–1,205,000. However, if an incubation period with a median of 9 years instead of 10 years is used, the estimated cumulative number of infections is 15% lower.

It was also found that estimates of the infection rates before 1987 are not nearly as sensitive to the choice of the smoothing parameter as are estimates after 1987, which were quite sensitive. The estimates are also sensitive to the assumed treatment effects (treatment relative risk and proportions in treatment) that modify the incubation period. Figure 8.12 depicts a sensitivity analysis of the estimated cumulative infections by April 1990 to various assumptions about treatment. For example, an analysis in which a treatment effect is not incorporated yields an estimate of cumulative number infected of only 715,000 and an earlier peak in the infection curve.

As previously mentioned, it is possible to estimate the number of individuals in different stages of HIV disease by propagating forward the number infected from stage to stage (Figure 8.9) (Brookmeyer and Liao, 1990a). Estimates of the numbers of AIDS-free patients with advanced HIV disease (i.e., stage 2 with CD4+ T cells below $200/\mu l$)

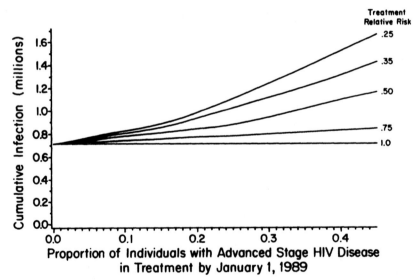

Figure 8.12 Sensitivity analysis of estimated cumulative HIV infections by April 1, 1990, to assumptions about the efficacy of treatment and the proportions of individuals with fewer than 200 CD4+T cells/mm^3 and without an AIDS diagnosis who were in treatment. (Source: Brookmeyer, 1991.)

indicate progressive increases from 1991 to 1996 (Table 8.3). However, these estimates are very sensitive to the assumed median duration of the advanced stage of HIV disease. The longer this duration, the more individuals one would expect to find prevalent in the advanced stage. This phenomenon is related to the well known epidemiological fact that the steady state prevalence of a disease is equal to the incidence multiplied by the mean duration.

Projections of AIDS incidence can be obtained by applying the incubation distribution to the infection rates in Figure 8.11. Projections of AIDS incidence on a log scale suggest that overall AIDS incidence will plateau over the next several years (Figure 8.13).

Rosenberg, Gail, and Carroll (1992) used the time-since-infection model (Section 8.6) to account for treatment effects and changes in the surveillance definition in 1987. They obtained estimates of cumulative infections about 27% smaller than Brookmeyer (1991), but, like Brookmeyer, they predicted a plateau in AIDS incidence from 1991 through 1994. The difference in results between the two approaches are due primarily to different assumptions about the efficacy of treatment and the proportions of infected individuals in treatment (Gail and Rosenberg, 1992).

Back-calculation results for specific transmission groups in the United States are discussed in Section 10.2. Public Health Service projections for the United States based on various back-calculation

Table 8.3 Sensitivity of Estimates of U.S. Prevalence (thousands) of Advanced Stage HIV Disease (stage 2)

Year	Median Duration (in years) in Stage 2			
	1.5	2.5	3.5	Range
1991	158	265	366	152–380
1992	180	304	412	169–440
1993	197	333	448	182–492
1994	209	354	470	186–510
1995	216	365	480	185–524
1996	218	370	482	178–594

Notes: Prevalence refers to numbers of AIDS-free individuals who are alive and have CD4+ T cell levels below 200 cells/μl (stage 2). The incubation distribution is defined by a three stage model: infected (stage 1), advanced HIV disease (stage 2), and AIDS (stage 3). The sojourn distribution in stage 2 is exponential with median 1.5, 2.5, or 3.5 years. The sojourn distribution in stage 1 is Weibull with shape parameter 2.08 and scale parameter chosen so that the median of the total incubation period was fixed at 10.0 years. Estimates are adjusted for a continuous infection rate of 30,000 per year in 1990 and thereafter. Further details are in Brookmeyer (1991).

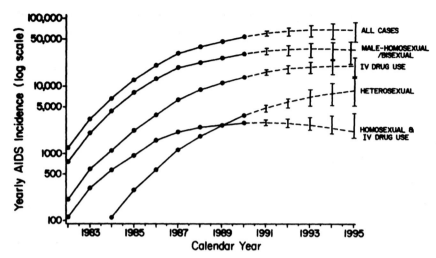

Figure 8.13 Projections of annual AIDS incidence 1991 to 1995 (log scale) for the entire United States and for four transmission groups. Projections corrected for 10% underreporting. (Source: Brookmeyer, 1991.)

methodologies have been described in CDC (1992c). Back-calculation methods have also been applied to AIDS surveillance data in many other countries, including Australia (Solomon, Fazekas de St Groth, and Wilson 1990), Canada (Marion and Schechter, 1991), New Zealand (Sharples, Carlson, Skegg, and Paul, 1991) and the United Kingdom (Day and Gore, 1989).

8.8 TECHNICAL NOTES

8.8.1 Generalized Least Squares Algorithms

An alternative approach to maximum likelihood estimation for estimating the infection curve (Section 8.3) is to use regression methods based on quasi-likelihood (McCullagh and Nelder, 1989). The algorithm is based on generalized least squares (Carroll and Ruppert, 1988). This procedure yields consistent estimates even if the Poisson assumption is violated, provided models for the mean and variance are correctly specified. The models for the mean and variance of Y_i are

$$E(Y_i) = \mu_i = \int_0^{T_i} g(s; \boldsymbol{\beta})\{F(T_i - s) - F(T_{i-1} - s)\}ds \quad (8.9.\text{a})$$

and

$$\text{Var}(Y_i) = \sigma^2 V(\mu_i), \quad (8.9.\text{b})$$

where $V(\mu)$ is some specified (known) function of the mean μ, and σ^2 is called an overdispersion parameter. If σ^2 is assumed to be 1 and $V(\mu) = \mu$, we have the usual Poisson model. Rosenberg and Gail (1991) introduced this algorithm for step function and spline models with Poisson variation $V(\mu) = \mu$. If $V(\mu) = \mu$ but σ^2 is arbitrary, the model can accommodate extra-Poisson variation (Brookmeyer and Liao, 1990a).

The generalized least squares algorithm begins with an initial estimate of β, called $\hat{\beta}^o$. Suppose at the jth iteration, the current estimate is $\hat{\beta}^{(j)}$. The algorithm proceeds as follows: First, the updated estimates, $\hat{\beta}^{(j+1)}$, are obtained by minimizing

$$\sum_{i=1}^n \frac{[Y_i - \mu_i(\hat{\beta}^{(j+1)})]^2}{V(\mu_i(\hat{\beta}^{(j)}))} \tag{8.10}$$

over all possible values for $\hat{\beta}^{(j+1)}$ where $\mu_i(\hat{\beta})$ is the estimate of $\mu_i = E(Y_i)$ obtained by substituting $\hat{\beta}^{(j)}$ into equation 8.9a.

Second, continue updating the estimates until convergence. At convergence, the generalized least squares estimates, $\hat{\beta}$, are called the quasi-likelihood estimates (Carroll and Ruppert, 1988; McCullagh and Nelder, 1989). For some probability distributions (e.g., Poisson), the quasi-likelihood estimates are actually the maximum likelihood estimates.

The overdispersion parameter σ^2 is often estimated by

$$\hat{\sigma}^2 = \frac{1}{n-p} \sum_{i=1}^n \frac{(Y_i - \mu_i(\hat{\beta}))^2}{V(\mu_i(\hat{\beta}))}$$

where p is the dimension of β.

The minimization step in expression (8.10) is especially easy for the piecewise constant step function model. This is because the expected value, $E(Y_i) = \mu_i$, is linear in the unknown parameters

$$\mu_i = \sum_{j=1}^p \beta_j Z_{ij},$$

where

$$Z_{ij} = \int_{c_{j-1}}^{c_j} \{F(T_i - s) - F(T_{i-1} - s)\}ds. \tag{8.11}$$

Then, the updated estimates $\hat{\beta}_{(m+1)}$ are given by

$$\hat{\beta}_{(j+1)} = (Z'\hat{W}Z)^{-1}Z'\hat{W}Y,$$

where Z is an $n + p$ matrix with (i,j) element given by equation (8.11), and $\hat{W}$ is the $n \times n$ diagonal weight matrix with diagonal elements given by the reciprocal of the mean, estimated by using the parameter values at the jth iteration. The ith diagonal element of $\hat{W}$ is

$$(\hat{\mu}_i)^{-1} = \left(\sum_{j=1}^{P} \hat{\beta}_j^{(j)} Z_{ij} \right)^{-1}$$

At convergence the variance-covariance matrix of $\hat{\beta}$ is

$$\text{Var}(\hat{\beta}) = (Z'\hat{W}Z)^{-1}\hat{\sigma}^2$$

where

$$\hat{\sigma}^2 = \frac{1}{n-p} \sum_{i=1}^{n} \frac{(Y_i - \hat{\mu}_i)^2}{\hat{\mu}_i}.$$

This algorithm is computationally simple and fast and is the method of choice for fitting piecewise constant step function models (Rosenberg and Gail, 1991). If negative values are produced, constrained optimization procedures are required (see Waterman, 1974; Gerig and Gallant, 1975). The constrained maximum likelihood estimates satisfy the Kuhn–Tucker conditions (McDonald and Diamond, 1990). Gail, Rosenberg, and Goedert (1990a) obtained nonnegative step function estimates for the infection curve by examining models obtained by deleting various steps from the full model until a nonnegative submodel satisfying the Kuhn–Tucker conditions was found. If there are p steps, one must examine $2^p - 1$ submodels, at most, until the appropriate nonnegative solution is found. The rapidity of the generalized least squares algorithm makes such a search feasible. Alternatively, an EM algorithm can be used to fit the piecewise constant step function model. This algorithm ensures positive values for the parameter estimates (Brookmeyer and Gail, 1988), but it is computationally slow.

8.8.2 The Poisson Assumption and Alternative Formulations

The statistical framework for back-calculation described in Section 8.3 used the assumption that infections arrive according to a nonhomogeneous Poisson process. However, this assumption is not crucial to the development.

An alternative formulation is to view the total number of infections that occurred up to calendar time T_n as a parameter, N, which is to be estimated (Brookmeyer and Gail, 1988). Suppose infections arrive according to a point process (not necessarily Poisson). The realized intensity function for the process is $g(s; \beta)$. Then, given that N infections have occurred, the N infection times can be viewed as independent identically distributed random variables with probability density

$$g^*(s; \beta) = \frac{g(s; \beta)}{\int_0^{T_n} g(s; \beta)ds}.$$

The above statement can be justified by assuming the point process for infections has the order statistic property (Deffner and Haeusler, 1985), or alternatively by assuming that the N infection times are exchangeable.

The number of individuals infected before T_n but not yet diagnosed is called $Y_{n+1} = N - Y.$ where

$$Y. = \sum_{j=1}^{n} Y_j .$$

Then $\mathbf{Y} = (Y_1, Y_2, \ldots, Y_n, Y_{n+1})$ has a multinomial distribution with unknown sample size N and cell probabilities $p_1, p_2, \ldots, p_n, p_{n+1}$ where

$$p_j = \int_0^{T_j} g^*(s; \beta)\{F(T_j - s) - F(T_{j-1} - s)\}ds.$$

One then proceeds to compute the maximum likelihood estimates of the parameters N and β from the multinomial log-likelihood function

$$LL(N; \beta; \mathbf{Y}) = \log(N!) - \sum_{i=1}^{n+1} \log(Y_i!) + \sum_{i=1}^{n+1} Y_i \log p_i .$$

Estimation of the size of a multinomial population has been considered in a number of different contexts (see Bishop, Fienberg, and Holland, 1975).

An alternative approach is to maximize the conditional log-likelihood, LL_c, which is conditional on the observed number of AIDS cases

$$Y. = \sum_{i=1}^{n} Y_i .$$

This also has multinomial structure:

$$LL_c(\beta; \mathbf{Y}) = \log(Y.!) - \sum_{i=1}^{n} \log(Y_i!) + \sum_{j=1}^{n} Y_i \log p_{c_j},$$

where p_{c_j} are the conditional probabilities of diagnosis in the jth interval given that diagnosis occurred before T_n,

$$p_{c_j} = \frac{\int_o^{T_j} g^*(s; \boldsymbol{\beta}) \{F(T_j - s) - F(T_{j-1} - s)\} ds}{\int_o^{T_n} g^*(s) F(T_n - s) ds}.$$

Sanathanan (1972) has shown that the conditional and unconditional likelihoods are asymptotically equivalent.

Rosenberg and Gail (1991) have shown that the Poisson and multinomial approaches give identical estimates of $\boldsymbol{\beta}$ and that estimated variances of $\hat{\boldsymbol{\beta}}$ are the same up to terms of order $(1/N)$. This result should not be surprising given the close connection between the multinomial and Poisson likelihood (McCullagh and Nelder, 1989, page 318).

The multinomial framework is more appealing than the Poisson framework from the point of view that we wish to reconstruct the infection rate in *this* AIDS epidemic, which has already occurred, rather than draw inferences about the infection rate that could be expected based on realizations of many AIDS epidemics. In this sense, it is more natural to view the cumulative number of infections that have occurred, N, as a parameter rather than a random variable.

While the Poisson and multinomial likelihoods yield essentially equivalent inferences, the stronger Poisson assumption would allow one to draw inferences about the HIV infection rates in other epidemics in similar settings. However, for the purpose of back-calculation we are only concerned with reconstructing the infection rate for *this* AIDS epidemic.

9

Epidemic Transmission Models

9.1 INTRODUCTION

Even though AIDS incidence data are reliable enough to make useful short-term projections of AIDS incidence (Chapters 7 and 8), such data lag the course of infection by several years and give much less reliable information on underlying infection trends in HIV prevalence and incidence. Even serial survey of seroprevalence in selected populations (Chapter 3) provide only uncertain evidence as to the general course of HIV prevalence and incidence. Yet it is precisely the trends in HIV prevalence and incidence that will determine the long-range impact of HIV infection. In this chapter, we discuss mathematical models of epidemic transmission in an effort to gain insight into plausible trends in HIV infection curves, $g(s)$.

Although Gonzales and Koch (1987) found that the exponential growth rate of AIDS incidence can transiently decrease at the beginning of an epidemic—even though the underlying infection curve $g(s)$ is increasing exponentially—as a result of convolution with the incubation period delay, we have calculated these theoretical transient effects to be small. Thus, the subexponential growth of AIDS incidence in the United States (Figure 1.1) mainly reflects earlier subexponential growth in the infection curve, $g(s)$. In this chapter we discuss epidemic transmission models that account for subexponential growth in the infection curve. Possible factors include diffusion of the epidemic from high risk to low risk subgroups, saturation with infection of high risk subgroups, behavioral changes that reduce the chance of HIV transmission, and aggregation of temporally separated subepidemics.

Realistic epidemic models are quite complex. For example, Figure

9.1 depicts lines of transmission among major risk groups. Each risk group is divided into susceptible (S) and infected (I) individuals. Even this diagram is simplified, because it does not take hemophiliacs and transfusion recipients into account nor allow for new individuals to enter the population (immigration) and others to leave the population alive (emigration) or die. At any point in time, each member of this population is in only one compartment. An individual may move from the compartment representing susceptible individuals to the compartment representing infected individuals in any box, according to transition laws that depend on the frequency and types of exposure among individuals in various compartments, the probabilities of viral transmission corresponding to these types of exposure, and the prevalence of infection in each of the interacting subpopulations.

If one knows the initial numbers in each compartment, the law governing rates of transmission from susceptible to infected status in a given time increment, and the parameters governing frequency of contacts and rates of transmission, one could project future HIV prevalence and infection rates deterministically from this model. Unfortunately, so many parameters are required, and the projections are so sensitive to correct specification of some of these parameters, that one can put very little credence in quantitative projections based on models of this complexity (Anderson, 1988a; and Isham, 1988). For this reason we emphasize qualitative findings from studies of epidemic models. These include: (1) insights into possible patterns for the infection curve, $g(s)$; (2) statements of conditions under which the epidemic is likely to grow; (3) some understanding of the effects of heterogeneity in the population and the role of preferential mixing within homogeneous subgroups on the infection curve, $g(s)$; (4) the use of compartmental models to evaluate possible prevention strategies; and (5) insight into the difficulties of interpreting studies of risk factors for infection.

Attempts to define epidemic transmission models also help one organize available epidemic information and identify parameters that have a major impact on projections of epidemic growth. Such parameters frequently warrant special epidemiologic studies to obtain improved estimates.

In Section 9.2 we discuss a simple two-compartment model, and some simplifying assumptions are relaxed in Section 9.3 to examine the effects of behavioral change, for example. The profound effects of various mixing patterns among several subgroups with differing risk behaviors are discussed in Section 9.4, and some models used to assess prevention activities are presented in Section 9.5. Stochastic models are

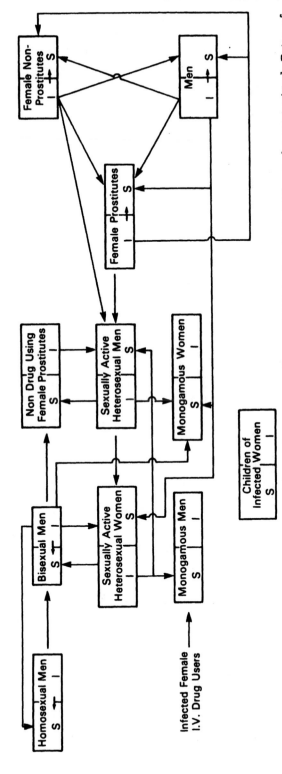

Figure 9.1 Compartmental model for spread of AIDS. Arrows indicate directions in which HIV may be transmitted. Rates of transmission from susceptible to infected status are governed by complex laws that depend on frequency and types of contact among various compartments, transmissibility of virus for corresponding behaviors, and prevalence of infection in each of the interacting boxes. (Source: Adapted from a presentation by Hethcote, 1987, and copied, with permission, from Gail and Brookmeyer, 1988.)

mentioned briefly (Section 9.6). Empirical parameter estimates are compared with estimates from epidemic models in Section 9.7. Three recent books cover many of these topics (Castillo-Chavez [ed.], 1989; Tan, 1992; Hethcote and Van Ark, 1992a).

9.2 A CLOSED TWO-COMPARTMENT MODEL

9.2.1 Model Definition and Properties

Suppose a large number of individuals, N_o, are engaging in behaviors that can transmit HIV, and that the chance of transmission per infected partner contacted is β. To be precise, we are assuming that all contacts with a partner are concentrated into an instant and that β is the probability that a susceptible partner is infected by having a partnership with an infected partner, without regard to the number or type of sexual acts during the partnership. Suppose the average rate of formation of new partnerships is μ per unit time and that each person is equally likely to form a new partnership with any other person. If $y(t)$ is the fraction infected with HIV at time t, then in the time interval $(t, t + dt)$ each susceptible individual is expected to form partnerships with $\mu y(t)dt$ infected individuals. The corresponding chance of infection is $\beta\mu y(t)dt$. Assuming that the hazard of death among infecteds is constant at α, so that $\alpha y(t)N(t)$ infecteds die of HIV related illness in this time interval, the rate of change of infecteds is

$$\frac{d\{N(t)\,y(t)\}}{dt} = \beta\mu y(t)N(t)\{1 - y(t)\} - \alpha N(t)\,y(t).$$

If the only losses from the population are HIV related deaths, so that

$$\frac{dN(t)}{dt} = -\alpha N(t)\,y(t),$$

then the left hand side of the previous equation becomes

$$N(t)\frac{dy}{dt} + \{y(t)\}^2\{-\alpha N(t)\},$$

and, after rearrangement and division by $N(t)$, (see Bremermann and Anderson, 1990), one obtains

$$\frac{dy}{dt} = (\beta\mu - \alpha)\,y(1 - y). \tag{9.1}$$

This equation has the solution

$$y(t) = y_o e^{k^* t}\{1 + y_o(e^{k^* t} - 1)\}^{-1}, \tag{9.2}$$

where $k^* = \beta\mu - \alpha$ and $y_o = y(0)$ is the prevalence at $t = 0$. Equation (9.2) is a logistic function.

The infection curve is the number of new infections per unit time and is given by

$$g(t) = \mu\beta y(t)N(t)\{1 - y(t)\}. \tag{9.3}$$

The infection curve describes the time course of incident infection, which is useful in planing prevention activities in various risk groups and figures prominently in the method of back-calculation for projecting AIDS incidence and estimating cumulative infections (Chapter 8). In a closed population with negligible mortality apart from AIDS related deaths, and assuming $dN/dt = -\alpha N(t)y(t)$ as previously, the solution for $N(t)$ is

$$N(t) = N_o\{y_o(e^{k^*t} - 1) + 1\}^{-\alpha/k^*}. \tag{9.4}$$

From equations (9.2), (9.3), and (9.4), the infection curve is given by

$$g(t) = \frac{N_o y_o(1 - y_o)\mu\beta e^{k^*t}}{\{1 + y_o(e^{k^*t} - 1)\}^{\alpha/k^* + 2}}. \tag{9.5}$$

At the beginning of the epidemic (t near zero), equations (9.2), (9.4) and (9.5) are approximately

$$y(t) \doteq y_o e^{k^*t}, \tag{9.6}$$

$$N(t) \doteq N_o e^{-\alpha y_o t} \doteq N_o, \tag{9.7}$$

and

$$g(t) \doteq N_o \mu\beta y_o e^{k^*t}, \tag{9.8}$$

respectively. Thus $y(t)$ and $g(t)$ grow exponentially initially, each with the same exponential growth constant $k^* = \mu\beta - \alpha$. During this period of exponential growth, the time it takes for both $y(t)$ and $g(t)$ to double is

$$t_d = \log_e(2)/k^*. \tag{9.9}$$

The "doubling time," t_d, can be estimated by graphing either $\log_e\{y(t)\}$ or $\log_e\{g(t)\}$ against t. The slope of this locus is k^*, which yields an estimate of t_d from equation (9.9).

Basic Reproductive Ratio, R_o

As is evident from equation (9.1), the seroprevalence $y(t)$, will only grow if $k^* = \mu\beta - \alpha > 0$. This requirement can be reexpressed as

$$R_o = \mu\beta/\alpha > 1. \tag{9.10}$$

More generally, one defines the basic reproductive ratio, R_o, as the expected number of infections that a single infected individual would produce in a large population of susceptibles during the average duration of infectiousness, D. In terms of this more general definition,

$$R_o = \mu\beta D. \tag{9.11}$$

In the simple two-compartment model, we have assumed that an infected individual remains infectious as long as he survives, and because the distribution of survival times is exponential with mean $D = 1/\alpha$, equation (9.10) follows from equation (9.11).

Numerical Examples

As an example, we consider a homosexual male population with $\mu = 15$ new partners per year. We assume $\beta = 0.1$ is the chance of transmission per infected partner (Chapter 2). The value α is chosen to match the mean time of the AIDS incubation distribution. The Weibull AIDS incubation distribution (Chapter 4) has a mean and median near 10 years. Thus we take $\alpha = 0.1$ per year. If treatments prolong survival beyond AIDS diagnosis substantially (Chapters 8 and 11), or if the mean AIDS incubation distribution is longer than predicted by the Weibull model, then smaller values of α would be appropriate. But α has little impact on the epidemic provided $\mu\beta \gg \alpha$.

Under this model with initial prevalence $y_o = 0.01$, half the population is infected in 3.3 years (Figure 9.2) and over 99% is infected by 6.6 years. The infection curve enters a subexponential phase as saturation is approached and is maximal at 3.23 years (Figure 9.3). By differentiating equation (9.5), this maximal time point is found to be

$$t_{\text{maximal}} = \frac{1}{k^*} \log_e\left\{\left(\frac{1-y_o}{y_o}\right)\left(\frac{k^*}{\mu\beta}\right)\right\}. \tag{9.12}$$

For explosive epidemics with $\mu\beta \gg \alpha$, this expression mainly depends on the product $\mu\beta$ and the initial prevalence y_o. If, instead of $y_o = 0.01$, the initial prevalence is $y_o = 0.03$, half the population is infected in 2.5 years, and the infection curve peaks 0.8 years earlier at 2.43 years. Such explosive growth was seen in HIV seroprevalence in several homosexual cohorts in the United States (CDC, 1987b).

In a rapidly growing epidemic with $\mu\beta \gg \alpha$, the initial exponential growth rate k^* depends mainly on $\mu\beta$. Thus any intervention that reduces $\mu\beta$ can slow the epidemic dramatically. For example, if the transmission probability is reduced from $\beta = 0.1$ to $\beta = 0.05$, as might be achieved by modifying sexual practices, the initial exponential growth rate is nearly halved (Figures 9.2 and 9.3). Reducing μ also slows the epidemic dramatically, as indicated for the case $\mu = 3$ new partners/years (Figures 9.2 and 9.3).

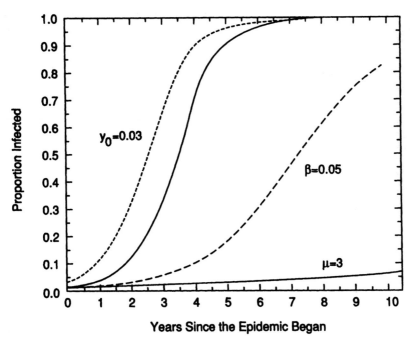

Figure 9.2 Seroprevalence curves for four epidemic models conforming to equation (9.2). Except where otherwise indicated, $\mu = 15$ partners per year, $\beta = 0.1$ per partner, $\alpha = 0.1$ per year, and $y_o = 0.01$.

Some Implications for Projecting HIV Infections

These examples demonstrate the extreme sensitivity of $y(t)$ and $g(t)$ to y_o, μ and β. Estimates of the infection curve also depend directly on N_0, the initial size of the population, which is usually uncertain. Because these parameters are seldom known with precision, quantitative projections of HIV prevalence and incidence from such an epidemic model are quite uncertain. However, a less contentious use of such models might be to suggest a functional form, such as equation (9.2), for short term extrapolation of trends (Chapter 7).

Implications for Studies of Risk Factors for Infection

The sensitivity to parameter values exhibited in Figures 9.2 and 9.3 also indicates the importance of adequate control for initial prevalence rates, y_o, and for μ in studies designed to detect factors that influence the chance of transmission, β. For example, assume that an exposed population (e) of persons who engage in a possibly risky behavior has an initial prevalence $y_o = 0.03$, whereas a control population (c) of persons who do not engage in this behavior has initial prevalence $y_o = 0.01$. Then, even if the possibly risky behavior conveys no

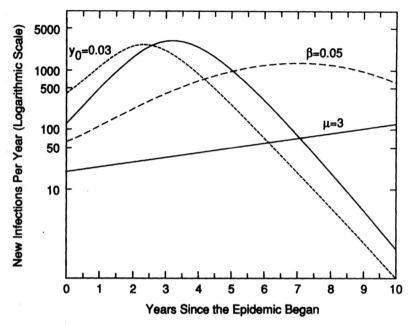

Figure 9.3 Infection curves on a logarithmic scale in a closed population of 10,000 persons for the four epidemics in Figure 9.2.

additional risk, so that $\beta_e = \beta_c = 0.1$ and $\mu_e = \mu_c = 15$ per year, the HIV prevalence odds ratio in a study conducted 2 years later would be $[y_e(2)/\{1 - y_e(2)\}]$ $[y_c(2)/\{1 - y_c(2)\}]^{-1} = [.330/.670]$ $[.141/.859]^{-1} = 3.00$, and the incidence rate ratio, $[g_e(2)/N_e(2)$ $\{1 - y_e(t)\}]$ $[g_c(2)/N_c(2)\{1 - y_c(2)\}]^{-1}$ $= \mu_e\beta_e y_e(t)/\mu_c\beta_c y_c(t)$ $=$ $y_e(t)/y_c(t) = .330/.141 = 2.34$. Thus, without adequate control for y_o, prevalent HIV case-control studies, which estimate the prevalence odds ratio, and incident HIV case-control studies, which estimate the incidence rate ratio, can be seriously misleading (Section 2.3.1). Similar arguments demonstrate the need to control for μ in such studies. De Gruttola and Mayer (1988); Koopman, Simon, Jacquez, et al. (1988); and Koopman, Longini, Jacquez, et al. (1991) point out that quantities like prevalence odds ratios and incidence rate ratios are difficult to interpret because they change rapidly during the course of an evolving epidemic (Section 2.3.1).

Summary of Results from the Two-Compartment Model
This simple two-compartment model is instructive in several respects. First, it indicates the quantitative sensitivity to the parameters μ, β, y_o

and $\mathcal{N}_o$. This sensitivity complicates the use of such models for projecting the course of the epidemic as well as the interpretation of studies of factors affecting transmission. Second, this model leads to consideration of $R_o = \beta \mu D = \beta \mu / \alpha$, the basic reproductive ratio, as a guide to whether the epidemic will grow or not. Third, the model predicts an initial exponential growth phase for prevalence $y(t)$ and for the infection curve, $g(t)$, followed by subexponential growth as the infection saturates the population and, finally, a rapidly decreasing infection curve (Figures 9.2 and 9.3). Such saturation effects may contribute to the subexponential growth in national AIDS incidence rates (Figure 1.1; Chapter 8) as well as to the reductions in the rates of new infection documented in homosexual cohorts in San Francisco (Winkelstein, Wiley, Padian, et al., 1988) and elsewhere (CDC, 1987b).

9.2.2 The Need for More General Models

However, this model is oversimplified in several respects, some of which may contribute importantly to the AIDS incidence trends seen so far and to the course of the underlying epidemic. In particular, the model makes the following unrealistic assumptions:

1. All persons in a given population have the same μ and β parameters (homogeneity).
2. There is free maxing in selecting partners. In particular, an uninfected individual is as likely to select an infected partner as an uninfected partner.
3. The population is closed. That is, there is no linkage to other populations, no immigration of susceptibles, no emigration, and no deaths of susceptibles.
4. The quantities α and β are assumed to be constant on the scale of time since infection. In fact, we know that the hazard of AIDS, and hence the hazard of death, increases with time from infection (Chapter 4) so that α is not truly constant, and some data suggest that the infectiousness is greatest early and late in the course of infection (Chapter 2) so that β may also vary.
5. It is assumed that μ, α and β are constant in calendar time. However, empirical evidence demonstrates that behavioral changes have occurred in homosexual populations (McKusick, Horstman, and Coates, 1985, and Pickering, Wiley, Padian, et al., 1986), and HIV incidence rates have decreased (Winkelstein, Wiley, Padian, et al., 1988), implying potential decreases in μ and β. Treatments have prolonged the AIDS incubation distribution and improved survival (Chapters 8 and 11), implying that α has been decreasing in calendar time.

That more general models might be required is indicated in Figure 9.4 in which we have plotted the logarithm of the infection curve estimated by Bacchetti (1990) for homosexual men in San Francisco together with a simple two-compartment model ($\mu = 15$, $\beta = 0.1$, $\alpha = 0.1$, $y_o = 0.005$ and $N_0 = 16,195$) chosen to match the infection curve of Bacchetti in the third quarter of 1981. Bacchetti's estimated infection curve, which was derived from empirical data on dates of seroconversion in selected cohorts, exhibits subexponential growth from the very beginning of the epidemic, as indicated by the initial curvature of this locus in Figure 9.4, whereas the simple two-compartment model predicts exponential growth initially. After the maximum rate of HIV incidence is reached, the two-compartment model predicts exponential decay of the infection curve, as indicated by the descending straight line in Figure 9.4, whereas the infection curve estimated by Bacchetti declines more gradually. In Section 9.3 and 9.4 we examine the effects of various modifications of the assumptions in the simple two-compartment model to gain greater insight into the behavior of real infection curves. Some of these modifications, such as

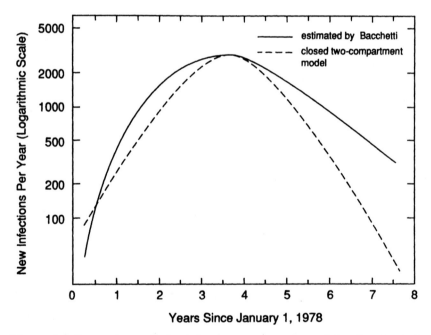

Figure 9.4 Comparison of the infection curve estimated by Bacchetti for homosexual men in San Francisco with the infection curve given by equation (9.5) with $\mu = 15$, $\beta = 0.1$, $y_o = 0.005$, $\alpha = 0.1$ and $N_o = 16,150$. The ordinate is on a logarithmic scale.

allowance for immigration, can be made in the context of a two-compartment model (Section 9.3), whereas other modifications require general models that allow for heterogeneity in risk behaviors (Section 9.4).

9.3 GENERALIZATIONS OF THE CLOSED TWO-COMPARTMENT MODEL

9.3.1 Immigration and Emigration

Somewhat more realistic models take into account the fact that the population is not closed. Rather, new susceptibles immigrate into the population each year, susceptibles may emigrate or die of causes unrelated to HIV infection, and infecteds may die of HIV-related or unrelated causes or emigrate. Typically, the population size will vary in these circumstances and equations (9.1) and (9.4) would need to be modified accordingly (Bremermann and Anderson, 1990). For example Gail and Brookmeyer (1988) considered a hypothetical population of 10,000 individuals between the ages of 20 and 39 years. In line with demographics from the United States, they assumed that $c = 410.7$ uninfected new 19-year-olds enter the population each year and that the annual probabilities of death were $\lambda_0 = 0.0013$ for susceptibles and $\lambda_1 = 0.05$ for infecteds. To achieve a steady state population size, they assumed a proportion $\pi = .04037$ emigrated alive each year. Gail and Brookmeyer modeled the epidemic in discrete yearly time intervals. At time t, $S(t)$ subjects are alive and susceptible and the remaining $I(t)$ living subjects are already infected with HIV. The chance that a susceptible would be infected by M randomly selected contacts in year t is

$$1 - \{1 - \beta y(t)\}^M. \tag{9.13}$$

Here $y(t) = I(t)/\{I(t) + S(t)\}$ is the proportion of living persons in the population who are infected at year t, and equation (9.13) follows from the fact that $\beta y(t)$ is the chance that any individual partner will be infected and will transmit HIV during the relationship. Equation (9.13) is very nearly equal to

$$\gamma(t) \equiv 1 - \exp\{-\beta\mu y(t)\}. \tag{9.14}$$

Indeed, equation (9.14) is exactly equal to the expected value of equation (9.13) if M follows a Poisson distribution with mean μ (Dietz and Schenzle, 1985) and is numerically very close to equation (9.13) more generally (Gail, Preston, and Piantadosi, 1989). From equation (9.14) we see that the probability of transmission depends on the product $k = \beta\mu$, which mainly determines the initial rate of growth of the epidemic, as in model (9.1).

Annual increments in the susceptible and infected groups are given by the following difference equations:

$$S(t + 1) - S(t) = - S(t)\{\lambda_0 + (1 - \lambda_0)\pi$$
$$+ (1 - \lambda_0)(1 - \pi)\gamma(t)\} + c \qquad (9.15)$$

and

$$I(t + 1) - I(t) = S(t)\{(1 - \lambda_0)(1 - \pi)\gamma(t)\}$$
$$- I(t)\{\lambda_1 + (1 - \lambda_1)\pi\}. \qquad (9.16)$$

This discrete time formulation of the epidemic model is easy to study, because equations (9.15) and (9.16) can be used to propagate the epidemic forward recursively, beginning at the initial values $S(0)$ and $I(0)$. Of course, this model is closely related to the continuous time model embodied in equation (9.1), and continuous time models can easily be generalized to allow for immigration and emigration. The strong analogy between equation (9.16) and equation (9.1) is evident if one identifies $\gamma(t)$ with $\beta\mu y(t)$, $S(t)$ with $N(t)(1 - y(t))$, $I(t)$ with $N(t)y(t)$, and λ_1 with α in the development leading to equation (9.1). Even though the same notation for β and μ has been used for epidemic models in continuous time (Section 9.2) and discrete time (Section 9.3) to emphasize the similarities, the actual values of these parameters needed to model a given epidemic differ, because the epidemic compounds continuously in the former models but only at discrete times in the latter models.

Because of the close analogy between continuous and discrete time models, it is not surprising that the logarithm of the discrete time infection curve,

$$g(t) = S(t)\{(1 - \lambda_0)(1 - \pi)\gamma(t)\}, \qquad (9.17)$$

resembles the infection curves in Figure 9.3. As an example, Gail and Brookmeyer (1988) considered a hypothetical population of 10,000 persons with initial prevalence of 5%, namely $I(0) = 500$ and constant growth constant $k = 0.8$, which is smaller than the value $k = \beta\mu = 0.1 \times 15 \doteq 1.5$ used in Section 9.2. The initial exponential growth followed by saturation seen with this model (Figure 9.5) resembles that seen with the close two-compartment models (Figures 9.3 and 9.4). However, unlike the closed population model in Section 9.2, which projects a rapid exponential decay of new infections after saturation (Figures 9.3 and 9.4), this open population model allows for an indefinite continuation of infections as new persons enter the

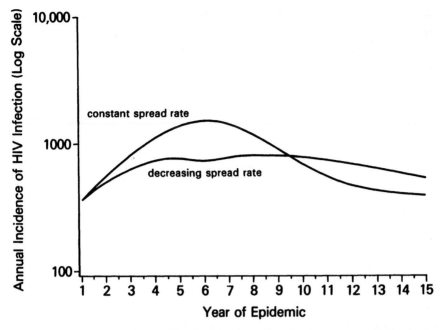

Figure 9.5 Annual AIDS incidence (the infection curve) on a logarithmic scale for an open high risk population $(k=0.8)$ of 10,000 persons as described in Section 9.3 and for an identical population with spread rate decreasing over five successive years in the sequence $k=0.8$, 0.7, 0.6, 0.5, 0.4 and remaining constant at 0.4 thereafter. (Source: Gail and Brookmeyer, 1988.)

population (Figure 9.5). This is, unfortunately, a very real possibility, in view of studies showing a continuing risk of infection among young homosexuals entering the homosexual population (San Francisco Department of Public Health, 1991). However such immigration does not account for the relatively slow decreases in $\log_e\{g(t)\}$ seen in Bacchetti's estimated locus (Figure 9.4), because Bacchetti's infection curve was estimated from closed cohorts.

9.3.2 Secular Changes in the Rate of Contact and Transmission Probability

Gail and Brookmeyer (1988) also used this discrete time model to study the effect of secular reductions in the spread constant $k = \mu\beta$. Such reductions might result either from reductions in the rate of acquiring partners, μ, or from specific behavioral changes, such as avoidance of anal sex, that reduce the chance of transmission per partnership, β. There is evidence that both such protective changes occurred in San Francisco during the 1980s (Winkelstein, Wiley, Padian, et al., 1988;

McKusick, Horstman, and Coates, 1985; Pickering, Wiley, Padian, et al., 1986). To mimic those improvements, Gail and Brookmeyer let $k = 0.8$ in year 1, 0.7 in year 2, 0.6 in year 3, 0.5 in year 4 and 0.4 in year 5 and thereafter (Figure 9.5). After an initial subexponential phase, the infection curve remained nearly flat for over 10 years. Anderson, Blythe, Gupta, and Konings (1989) and Anderson (1989) discuss the effects of behavioral changes using continuous time epidemic models.

9.3.3 Nonconstant Mortality Rate

To study the impact of the assumption that α remains constant on the scale of time since infection, Anderson, Medley, May, and Johnson (1986) compared this model with a more realistic model of the AIDS incubation distribution that allowed the hazard of AIDS to be small initially and to increase with time since infection. To make the models comparable, each was chosen to have the same mean AIDS incubation period, D. The model with increasing hazard exhibited a slight acceleration of the epidemic, compared to the simple model with the exponential AIDS incubation distribution. This result is plausible because the initial exponential growth rate of the model with constant AIDS hazard, α, is $k^* = \mu\beta - \alpha$, which is slightly smaller than the initial exponential growth rate for the model with increasing AIDS hazard. The latter model has a very small initial hazard of AIDS, resulting in an initial growth rate of about $\mu\beta$. Note, however, that the reproductive rate, $R_o = \mu\beta D$, is the same for both models. Castillo-Chavez, Cooke, Huang, and Levin (1989a, 1989b) provide further details.

9.3.4 Nonconstant Infectivity

The simple model in Section 9.2 also assumes that the per partner infectivity, β, does not depend on the duration of infection in the infected partner. Hyman and Stanley (1988); Anderson (1988b); and Anderson, Blythe, Gupta, and Konings (1989) studied models in which the infectivity, β, was regarded as a function of time since infection. Holding the average value of β constant, these authors found that models with higher initial infectivity led to accelerated epidemics compared to models with higher infectivity later in the course of infection. This result is again plausible because the initial exponential growth rate $k^* = \mu\beta - \alpha$ would be higher, initially, in the models with higher initial infectivity.

9.4 HETEROGENEOUS SUBGROUPS AND THE IMPORTANCE OF MIXING PATTERNS

9.4.1 The Role of Selective Mixing

The simple two-compartment models in Sections 9.2 and 9.3 ignore the fact that real populations are not homogeneous. It is usually more realistic to regard populations as consisting of subgroups with various levels of risk behavior and to study the impact of such heterogeneity of risk behavior and of various possible mixing patterns that describe how frequently members of these subpopulations interact to transmit infection. Such subgroups could differ not only in their rates of new partnership formation, μ, but in their transmission probabilities per partnership, β, and in their initial infection prevalences, y_o.

May and Anderson (1987) cite data documenting the enormous variability in the numbers of sexual partners per year found among homosexual or bisexual men, both in the United States and in the United Kingdom. For example, unpublished data from London in 1984 indicated that nearly half the men surveyed had reported between 6 and 50 partners per year. However, about 3% reported no partners and about 5% reported more than 100 partners per year.

Ignoring such heterogeneity and using the simple two-compartment model with average values of μ and β is misleading in two respects. This "average" model underestimates the early growth rate of the epidemic. Over the longer term the average model mistakenly implies exponential growth and overestimates the rate of rise of seroprevalence in the population as a whole. In fact, heterogeneity induces subexponential growth of the epidemic, especially if members of various subgroups selectively form most new partnerships with members of their own subgroups.

To see how ignoring heterogeneity can yield an unrealistic model of the epidemic, consider the instructive case in which the entire population of size N is composed of "unlinked" subgroups, with sizes N_i, contact rates μ_i, common transmission possibilities $\beta_i = \beta$ and common initial prevalences $y_i(0) = y_o$. By "unlinked" we mean that contacts are completely confined within subgroups. This is an example of complete "selectivity", because no contacts occur among subgroups. If we ignored this structure and assumed that the epidemic would grow like a simple two-compartment epidemic with mean contact rate $\bar{\mu} = (\Sigma N_i \mu_i)/N$ and size $N = \Sigma N_i$, we would calculate from equation (9.8) that the initial infection curve would grow exponentially according to

$$N\beta y_o \bar{\mu} \exp\{(\bar{\mu}\beta - \alpha)t\}. \tag{9.17}$$

In fact, from (9.8), the composite epidemic will have an initial infection curve

$$\Sigma \, \mathcal{N}_i \beta y_o \mu_i \exp\{(\mu_i \beta - \alpha)t\}.$$

For small t, the exponential term can be expanded in Taylor series and the values $\bar{\mu} = (\Sigma \mathcal{N}_i \mu_i)/\mathcal{N}$ and $\sigma^2 = \{\Sigma(\mu_i - \bar{\mu})^2 \mathcal{N}_i\}/\mathcal{N}$ substituted to yield the approximation

$$\mathcal{N}\beta y_o \bar{\mu} \exp[\{\beta(\bar{\mu} + \sigma^2/\bar{\mu}) - \alpha\}t]. \tag{9.18}$$

The ratio of equation (9.18) to equation (9.17) is $\exp(t\beta\sigma^2/\bar{\mu})$, which exceeds unity and indicates that heterogeneity accelerates the earliest phases of the infection curve, compared to a homogeneous population with the average contact rate, $\bar{\mu}$. In essence, the promiscuous subgroups have a profound effect on the earliest portions of the composite infection curve. Anderson, Medley, May, and Johnson (1986) obtained the result in equation (9.18) for the case of free mixing (proportionate mixing) across subgroups.

Over the longer term, heterogeneity tends to retard aggregate epidemic growth. For example, in the previous case of unlinked subgroups, the rate of growth of the aggregate epidemic decreases progressively as the subgroups with high contact rates saturate and the subsequent new infections arise in subgroups with lower contact rates. This pattern results in markedly subexponential growth of the infection curve and lower composite seroprevalence rates than a homogeneous population with the same mean contact rate, $\bar{\mu}$. Indeed, the epidemic would die out in those subgroups with reproductive rates less than unity, resulting in final seroprevalences less than 100%.

Even though the simple model with completely unlinked subgroups is unrealistic, the results it yields regarding early acceleration of the epidemic and subsequent retardation are found with more realistic models of mixing. Koopman, Simon, Jacquez, et al. (1988) studied composite AIDS incidence as a function of "selectiveness", which they defined as the proportion of new partnerships reserved exclusively within subgroups of the population. A population of homosexual men was partitioned into five subgroups with differing rates of new partnership formation, μ. New partnerships that were not reserved exclusively within subgroups were allocated at random among members of the entire population. If the selectiveness is 1.0, the subgroups are completely unlinked, and if the selectiveness is 0.0, there is free mixing. Koopman, Simon, Jacquez, et al. (1988) showed that increasing selectivity accelerated AIDS incidence in the earliest phase of the epidemic in this heterogeneous population but reduced AIDS incidence rates later. Thus the selective mixing model used by Koopman, Simon, Jacquez, et al. (1988), which was developed by Jacquez, Simon, Koopman, et al. (1988), accounts for the early subexponential growth seen, for example, in the infection curve estimated by Bacchetti for homosexuals in San Francisco (Figure 9.4).

Other theoretical models of structured mixing are obtained by partitioning the contacts of various subgroups into social "activity groups" (Jacquez, Simon, and Koopman, 1989; Koopman, Simon, Jacquez, and Park, 1989; Sattenspiel, 1987). Dietz (1988) and Dietz and Hadeler (1988) consider a very important related idea of high selectivity within heterosexual pairs by dividing the heterosexual population into eight compartments according to whether an individual is male or female, infected or not infected, and paired in a sexual relationship with a member of the opposite sex or not. The durability of pairings has an important influence on the spread of the epidemic because durable pairs of uninfected partners are not at risk of infection.

If many risk groups are indexed by a continuous variable, such as the number of new partnerships formed per unit time, and if new partnerships are highly concentrated within the same or adjacent risk groups only, one can think of the epidemic as a "saturation wave of infection among risk groups moving from high to low risk" (Colgate, Stanley, Hyman, et al., 1988; Hyman and Stanley, 1988). Such a model accounts for subexponential growth from the beginning of the epidemic. This idea would also seem to be very important in taking age structure into account in demographic studies, because new partnership formation tends to be restricted to persons with similar ages in many societies. However, an analysis of this type suggests that sex between older men and younger women contributes importantly to the spread of AIDS in Africa (Knolle, 1990).

9.4.2 General Mixing Patterns and Other Effects of Heterogeneity

A general approach to modeling heterogeneity in discrete time is to divide the population into sub-groups of size N_i, to let μ_{ij} be the average number of new partnerships that a member of population i will form with members of population j each year, and to let β_{ij} be the probability that a susceptible person in population i will be infected during the period of an average relationship with an infected member of population j. Note that μ_{ij} and β_{ij} need not be symmetric, although the average annual number of new partnerships formed between members of populations i and j, namely $c_{ij} = N_i\mu_{ij} = N_j\mu_{ji}$ is symmetric. The probability that a member of population i will become infected in year t is given by

$$\gamma_i(t) = 1 - \exp\left\{\sum_j \mu_{ij}\beta_{ij}y_j(t)\right\}, \tag{9.19}$$

in an extension of the notation used in equation (9.14) (see also Gail and Brookmeyer, 1988; and Gail, Preston, and Piantadosi, 1989). A high risk subgroup, i, has large values of $\mu_{i+} = \Sigma_j\mu_{ij}$ and/or large values of β_{ij}.

Gail and Brookmeyer (1988) studied the effects of mixing a high-risk population of 10,000 persons with initial prevalence 5% with a much larger low risk population of 90,000 persons with initial prevalence 1%. They assumed $\beta_{11} = 0.05$ and $\beta_{12} = \beta_{21} = \beta_{22} = 0.1$, on the grounds that relationships involving the low-risk population might last longer and have greater chances of transmission. This assumption is open to debate, however (Chapter 2). Other parameters are defined in the legend to Figure 9.6. Rather than assume selective mixing, Gail and

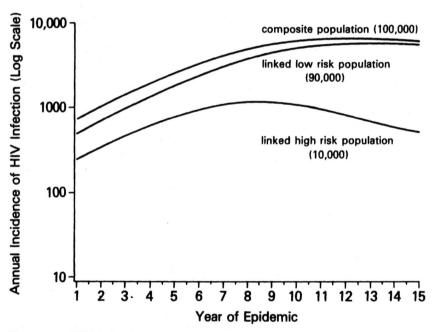

Figure 9.6 HIV infection curves in a composite population consisting of 10,000 high risk individuals with 5% initial HIV prevalence and a low risk population of 90,000 individuals with 1% initial prevalence. Assumed parameter values are $I_1(0)=500$, $S_1(0)=9500$, $\mu_{11}=7.529$, $\mu_{12}=8.471$, $I_2(0)=900$, $S_2(0)=89,100$, $\mu_{21}=0.941$, $\mu_{22}=1.059$, $c_1=411$ per year, $c_2=3696$ per year, $\beta_{11}=0.05$ and $\beta_{12}=\beta_{21}=\beta_{22}=0.1$.

Brookmeyer assumed free mixing between the low- and high-risk populations. This assumption has been termed "proportionate mixing" (Nold, 1980) because the μ_{i+} contacts from subgroup i are allocated to group j in proportion to the total contacts among members of subgroup j, namely

$$\mu_{ij} = \mu_{i+}(\mu_{j+}N_j)\left(\sum_{l=1}^{I} \mu_{l+}N_l\right)^{-1}. \tag{9.20}$$

An equivalent definition of proportionate mixing is

$$c_{ij} = c_{i+}c_{+j}/c_{++}. \tag{9.21}$$

Under these assumptions, we note from Figure 9.6 that the infection curve of the high-risk population grows more slowly than when the high-risk population was isolated (Figure 9.5) because about half of its contacts are with the low-risk population. Nonetheless, the infection curve of the linked high risk population reaches a maximum value by year 8, after which its contribution to the aggregated annual incidence declines. The infection curve of the low-risk linked population exhibits rapid exponential growth because it is driven by contact with the high-risk population. The composite annual incidence rate shows a growth pattern similar to that of the low-risk subgroup, namely initial exponential growth followed by a subexponential growth phase. This pattern is very similar to that seen for the aggregated epidemic of AIDS cases in the United States (Figure 1.1). Compared to models that allow for selective mixing, models with proportional mixing lead to more rapid involvement of low-risk subgroups and a longer exponential growth phase of the aggregate epidemic (Koopman, Simon, Jacquez, et al., 1988; Colgate, Stanley, Hyman, et al., 1988; Hyman and Stanley, 1988). Even under proportionate mixing, however, the composite prevalence of infection rises more slowly, the greater the heterogeneity in risk behavior (Anderson, Medley, May, and Johnson, 1986).

Another type of heterogeneity consists of variation in the stage of the epidemic in different subpopulations. For example, different geographic areas may have different prevalences at the time when the epidemic begins to be observed. This phenomenon is illustrated by a high-risk population with initial prevalence 5% linked to a similar high-risk population with 0% initial prevalence (Figure 9.7). See the legend to Figure 9.7 for precise parameter values. The epidemic in the first population saturates while the epidemic in the second population is entering its subexponential phase. The composite epidemic grows subexponentially and then undulates. This example illustrates that the

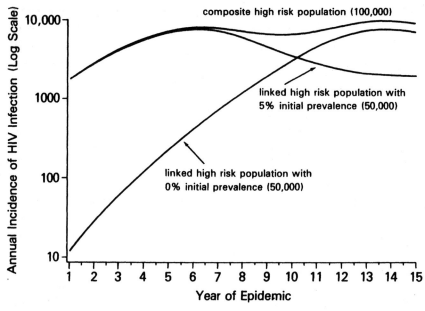

Figure 9.7 HIV infection curves in a composite population consisting of two linked high risk subpopulations at different stages of epidemic development. Each subpopulation contains 50,000 members, but one subpopulation has initial HIV prevalence 5%, whereas the other has initial prevalence 0%. The assumed parameter values are $I_1(0)=2500$, $S_1(0)=47,500$, $I_2(0)=0$, $S_2(0)=50,000$, $\mu_{11}=16$, $\mu_{12}=0.1$, $\mu_{21}=0.1$, $\mu_{22}=16$ and $\beta_{11}=\beta_{12}=\beta_{21}=\beta_{22}=0.05$.

composite infection curve can be hard to predict when subpopulations at various stages of the epidemic are aggregated. Some work has been done on the effects of aggregating spatially and temporally distinct epidemics and of studying linkages between epidemics in different locations (Gould, 1988; Golub and Gorr, 1990). The models of Blower, Hartel, Dowlatabadi, et al. (1991) suggest that temporary stabilization of HIV seroprevalence rates in populations of intravenous drug users in New York City may have resulted from interactions with the heterosexual population and from heterogeneity of risk behaviors among intravenous drug users.

9.5 EVALUATING PREVENTION STRATEGIES

A good model of epidemic growth could be used to determine which parameters had the greatest impact on the course of the epidemic and to evaluate prevention strategies to change those parameters. Even though quantitative projections of the course of the epidemic are sensitive to many unknown parameters (Section 9.2), a particular prevention strategy may yield good benefits over a wide range of assumptions and parameter values. As part of an evaluation of potential prevention strategies based on epidemic models, it is important to determine whether the proposed strategies are, in fact, robust, to model assumptions.

Simply sketching out a compartmental model as in Figure 9.1 can be a useful step in identifying possible points for prevention activities. Steps to reduce probabilities of transmission, β_{ij}, and to reduce new exposure encounters, μ_{ij}, especially among high-risk groups, can retard the epidemic. Steps to sever linkages between high- and low-risk groups by reducing contacts, μ_{ij}, can prevent spread to the low-risk groups.

One can gain additional insight into prevention strategies by examining conditions required for epidemic growth in linked subpopulations. Suppose there are I subpopulations with prevalences y_i. The epidemic will be farthest from saturation and will have its greatest potential for growth if all y_i are near zero, in which case the generalization of equation (9.1) to multiple populations (Bremermann and Anderson, 1990; Hethcote and Yorke, 1984) is

$$\frac{dy_i}{dt} = (\mu_{ii}\beta_{ii} - \alpha)y_i(1 - y_i) + (1 - y_i)\sum_{j \neq i} \mu_{ij}\beta_{ij}y_j \qquad (9.22)$$

$$\doteq (\mu_{ii}\beta_{ii} - \alpha)y_i + \sum_{j \neq i} \mu_{ij}\beta_{ij}y_j. \qquad (9.23)$$

Equation (9.23) is zero for all $i = 1, 2, \ldots, I$ and for $y_i \neq 0$ only when the y_i are eigenvectors corresponding to the eigenvalues of the $I \times I$ matrix of coefficients of y_i in (9.23). In fact, the epidemic will grow if the dominant eigenvalue of the matrix $\{\mu_{ij}\beta_{ij}\}$ exceeds α, and the basic reproductive ratio of the epidemic can be defined as $R_o = \{\text{maximal eigenvalue of } (\mu_{ij}\beta_{ij})\}/\alpha$.

As an illustration, consider a population containing $n_1 = 1000$ heterosexuals with $\mu_{1+} = 5$ and $n_2 = 9000$ heterosexuals with $\mu_{2+} = 1$, and assume $\beta = \beta_{11} = \beta_{12} = \beta_{21} = \beta_{22} = 0.05$ and $\alpha = 0.1$. Assume proportionate mixing. Then one calculates $c_{11} = 1785.7$, $c_{12} = c_{21} = 3214.3$ and $c_{22} = 5785.7$. It follows that $\mu_{11} = 1.786$, $\mu_{12} = 3.214$, $\mu_{21} = 0.357$ and $\mu_{22} = 0.643$. For arbitrary β, the eigenvalue equation is $(1.786\beta - \lambda)(0.643\beta - \lambda) - (3.214\beta)(0.357\beta) = 0$, which yields maximum eigenvalue $\lambda = 2.429\beta$. For $\beta = 0.05$ and $\alpha = 0.1$, $R_o = 2.429\beta/\alpha = 1.214$, indicating that the epidemic will grow initially.

Now suppose two prevention strategies are being considered. One is a wide-ranging publicity campaign to encourage the use of condoms. If the effects of this campaign were to reduce β from 0.05 to 0.04, R_o would be reduced to $2.429 \times 0.04/0.1 = 0.97$, just below the level needed for epidemic growth. An alternative strategy is to focus the campaign on the 1000 members of the higher risk subgroup in an effort to reduce μ_{1+} to 4 and $\beta_{11} = \beta_{12} = \beta_{21}$ to 0.04. Under this strategy, $\mu_{2+} = 1$ and $\beta_{22} = 0.05$ are unaffected. Then, under proportionate mixing, $\mu_{11} = 1.231$, $\mu_{12} = 2.769$, $\mu_{21} = 0.308$ and $\mu_{22} = .692$, and the largest eigenvalue of $(\mu_{ij}\beta_{ij})$ is $\lambda = 0.0796$, leading to a basic reproductive ratio of $R_o = \lambda/\alpha = .796$. Under these assumptions, this strategy would be more effective in preventing the initial spread of the epidemic than the previous strategy. Note that a strategy that severed all linkage between the two subgroups could stop the epidemic in the lower risk subgroup for which $R_o = \mu\beta/\alpha = 1 \times 0.05/0.01 = 0.5$, but this strategy would allow rapid initial spread in the high-risk subgroup for which $R_o = 5 \times .05/0.1 = 2.5$. Diekmann, Heesterbeek, and Metz (1990) give very general methods for computing the basic reproductive ratio for complex epidemic models.

The previous examples only dealt with the initial growth phase and included no sensitivity analyses. By contrast, Gail, Preston, and Piantadosi (1989) evaluated the effects of a voluntary confidential screening program for HIV by carrying out projections in hypothetical populations of 100,000 persons over a 15-year time span and by considering a wide range of model assumptions and parameter values. They considered several measures of the effectiveness of intervention, including the absolute numbers of infections prevented over given time spans and the *economic ratio* (ER), which is defined as the number of HIV screening tests required to prevent one infection. The methods used allowed for selective mixing among subgroups, and for migration into and out of the study population. Compartmental models were adapted to evaluating potential screening programs by dividing susceptible and infected populations into three compartments: Those who had been tested as HIV positive previously; those who had been tested as HIV negative in the preceeding year; and those who had never tested positive and were untested in the preceeding year. Under a wide range of assumptions on the behavioral changes induced by knowledge of a positive HIV test, including some special studies allowing for perverse reactions to this information, Gail, Preston, and Piantadosi found that hundreds or thousands of infections could be prevented in high-risk populations, with economic ratios of 100 or less. In isolated low-risk populations with 0.1% initial prevalence, ER values of 2000 or more were found and only a few infections were prevented. In a mixed population of very active gays, other gays, bisexuals, and male and female heterosexuals, it was found that a voluntary confidential testing program aimed primarily at the gay and bisexual subgroups prevented more disease in the heterosexual population and had lower ER values than a program that tested all subpopulations equally. Although it may not be possible to make precise estimates of the gains from a voluntary confidential testing program by using epidemic models, the broad conclusions remain valid over a wide range of parameter values and model assumptions and seem to accord well with the experience and policies adopted by public health experts (Institute of Medicine, 1988).

Van Druten, Reintjes, Jager, et al. (1990) studied the effects of programs to prevent needle sharing among intravenous drug abusers in linked populations of highly promiscuous homosexual and bisexual men, less promiscuous homosexual and bisexual men, intravenous drug abusing men and women, and heterosexual men and women. This analysis requires replacing terms like $\mu_{ij}\beta_{ij}$ in equation (9.22) with sums of such terms over various modes of HIV transmission, such as sexual transmission and transmission via shared drug paraphernalia. The results from this model suggest that blocking needle sharing may benefit both intravenous drug abusers and promiscuous heterosexual men and women. Peterson, Willard, Altmann, et al. (1990) developed models that focus on various subpopulations of intravenous drug abusers defined by frequency of use. They found that interventions to reduce needle sharing produce good benefits within five years in heavy users with substantial initial prevalence rates. Thus, as for voluntary confidential testing, the quantitative benefits of the intervention depend on the stage of the epidemic. Kaplan (1989) developed a detailed model of how injection equipment is shared in "shooting" galleries and described calculations to determine the effectiveness of programs to encourage cleansing or disinfecting the injection equipment.

9.6 STOCHASTIC EPIDEMIC MODELS

The previous models (except for Peterson, Willard, Altmann, et al., 1990) are deterministic in the sense that once the initial conditions and parameters are specified, the prevalence function and infection curves are uniquely determined and can be found by recursive methods, as for example in equations (9.15) and (9.16). Such models adequately describe the course of an epidemic in large populations with large numbers infected, because in such populations statistical variations in the occurrence of events for particular individuals have little influence on the epidemic as a whole. By contrast, the random timimg and occurrence of events in small populations or populations with small numbers infected can induce substantial unpredictability as to how the epidemic will develop, even given exact initial conditions, and much theoretical effort has been devoted to the development of stochastic epidemic models (Bailey, 1975; Becker, 1989). From such models one can calculate the probability that the epidemic will die out, the expected value of the prevalence function, and a prediction interval for the prevalence function. In large populations with large numbers infected, the mean prevalence function from a stochastic model will converge to the corresponding deterministic prevalence function. Tan and Hsu (1989) studied the effects of stochastic variation in a population of 100,000 individuals. If only 10 individuals have been infected initially, the expected number infected at 20 months was computed to be 160 with variance 1600 and coefficient of variation $1600^{1/2}/160 = .25$. If, instead, 10,000 persons were infected initially, the expected number infected at 20 months was calculated as 30,000 with variance 60,000 and coefficient of variation $60,000^{1/2}/30,000 = 0.008$. Thus, there is negligible variation about the expected prevalence at 20 months if larger numbers are infected initially, but considerable uncertainty if only 10 are infected initially. Tan (1992) discusses such stochastic models in detail.

Although stochastic epidemic models may be useful for special studies in limited geographic areas or subgroups, such as the study of Peterson, Willard, Altmann, et al. (1990) on the variability of epidemics in small drug-using communities, these models require additional assumptions on probability structure, and calculations are more difficult than for deterministic models. In addition, most interest centers on determining the expected prevalence function and infection curve in large populations. For these reasons, most of the literature on AIDS modeling has focused on deterministic models that are elaborate enough to describe important features of the prevalence function and infection curve.

9.7 COMPARING PARAMETERS IN EPIDEMIC MODELS WITH EMPIRICAL ESTIMATES OF DOUBLING TIMES AND HIV PREVALENCE RATIOS

9.7.1 Homosexual and Bisexual Males

The San Francisco infection curve for homosexual men (Figure 1.5) estimated by Bacchetti (1990) has a doubling time of about 3 months in

July 1978, 5 months in January 1979, and 8 months in July 1979. Data from the San Francisco City Clinic Cohort also indicate a doubling time of about 8 months in early 1979 (Winkelstein, Samuel, and Padian, 1987). We shall try to use this information to obtain an indirect estimate of the probability of transmission per partnership, β.

Winkelstein, Lyman, Padian, et al. (1987) obtained information from a probability sample in June 1984 through January 1985 on the numbers of male sexual partners that each sampled gay man had had in the previous 2 years. Of 796 sampled gay men, 17 had had 0 partners, 66 had had 1 partner, 206 had had 2–9 partners, 312 had had 10–49 partners and 195 had had 50 or more partners. If we assume that the average numbers of contacts were 5.5 for the 2–9 category, 29.5 for the 10–49 category and 60 for the 50+ category, the mean number of contacts is 27.77 and the variance is 459.89. On a per-year basis, the mean and variance are $\bar{\mu} = 13.88$ and $\sigma^2 = 114.97$.

Because there is substantial heterogeneity in sexual behavior, it could be misleading to simply apply equations like (9.6) or (9.8) with the mean number of contacts per year $\bar{\mu} = 13.88$ in place of μ. One approximation is to assume that the rapid early phase of the epidemic represents infections in a homogeneous isolated high risk subpopulation with a contact rate μ substantially greater than $\bar{\mu}$. Letting $\mu = 100$ or 50 yields a range of estimates of β from 0.008 to 0.055, depending on μ and the doubling time (Table 9.1). If one further assumes that risk of infection only derives from partners who engage in anal/genital sex, estimates of β increase. Available data suggest that about one-third of partnerships result in anal/genital sex (McKusick, Horstman, and Coates, 1985; Winkelstein, Samuel, and Padian, 1987). Multiplying the previous estimates by 3 yields values of β ranging from 0.025 to 0.166, in reasonable agreement with the value 0.102 obtained from a prospective evaluation of gay men who engage in anal/genital sex (see Section 2.5.4, and Grant, Wiley, and Winkelstein, 1987).

The previous calculation was based on the assumption that the early doubling time is determined by an isolated high risk subpopulation. This is an extreme example of selectivity in a heterogeneous population. An alternative approach is to assume proportionate mixing in a heterogeneous population (Anderson, Medley, May, and Johnson, 1986; May and Anderson, 1987; Anderson and May, 1988). The "effective" rate of contact becomes $(\bar{\mu} + \sigma^2/\bar{\mu})$ instead of $\bar{\mu}$, just as in equation (9.18). Using the value $\bar{\mu} = 13.9$ and $\sigma^2 = 115$ from Winkelstein, Lyman, and Padian (1987), one estimates β to be between 0.038 and 0.125 for all partnerships. Setting $\mu = 13.9/3$ and $\sigma^2 = 115/9$ for partnerships involving anal/genital sex, one estimates β to be between 0.112 and 0.375 (Table 9.1).

Table 9.1 Estimates of the Transmission Probability per Partnership (β), Based on Doubling Times in the Infection Curve in Gay Men in San Francisco

	Range of Doubling Times (months)		
	3	8	10
All partnerships			
Epidemic model			
Homogeneous high risk population[a]			
$\mu = 100$ partners/yr	.028	.010	.008
$\mu = 50$ partners/yr	.055	.021	.017
Proportionate mixing[b]			
$(\bar{\mu} + \sigma^2/\bar{\mu}) = 13.9 + 115/13.9$	.125	.047	.038
Only partnerships involving anal/genital sex			
Epidemic model			
Homogeneous high risk population[a]			
$\mu = 100/3$ partners/yr	.083	.031	.025
$\mu = 50/3$ partners/yr	.166	.062	.050
Proportionate mixing[b]			
$(\bar{\mu} + \sigma^2/\bar{\mu}) = 4.63 + 12.8/4.63$	.375	.141	.112

[a]Calculation is based on equation (9.9) except that $k = \mu\beta$ is used instead of $k^* = \mu\beta - \alpha$, because mortality is very low shortly after infection.

[b]Based on equation (9.9) except that $k = (\bar{\mu} + \sigma^2/\bar{\mu})\beta$ is used in place of k^*.

It is clear that both of these approaches are very approximate, not only because key parameters are imprecisely known, but also because the models themselves are oversimplified in their treatment of heterogeneity and selectivity. It is encouraging that an approach based on complete selectivity and an approach based on proportionate mixing both yield estimates of β in reasonable accord with empirical data for homosexual partnerships involving anal/genital sex. By contrast, ignoring heterogeneity would lead to serious overestimates of β. For example, if one assumed a homogeneous population with $\bar{\mu}/3 = 4.63$ partnerships per year involving anal/genital contact, estimates of β in Table 9.1 would range from .18 to .60, depending on the assumed doubling time. These estimates substantially exceed the value 0.10 estimated by prospective follow-up of gay men (Grant, Wiley, and Winkelstein, 1987),

9.7.2 Heterosexual Populations

In the United States and other developed countries, it is misleading to interpret doubling times for people infected through heterosexual sex using calculations such as those in Table 9.1, because many infections in heterosexuals arise from contact with bisexual men and with intravenous drug users. Simple epidemic models might be more applicable in regions such as Africa, where most transmission is thought to be related to heterosexual contact (Anderson, May, Boily, et al., 1991).

Equation (9.23) defines a simple epidemic model for initial heterosexual spread, where $i = 1$ corresponds to the male and $i = 2$ to the female subpopulation. Note that $\mu_{11} = \mu_{22} = 0$. Letting $\phi = (\mu_{12}\beta_{12}/\mu_{21}\beta_{21})^{1/2}$ and $k = (\mu_{12}\beta_{12}\mu_{21}\beta_{21})^{1/2}$, we can write the solution for males as

$$y_1(t) = 0.5(y_{10} + \phi y_{20}) \exp\{(k - \alpha)t\}$$
$$+ 0.5(y_{10} - \phi y_{20}) \exp\{- (k + \alpha)t\}, \qquad (9.24)$$

where y_{10} and y_{20} are the initial prevalences in males and females respectively. The prevalence for females is given by equation (9.24) with y_{20}, y_{10} and ϕ^{-1} replacing y_{10}, y_{20} and ϕ respectively.

Equation (9.24) has several implications:

1. After a short period, the second term becomes negligible, and the epidemic enters an exponential phase with growth constant $(k - \alpha)$ in both males and females (May and Anderson, 1987).
2. The epidemic will only grow if $k > \alpha$. Indeed, the basic reproductive ratio $R_o = k/\alpha$, because the maximal eigenvalue of $\{\mu_{ij}\beta_{ij}\}$ is k.
3. During the exponential growth phase, the prevalence ratio is $y_1(t)/y_2(t) = \phi$.

Extensions of this model to allow for heterogeneity in the rate of forming new partnerships show that one should replace μ_{12} and μ_{21} by "effective" contact rates such as $\mu_{12}^* = \bar{\mu}_{12} + \sigma_{12}^2/\bar{\mu}_{12}$ as in the previous section (May and Anderson, 1988; Diekmann, Heesterbeek, and Metz, 1990).

We apply these ideas to data on sexual practices and HIV prevalence among men and women attending outpatient clinics in rural Uganda (Hudson, Hennis, Kataaha, et al., 1988). Men attending outpatient clinics claimed to have had 2.8 sexual partners on average in the last 5 years compared to 1.5 for women. We shall assume that the corresponding annual rates of acquisition of new partners are $2.8/5 = 0.56$/year and $1.5/5 = 0.30$/year, even though specific data on numbers of new partners were not reported. Of 81 males over age 20, 4 (4.9%) had antibodies to HIV compared to 6 of 83 females (7.2%), yielding a male-to-female prevalence ratio of 0.68. This is similar to the sex ratios 0.70, 0.64 and 0.85 observed in three other rural areas of Uganda (Berkley, Naamara, Okware, et al., 1990). In two of those

These limitations arise because quantitative projections are very sensitive to initial sizes and HIV prevalences in subpopulations, to transmission probability parameters β_{ij}, and to the rates and distributions of new exposure-producing contacts among and within subpopulations. This sensitivity also affects the reliability of studies of risk factors for HIV transmission, because odds ratios and relative risks depend on the stage of the epidemic, and because many potentially important confounders must be controlled.

Although simple epidemic models for isolated populations and for linked populations with proportional mixing suggest that the aggregate epidemic will grow exponentially initially before entering a subexponential phase, more realistic models that allow both for substantial heterogeneity of risk behavior and for selectivity in mixing predict subexponential growth from the beginning of the epidemic. This subexponential pattern was observed among homosexual men in San Francisco, for example (Figure 9.4).

There is rough agreement of quantities such as the doubling time and the ratio of the prevalence of HIV among males to that in females, which are observable in studies of populations, with estimates of these quantities from epidemic models that incorporate data on contact rates and transmission probabilities.

The shape of the epidemic curve over the longer term is hard to predict, especially if incident cases from temporally separated subepidemics are aggregated or if behaviors change over time. The pattern of exposure linkages among subpopulations can have an important impact on the course of the epidemic. A high degree of segregation among heterogeneous subpopulations tends to accelerate the earliest phases of the epidemic but reduces the aggregate prevalence later.

Epidemic models may offer useful leads in planning intervention strategies. Outlining compartmental models such as Figure 9.1 may indicate potential interventions and highlight important missing information. More formal consideration of the basic reproductive ratio to evaluate the earliest phase of the epidemic and projections over a 15-year span may give qualitative insight as to which prevention strategies are most promising.

10

Synthesizing Data Sources and Methods for Assessing the Scope of the Epidemic

10.1 INTRODUCTION

In the preceeding chapters, we reviewed four methodological approaches for assessing the scope of the epidemic: surveys of HIV prevalence (Chapter 3); extrapolations of the AIDS incidence curve (Chapter 7); back-calculation methods (Chapter 8); and epidemic models of HIV transmission (Chapter 9). The objective of this chapter is to briefly review the strengths and limitations of these methodologies and to consider hybrid approaches that combine information from various sources. In particular, we review hybrid approaches that have been proposed for studying pediatric AIDS, for forecasting AIDS incidence in developing countries, and for forecasting in small geographic areas.

The selection of appropriate methodologies and data sources for tracking the epidemic depends on the specific objectives. These objectives could include: projections of AIDS incidence; estimating HIV prevalence either in the general population or in specific subgroups; estimating historical trends in infection rates; projecting future infection rates; and evaluating the impact of different prevention strategies. The best methodological approach depends on the specific objective.

For example, extrapolations of AIDS incidence data yield sensible short-term projections of AIDS incidence, but no information on infection rates. Back-calculation can be used to project AIDS incidence and provides information about past infection rates, but little information about recent infection rates and no information about future infection rates. Single cross-sectional seroprevalence surveys provide information only about current HIV prevalence, whereas serial seroprevalence surveys and ongoing follow-up studies of selected cohorts may provide useful information on recent trends in the infection rates. Transmission models provide insight into factors that can influence future infection rates.

In this chapter, we briefly review the strengths and limitations of various approaches for estimating HIV prevalence (Section 10.2) and illustrate approaches for combining data sources and methods in three examples: developing countries (Section 10.3); pediatric populations (Section 10.4); and small area estimation (Section 10.5).

10.2 COMBINING DATA AND METHODS

10.2.1 Review of Main Methodologies

HIV prevalence estimates can be obtained from either seroprevalence surveys, back-calculation methods, or epidemic models of HIV transmission. The sources of error and uncertainties with each of the approaches were reviewed in detail in the preceeding chapters (surveys, Chapter 3; back-calculation, Section 8.4; transmission models, Chapter 9). We have summarized the main sources of uncertainties with each methodology in Table 10.1 and starred (*) the most serious problems. The main problem with representative surveys is nonresponse bias. The main problem with surveys of selected populations are uncertainty about how representative these surveys are of the groups they purport to describe and uncertainty about the overall sizes of those groups (e.g., total number of IV drug users in the United States). The main problems with back-calculation are uncertainties in the incubation distribution, treatment effects that modify the incubation distribution, and inherent statistical imprecision for estimating recent infection rates. In many developing countries, surveillance systems to obtain counts of AIDS incidence are too unreliable for use with back-calculation. The main problems with epidemic models of transmission include uncertainties in the pattern of mixing, size of transmission groups, rates of contact, infectivity, initial HIV prevalence, and behavioral changes.

The suitability of an approach for estimating HIV prevalence depends on the risk (transmission) group. For example, back-calculation methods may be more reliable than surveys in both

Table 10.1 Sources of Error and Problems in Estimating HIV Prevalence Associated with Four Methodologies

Representative Surveys	Surveys of Selected Populations	Back-calculation	Epidemic Models of HIV Transmission
*Nonresponse bias	*Representativeness	*Incubation period	*Patterns of mixing
Expense	*Lack of data on the size of the population represented	*Treatment effects	*Rates of contact
Representativeness of survey (coverage bias)	Expense	*Imprecision of estimates of recent infection rates	*Size of transmission groups (compartments)
Assay errors	Assay errors	Errors in AIDS incidence data and reporting delay corrections	*Infectivity
		Changes in surveillance definition	*Initial HIV prevalence
		Model selection for the infection curve	*Behavioral changes
		Migration	Duration of infectiousness
			Incubation period
			Migration

Note: The items marked with a * are considered the most significant problems or sources of error.

263

homosexual and intravenuous drug using populations because of nonresponse bias and lack of representativeness of surveys in these populations and because of uncertainties in the sizes of these populations. On the other hand, nearly exhaustive HIV seroprevalence surveys among newborns provide the most valuable data for assessing the scope of the epidemic in infants and HIV prevalence in childbearing women (Section 10.4).

Fortunately, the sources of the error associated with each of these methodologies are different. Accordingly, confidence in the estimates is enhanced if the various methodologies produce consistent results.

10.2.2 Informal Approaches

The estimates obtained from these methodologies usually have been compared and combined informally. For example, based on HIV seroprevalence survey data, the CDC estimated that between 800,000 and 1.2 million Americans were infected in 1989 (Centers for Disease Control, 1990a). Estimates of HIV prevalence based on several back-calculation models ranged from 650,000 to 1.4 million. The fact that two different methodological approaches yielded estimates of seroprevalence centered at about 1 million led CDC to estimate that there were about 1 million infected Americans in 1989.

Theories of epidemic transmission offer qualitative insight into the shape of the infection curve and thus provide a check on the plausibility of back-calculated infection rates. For example, one reconstruction of the U.S. infection curve based on back-calculation with splines (Figure 8.11) showed that the epidemic quickly slowed to subexponential growth by the early 1980s. The doubling times of the epidemic (time for cumulative numbers infected to double) increased from 7.8 months in the beginning of 1981 to 12.7 months in the beginning of 1982 to 19.2 months in the beginning of 1983. According to epidemic theory this rapid increase in doubling times could result initially from diffusion of the epidemic from high to lower risk subgroups e.g., subgroups with fewer number of sexual partners) and, later, from favorable behavioral changes and also saturation effects (depletion of uninfected individuals).

Analyses similar to that in Figure 8.11 were performed for each of four transmission groups in the United States (Figure 10.1). Figure 10.1 displays reconstructed infection rates based on back-calculation with splines for homosexuals, intravenous drug users, heterosexuals, and homosexuals who use intravenous drugs (Brookmeyer, 1991). The sharp declines in infection rates among homosexual men, suggested in Figure 10.1, are corroborated by surveys and cohort studies that show

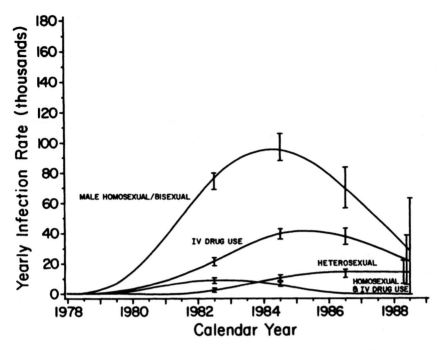

Figure 10.1 Reconstruction of infection curves in the U.S. for transmission groups based on back-calculation. (Source: Brookmeyer, 1991.)

declines both in rates of high-risk behaviors among homosexual men (McKusick, Horstman, and Coates, 1987) and in rates of rectal gonorrhea (Pickering, Wiley, Padian, et al., 1986). Surveys and cohort studies in the San Francisco homosexual population also provide direct estimates of the infection rates (see Section 3.5.1 and Table 3.8). These surveys suggest that the infection rate grew rapidly between 1977 and 1981, slowed between 1981 and 1982 and subsequently declined markedly (Winkelstein, Samuel, Padian, et al., 1987; Winkelstein, Wiley, Padian, et al., 1988; Hessol, Lifson, O'Malley, et al., 1989; Centers for Disease Control, 1987b; Bacchetti and Moss, 1989; Segal and Bacchetti, 1990). These direct surveys in San Francisco suggest that infection rates among San Francisco homosexual men peaked in late 1981 or 1982, almost 2 years earlier than the national reconstruction for the homosexual epidemic given in Figure 10.1. This difference could be explained by earlier behavioral changes or by earlier saturation and diffusion effects in San Francisco than in the rest of the nation. In any case, both the survey data from San Francisco and the reconstruction based on back-calculation suggest that the infection rate among homosexual men peaked in 1984 or even earlier and has subsequently declined markedly. However, current rates are uncertain, and there is disturbing evidence that young gay men continue to engage in high risk behaviors (San Francisco Department of Public Health, 1991).

Infection rates among intravenous drug users grew more rapidly before 1981 than after 1981 (Figure 10.1). This slowing could be explained either by behavior changes, such as reduced sharing of injection equipment, or by diffusion of the epidemic to subgroups with lower levels of high-risk behaviors. Figure 10.1 also indicates that the rapid initial phase of both the homosexual and intravenous drug user epidemic preceeded the heterosexual epidemic by several years. This finding is consistent with the fact that in the early 1980s the primary source of infection among heterosexuals was sex with a bisexual male or with an intravenous drug user. The estimated infection rate among heterosexuals remained relatively constant in the late 1980s (Figure 10.1), as is consistent with epidemic models that incorporate changes in high risk behavior (Gail and Brookmeyer, 1988).

Despite the encouraging trends estimated for infection rates in several risk groups (Figure 10.1), one should remember that information on current infection rates is subject to substantial uncertainty. Moreover, even if national trends in HIV incidence were reaching a plateau for heterosexual transmission or transmission among intravenous drug users, there are local areas where the rates of infection in these groups is still rapidly increasing (see Rosenberg, Levy, Brundage, et al. (1992) and Section 10.5). Further, one ought not be complacent even about risk groups like gay men that have exhibited decreases in infection rates. If the annual rate of seroconversion remains at 1% in this group (Table 3.8), perhaps 25,000 new HIV infections per year could result. Furthermore, one must consider the possibility that younger men who are now beginning to engage in homosexual behaviors are less likely to avoid risk behaviors than those who experienced the epidemic in the 1980s (San Francisco Department of Public Health, 1991).

10.2.3 Formal Approaches

It may be advantageous to combine information from various sources using formal statistical methods rather than by informal comparisons. For example, prior information about the shape of the infection curve could be introduced into back-calculation methods by selecting appropriate parametric models for the infection curve, $g(s; \beta)$. Epidemic theory of HIV transmission could suggest a family of parametric models for the infection curve (Chapter 9).

A formal approach for combining information from surveys and back-calculation was suggested by Brookmeyer and Liao (1990a). Suppose we have both AIDS incidence data and seroprevalence survey data. Let Y_j be the number of AIDS cases diagnosed in the jth calendar interval (T_{j-1}, T_j), Let $\hat{N}^*$ be an independent unbiased estimate of the number of HIV infected AIDS-free individuals in the population at calendar time T^* obtained from surveys. We also assume we have available a measure of precision of the estimate, $\hat{N}^*$, namely the variance, V^*. The AIDS incidence data and the survey data both provide information on the underlying infection rate $g(s; \beta)$, which we seek to estimate. For the survey data, the mean and variance of the $\hat{N}^*$ are (ignoring changes in the size of the population due to emigration or immigration and mortality)

$$E(\hat{N}^*) = \int_0^{T^*} g(s; \beta)\{1 - F(T^* - s)\}ds \qquad (10.1)$$

and

$$\mathrm{Var}(\hat{N}^*) = V^*.$$

Back-calculation (see equation 8.5) yields the relationships

$$E(Y_j) = \int_0^{T_j} g(s; \beta) \cdot [F(T_j - s)|s) - F(T_{j-1} - s|s)]ds$$

and

$$\mathrm{Var}(Y_j) = \sigma^2 E(Y_j).$$

Generalized least squares can be used to estimate the common parameters, β, of the infection curve $g(s; \beta)$ (Carroll and Ruppert, 1990).

10.3 FORECASTING IN DEVELOPING COUNTRIES

A main problem in assessing the scope of the epidemic in developing countries concerns the incompleteness of AIDS case reporting. The lack of reliable AIDS incidence data severely limits the usefulness of back-calculation or simple extrapolation methods. In these situations, HIV seroprevalence surveys rather than AIDS surveillance data become the cornerstone for forecasting.

The World Health Organization (WHO) has proposed a methodology for projecting AIDS incidence in developing countries. The

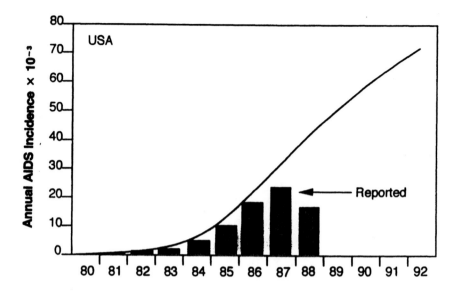

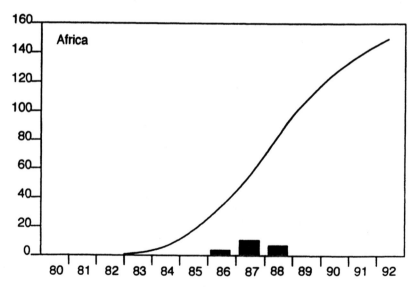

Figure 10.2 Reported and projected AIDS cases in United States, Europe, Africa and the world; the gap between the tops of the bars and the curve may reflect unreported cases. (Source: Chin and Mann, 1989. This material is reproduced by permission of the World Health Organization.)

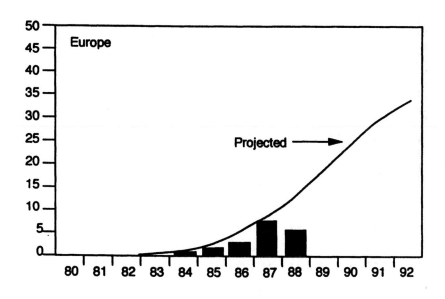

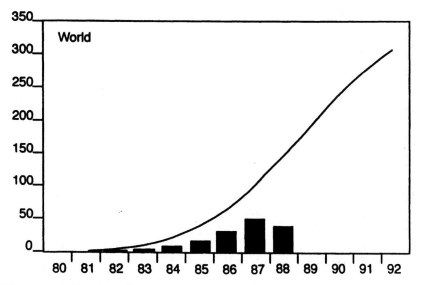

Figure 10.2 (Continued)

methodology involves back-calculating historical infection rates from seroprevalence surveys rather than from AIDS incidence data (Chin and Lwanga, 1991). The basic idea is to use survey estimates of HIV prevalence together with the incubation period distribution to reconstruct historical infection rates. These rates are then propagated forward to obtain short-term projections of AIDS incidence. Of course, many different infection curves can yield the same point prevalence estimate. The WHO methodology circumvents this problem of "nonidentifiability" by assuming a particular parametric family of infection curves. Their model assumes a unimodal infection curve of the form

$$g(s) = Kg_o(s) = K\frac{s^{p-1}e^{-s}}{(p-1)!},$$

where $g(s)$ is the infection rate at year s, and K and p are parameters. The peak of this infection curve occurs at time $t = (p-1)$. Both the calendar time of the start of the epidemic (corresponding to $s = 0$) and, the calendar time of the peak in infection rates are assumed known. These assumptions determine the shape of the infection curve, $g_o(s)$, and seroprevalence survey data are used to estimate the proportionality constant, K. It is assumed that an estimate of the number of infected AIDS-free individuals $\hat{N}$ in year T is available from seroprevalence surveys. Then, an estimate of K is

$$\hat{K} = \hat{N} \bigg/ \int_o^T g_o(s)\{1 - F(T-s)\}ds,$$

and the estimated infection curve is $g(s) = \hat{K}g_o(s)$.

The WHO obtains short-term projections of AIDS incidence by propagating forward the infection rates, $g(s)$, according to the incubation distribution. This approach has been termed *forward calculation*. For example, assuming 5 million HIV infected adults in SubSaharan Africa in 1990 (Chin, 1990; Chin and Lwanga, 1991), the WHO estimated there would be 700,000 cumulative adult AIDS cases by the end of 1990. This estimate is 10 times greater than the number of AIDS cases reported by the end of 1990 (Figure 10.2) and is indicative of substantial under-reporting of cases in parts of the developing world.

There are important sources of uncertainty in these estimates. First, the estimates strongly depend on the assumed HIV prevalence (e.g., 5 million HIV infected adults in SubSaharan Africa), which were partly based on HIV seroprevalence surveys and partly on expert opinion. Second, the estimates could be expected to be sensitive to the assumed parametric family of infection curves. Nevertheless the WHO procedure illustrates a hybrid approach to forecasting that combines different data sources (HIV seroprevalence surveys and incubation period distributions) and different analytical methods (estimation of prevalence from surveys and forward calculation).

10.4 FORECASTING PEDIATRIC AIDS

In this section, we review some methodological approaches for assessing the scope of the pediatric AIDS epidemic. The incubation period of perinatally transmitted HIV infection is somewhat shorter than for other transmission modes (Auger, Thomas, De Gruttola, 1988). Furthermore, in some settings one has access to nearly exhaustive HIV seroprevalence surveys among newborns. Thus, the preferred methodological approaches for assessing the scope of pediatric AIDS are different than for adult AIDS. Predictions for pediatric AIDS are best obtained by using several methodologies and data sources. We propose an approach for assessing the pediatric epidemic that combines empirical extrapolations, back-calculations, and HIV seroprevalence survey data. The methods are illustrated on the New York City pediatric AIDS epidemic.

Table 10.2 lists the various modes of transmission for pediatric AIDS cases in the United States. The vast majority (84%) of cases result from perinatal transmission (mother to child). Because of the shorter incubation period of pediatric AIDS, short-term forecasts of pediatric AIDS strongly depend not only on the numbers of newborns infected years ago but also on the current and future perinatal infection rates. In contrast, short-term projections of adult AIDS incidence depend

Table 10.2 Classifications of Pediatric AIDS by
Risk Group in the United States

1. Mother at risk for AIDS/HIV infection	84%
a. Mother is IVDU	42
b. Mother had sex with IVDU	17
c. Mother had sex with bisexual male	2
d. Mother born in pattern II country	8
c. Mother was transfusion recipient	2
d. Mother with other or unspecified risk	13
2. Child was recipient of blood transfusion, component or tissue	9
3. Child with hemophilia/coagulation disorder	5
4. Undetermined	2

Source: HIV/AIDS Surveillance Report, Centers for Disease Control, January 1991. Based on cases reported through December 1990.

primarily on the number of people infected several years earlier, because the risk of developing AIDS in the first few years following infection is small in adults. The annual number of perinatally infected newborns is given by (Chin, 1990),

$$\sum_i N_i f_i p, \tag{10.2}$$

where N_i is the number of infected women at age i; f_i is the proportion of women at age i who give birth in the year (i.e., the age specific fertility rate); and p is the probability of transmission from an infected mother to child. A number of different epidemiological studies have suggested that the transmission probability, p, is approximately one-third (Section 2.4.3).

A hybrid approach to forecasting AIDS in New York City, using pediatric AIDS incidence data through 1986, is summarized in four steps as follows:

1. Use pediatric AIDS incidence data through 1986, together with an estimate of the pediatric incubation period, to reconstruct perinatal infection rates for the period 1981–6, using back-calculation methods.
2. Use seroprevalence surveys among newborns in New York to estimate the perinatal infection rate in 1988.
3. Use simple regression methods to obtain a smoothed reconstruction of the perinatal infection curve for the period 1981–8. Use simple extrapolation to forecast perinatal infection rates in the short-term.
4. Propagate forward the perinatal infection rates derived in step 3 by using the incubation period to obtain projections of pediatric AIDS incidence.

Step 1.   Table 10.3 is a crossclassification of pediatric (perinatal) AIDS cases in New York City by birth year and incubation period. The incubation period for perinatally transmitted AIDS is defined as the age of AIDS diagnosis. The data in Table 10.3 are right truncated because AIDS cases with long incubation periods may not yet be diagnosed. The data structure of Table 10.3 is the same as the transfusion-associated AIDS data considered in Section 4.3 and the reporting delay data considered in Section 7.3. Methods for right truncated data outlined in Chapter 7 could be used to estimate both the incubation period distribution and the number of infected newborns by birth year.

Auger, Thomas, and De Gruttola (1988) give an estimate of the incubation period for pediatric AIDS (Table 10.4); we use this estimate to reconstruct the number of infected newborns. For example, by the end of 1987 there were 54 diagnosed AIDS cases who were born in 1986

Table 10.3 New York City Pediatric AIDS Incidence Data Crossclassified by Birth Year and Incubation Period (cases diagnosed by end of 1987)

Birth Year	Incubation Period (Years)							Cumulative Cases Diagnosed	Number Infected
	0–1	1–2	2–3	3–4	4–5	5–6	6–7		
1981	1	2	3	0	5	4	0	15	23
1982	1	4	3	1	1	0	—	10	18
1983	20	8	1	4	2	—	—	35	74
1984	20	2	3	4	—	—	—	29	75
1985	27	7	14	—	—	—	—	48	148
1986	42	12	—	—	—	—	—	54	225

Notes: Data adapted from Auger, et al. (1988). Cases include only those from perinatal transmission (i.e., mother at risk of HIV infection). Number infected is obtained by dividing cumulative cases by $F(T)$ where T is the truncation time, and F is the incubation distribution.

Table 10.4 Incubation Period for Pediatric AIDS

$F(1) = .18$	$F(6) = .60$
$F(2) = .30$	$F(7) = .70$
$F(3) = .35$	$F(8) = .85$
$F(4) = .42$	$F(9) = .92$
$F(5) = .52$	$F(10) \approx 1.00$

Source: Based on Auger, Thomas, and De Gruttola (1988).

Notes: $F(t)$ is the cumulative probability of AIDS diagnosis within t years of birth. Incubation distribution is the conditional distribution given diagnosis within 10 years. It is assumed $F(10) = 1.0$, which may be a reasonable assumption. Auger, Thomas, and De Gruttola estimate $F^*(t)$, the conditional distribution given diagnosis within 10 years. In this table it is assumed $F = F^*$, that is, $F(10) = 1.0$.

(for simplicity we assume they were all born in the middle of the year). The probability the incubation period is less than 1.5 years is approximately $F(1.5) = [F(2) + F(1)]/2 = .24$ (from Table 10.4). Thus, the estimated number of infected children born in 1986 is $54/.24 = 225$. The estimated numbers of infected children by year of birth is given in the last column of Table 10.3.

Step 2.   Novick, Berns, Stricof, et al. (1989) reported the results of an ongoing newborn seroprevalence study in New York state in the one-year period from November 30, 1987, to November 30, 1988. Blood was collected from every infant using heel-prick techniques as part of a mandatory program for the detection of hereditary disorders. Assays were performed on anonymous samples, and no identifying information was abstracted. During this period in New York City, 125,120 newborns were tested, of whom 1570 were HIV positive (1.25% HIV seropositive). Assuming a perinatal transmission rate of $p = 1/3$, one estimates $1570 \times 1/3 = 523$ perinatally transmitted infections in 1988.

Step 3.   In order to piece together the infection rates based on back-calculation (1981–6) and seroprevalence surveys (1988), the infection rates were graphically smoothed by eye (Figure 10.3). A more sophisticated analysis would regress the log infection rates on a polynomial in time, using a weighted least squares approach that accounts for the variance and covariances of the estimated infection rates. It was necessary to extrapolate Figure 10.3 to obtain future perinatal infection rates. The working assumption was that rates remained constant, at least for the very short term. Thus it was assumed there were about 523 new perinatal infections per year in 1988 and thereafter. In fact, more recent work of Novick, Glebatis, and Stricof (1991) has shown that the numbers of new seronegative infants

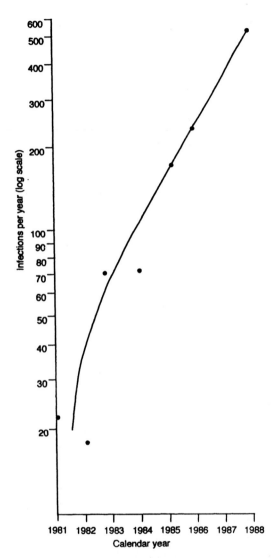

Figure 10.3 New York City pediatric (perinatal) infection rates. Estimates for 1981–86 based on back-calculation; estimate for 1988 based on seroprevalence surveys among newborns.

born each year in New York City has remained constant from November 30, 1987, to March 31, 1990.

Step 4.   The rates in Figure 10.3 were propagated forward using the incubation distribution to obtain AIDS incidence projections. For example, from the estimated 523 infections occurring in 1988 there are an expected $523 \times (.085) = 44$ AIDS cases diagnosed in 1990. The factor .085 arises by assuming that all 523 infections occurred in the middle of 1988. The probability an infant infected in the middle of 1988 would be diagnosed in 1990 is $F(2.5) - F(1.5)$, which is $[F(3) - F(1)]/2 = .085$ by linear interpolation. The results of these sorts of calculations are given in Table 10.5.

A more formal modeling approach for combining AIDS surveillance with HIV seroprevalence surveys of newborns for assessing the scope of the pediatric epidemic was described by De Gruttola, Tu, and Pagano (1992). By combining these two data sources, they estimated that approximately 10.0–12.0% of children born to infected mothers will develop AIDS by age 6. They concluded that pediatric AIDS incidence in New York City will continue to rise, but at rates smaller than those in Table 10.5, perhaps because their data suggest longer incubation periods than in Table 10.4. Their analysis suggested that the median age at diagnosis of a pediatric AIDS case will increase over the next several years.

To accurately forecast health care needs it is important to consider not only AIDS incidence but also AIDS prevalence. AIDS prevalence refers to the numbers of individuals who are alive with an AIDS diagnosis. In order to forecast AIDS prevalence, AIDS incidence would be "forward calculated" using the survival function for AIDS. Scott, Hutto, Makuch, et al. (1989) report a median survival of pediatric AIDS (time from AIDS diagnosis to death) of 38 months. Assuming an exponential survival distribution, this suggests that 80.3% of the cases that survive through the end of the current year would survive to the end of the next year. For each cohort of new AIDS cases, the factor 80.3% is successively applied to estimate the numbers of survivors by year following diagnosis. Applying such calculations to the annual AIDS incidence data in Table 10.5, one projects sharp increases in the prevalence of pediatric AIDS in New York City from fewer than 100 cases in 1985 to over 1500 cases in 1995.

This method of forecasting pediatric AIDS depends on a number of data sources and methods. The results are therefore subject to several sources of uncertainty. The results are sensitive to the estimated recent perinatal infection rate based on seroprevalence surveys (e.g., the estimated number of 523 perinatally transmitted infections in 1988 in New York City) and to the assumption that this rate persists. Second, the incubation period of perinatally transmitted HIV infection is uncertain. The results of Auger, Thomas, and De Gruttola (1988) were based on right truncated data and do not account for incubation periods associated with perinatal transmission longer than 10 years (see

Table 10.5 Forward Calculation of Perinatal Infection Rates to Obtain Pediatric AIDS Incidence

Year of Infection	Yearly Number Infected	Expected Yearly Number of AIDS Diagnoses								
		1987	1988	1989	1990	1991	1992	1993	1994	1995
1981	16	1.4	2.0	1.8	1.2	0	0	0	0	0
1982	35	3.2	3.2	4.4	3.9	2.6	0	0	0	0
1983	60	5.1	5.4	5.4	7.5	6.6	4.5	0	0	0
1984	95	5.7	8.1	8.6	8.6	11.9	10.5	7.1	0	0
1985	148	12.6	8.9	12.6	13.3	13.3	18.5	16.3	11.1	0
1986	225	33.8	19.4	13.5	19.1	20.3	20.3	28.1	24.8	16.9
1987	343	30.9	51.5	29.2	20.6	29.2	30.9	30.9	42.9	37.7
1988	523	—	47.1	78.5	44.5	31.4	44.5	47.1	47.1	65.4
1989	523	—	—	47.1	78.5	44.5	31.4	44.5	47.1	47.1
1990	523	—	—	—	47.1	78.5	44.5	31.4	44.5	47.1
1991	523	—	—	—	—	47.1	78.5	44.5	31.4	44.5
1992	523	—	—	—	—	—	47.1	78.5	44.5	31.4
1993	523	—	—	—	—	—	—	47.1	78.5	44.5
1994	523	—	—	—	—	—	—	—	47.1	78.5
1995	523	—	—	—	—	—	—	—	—	47.1
Totals		93	146	201	244	285	331	376	419	460

Note: Yearly number infected is obtained from Figure 10.3.

Table 10.4). The results also depend on the assumption that about one third of initially seropositive newborns are, in fact, infected with HIV (Section 2.4.3).

10.5 FORECASTING FOR SMALL AREAS

Forecasts for small geographic areas may be subject to considerable uncertainty because the type and amount of available data may be limited. In some areas, such as San Francisco, extensive information from HIV seroprevalence surveys can be used to produce forecasts. For example, Lemp, Payne, Rutherford, et al. (1990) projected AIDS incidence in San Francisco by forward projecting infection rates, g_i, according to equation (8.2). The estimated infection rates among homosexual and bisexual men in San Francisco were based on data from the San Francisco Men's Health Study and a random-digit telephone survey on the size of the homosexual population.

Extensive data on infection rates, like that in San Francisco, is seldom available. Typically, the data in small geographic areas are limited to a few reported AIDS cases and an occasional seroprevalence survey. Public health planners have used ad-hoc *ratio-type* methods to make projections for small geographic areas. The basic idea of these approaches is to obtain forecasts and estimates for a small area by multiplying forecasts and estimates from another larger area, where more reported AIDS cases or more extensive HIV seroprevalence surveys are available, by an appropriate ratio, such as the ratio of cumulative AIDS incidence in the small area to cumulative AIDS incidence in the larger area.

For example, in 1988 the New York City Department of Health estimated the number of infected New Yorkers based on an estimate of the number of infected individuals in San Francisco. The estimates of the number infected in San Francisco were obtained from extensive HIV seroprevalence surveys. The underlying assumption was that the cumulative numbers of AIDS cases in San Francisco and New York are in the same proportion as the cumulative numbers infected in San Francisco and New York (Brookmeyer, Dondero, Farber, et al., 1989). If α is the observed ratio of the cumulative AIDS cases in New York divided by the cumulative AIDS cases in San Francisco, then the assumption of the ratio approach is:

Cumulative infections in NYC =

$$\alpha \times \text{Cumulative infections in San Francisco.}$$

This equation is justified only if the infection curves in San Francisco, $g_1(s)$, and New York City, $g_2(s)$, are proportional, that is

$$g_2(s) = \alpha g_1(s). \tag{10.3}$$

The infection curves must have the same shape as illustrated in Figure 5.2. However, if the epidemic began earlier in New York City than San Francisco, the curves could differ by a translation as illustrated in Figure 5.3. The New York City calculations for white homosexual men were adjusted for such a translation by lagging the San Francisco epidemic behind the New York City epidemic by one year.

Equation (10.3) implies that the ratio, R, of cumulative infections to AIDS cases in area 1 is the same as the ratio in area 2, provided the incubation distributions are the same in the two areas. This ratio depends strongly on the shape of the epidemic curve. Table 10.6 gives the ratio of cumulative infections to cumulative AIDS cases for the nine epidemics illustrated in Figure 8.5. The ratio R varies from 4.6 (epidemic 4) to 38.7 (epidemic 3). Early in an HIV epidemic, the ratio is large, as a consequence of the long incubation period of HIV infection. As cases of AIDS begin to surface, the ratio will typically decrease (Brookmeyer, 1989). Thus, the ratio of cumulative infections to cumulative AIDS cases is not constant over time, and may vary among transmission groups. The variation in the ratio over time and among transmission groups can be illustrated empirically for homosexual men in San Francisco and persons with hemophilia in the United States, because historical information on infection rates in these two populations are available. Both groups exhibit sharp declines in the ratios (Table 10.7).

Table 10.6 Illustration of Variation in Ratio, R, of Cumulative Infections to Cumulative AIDS Cases

Epidemic Curve (From Figure 8.5)	Cumulative Number Infected	Cumulative AIDS Cases	Ratio
1	50,000	10,595	4.7
2	50,000	4,683	10.7
3	50,000	1,293	38.7
4	50,000	10,814	4.6
5	50,000	5,412	9.2
6	50,000	2,083	24.0
7	50,000	3,915	12.8
8	50,000	1,536	32.6
9	50,000	5,302	9.4

Note: Incubation distribution $F(t) = 1 - e^{-.0021t^{2.5}}$; Ratio = cumulative infections/cumulative AIDS.

Table 10.7 Illustration of Variation Over Time and Across Transmission Groups in the Ratio of Cumulative Infections to Cumulative AIDS Cases

	Homosexual Men in San Francisco			U.S. Patients with Hemophilia		
	Cumulative Infections	Cumulative AIDS	Ratio *R*	Cumulative Infections	Cumulative AIDS	Ratio *R*
1983	15,659	109	143.7	7,428	8	928.5
1984	19,033	373	51.0	8,563	23	372.3
1985	20,443	1740	11.7	9,932	82	121.1
1986	21,250	2881	7.4	10,052	202	49.8
1987	21,741	4281	5.1	10,052	391	25.7

Source: Adapted from Brookmeyer, 1989.

If assumption (10.3) holds even approximately, ratio methods may be useful in applying information from one area to a smaller area where fewer data are available. The simplicity of the ratio calculation also make it attractive.

Back-calculations can also be applied to small areas. However when the number of observed AIDS cases is small, stochastic error (error from parameter estimation) becomes as important as systematic sources of uncertainty, such as uncertainties in the incubation distribution. For example, consider two areas where the infection rates are proportional, that is, equation (10.3) holds. Under step function models for the infection curves, the coefficient of variation (CV equals standard error divided by the true value of the parameter) for any linear functional of the estimated infection rates (including cumulative infections, or projected AIDS incidence) for the two areas are related through

$$\text{CV in area } 2 = \frac{1}{\sqrt{\alpha}} \text{CV in area } 1.$$

For example, epidemic curve 1 in Figure 8.5 (for which we expect 10,595 cumulative AIDS cases after 10.5 years) gave a coefficient of variation generally less than 0.05 for a number of important functionals including estimated cumulative infections (Rosenberg, Gail, and Pee, 1991). If we had a smaller epidemic with similar shape where $\alpha = .01$, we would expect only about 106 AIDS cases and the coefficient of variation would be about $1/\sqrt{0.01} \times .05 = .50$. Epidemics with infection curves similar to curve 1 produce more reliable back-calculation estimates than some of the other infection curves. However if there are only 100 observed AIDS cases, even in this situation the stochastic component of the error will dominate. Nevertheless, back-calculations have been applied to a number of small areas. Sharples, Carlson, Skegg, and Paul (1991) used the methods on 213 cumulative AIDS cases diagnosed in New Zealand. Tango (1989) used back-calculation on 45 hemophilia-associated AIDS cases with known exact dates of AIDS diagnosis in Japan. Further extentions, such as an empirical Bayes formulation of back-calculation, may offer a fruitful approach for modelling many small subgroups. Zeger, See, and Diggle (1989) used an empirical Bayes approach to smooth surveillance data in small areas (Section 7.6.2).

In small areas, it is especially useful to try to validate results of back-calculation by analyzing multiple independent data sources. For example, Rosenberg, Levy, Brundage, et al. (1992) estimated the infection rates in the District of Columbia from back-calculation on

3246 AIDS cases. They compared these estimates with independent data on HIV seroprevalence measured directly in several selected populations, including exhaustive surveys of newborn infants, civilian applicants for military service, intravenous drug users in drug treatment settings, and hospital patients admitted for conditions unrelated to HIV infection. Back-calculation methods yielded an estimate of 11,784 people infected by January 1, 1991, of whom 9461 were still alive (plausible range 7544–20,844). To obtain race-sex specific estimates, the back-calculated estimates were multiplied by the proportion of AIDS cases in each race-sex stratum. These estimates were compared to estimates obtained from seroprevalence surveys. For example, based only on 247 cumulative AIDS cases among black women by January 1, 1991, back-calculation yielded an estimate of 2077 living infected black women. In comparison, serosurveys of newborns indicated that 1957 childbearing women were infected in the age range 15–44. Likewise, back-calculated estimates of 3823 living infected intravenous drug users were very similar to the prevalence estimate of 3552 obtained directly from serosurveys in drug treatment centers.

These back-calculation estimates indicate that AIDS incidence will increase by 34% in the District of Columbia during the period from 1990 to 1994, in contrast to flat national trends, and that the increase will be due almost entirely to increases among intravenous drug users and heterosexuals. Back-calculations indicate that these increases among intravenous drug users and heterosexuals reflect increases in infection rates that began in the mid-1980s. These trends in infection rates are consistent with survey data from newborns in the District of Columbia (HIV prevalence doubled from 1989 to 1991 among black childbearing women), with military applicant screening data, and with seroprevalence surveys among hospital patients admitted for conditions unrelated to HIV. Although national trends in infection rates in the United States may suggest a plateau among heterosexuals, these results for the District of Columbia indicate that the infection rates may still be growing rapidly in some urban areas.

11

Developing and Evaluating New Therapies and Vaccines

11.1 INTRODUCTION

In March of 1987, only 6 years after AIDS was defined, the U.S. Food and Drug Administration (FDA) approved the use of 3'-azido-2'-3' dideoxythymidine (AZT), now called zidovudine, for the treatment of severe HIV infection. This remarkable progress was based on the isolation of HIV in 1983 and 1984 and its characterization as a lymphotropic retrovirus (Chapter 1).

In this chapter we review the history of AZT development, in part to illustrate concrete problems encountered in designing, carrying out, and interpreting clinical trials for HIV disease (Section 11.2). Section 11.3 contains a discussion of approaches to the development of therapies based on an understanding of the pathophysiology of HIV infection. The role of observational studies and examples of such studies for evaluating therapy are considered in Section 11.4 and followed by a description of the special problems and design issues for controlled clinical trials of HIV disease (Section 11.5). We discuss aspects of vaccine development in Section 11.6.

11.2 HISTORY OF THE DEVELOPMENT OF AZT

11.2.1 Advanced HIV Disease

The development of AZT was based on an understanding of the biology of HIV. As previously reviewed by Newman (1990), AZT had been synthesized in 1964 as a possible anticancer agent (Horvitz, Chua, and Noel, 1964) and was later shown to be active against a mouse retrovirus called the Friend leukemia virus (Ostertag, Roseler, Krieg, et al., 1974). Researchers at the Burroughs Wellcome Company confirmed the activity of AZT against the Friend leukemia virus in 1984. AZT was then shown by Mitsuya, Weinhold, Furman, et al. (1985) to inhibit the infectivity and cytopathic effects of HIV in human cells.

Encouraged by this finding, Yarchoan, Klecker, Weinhold, et al. (1986) carried out a phase I study in 19 patients with AIDS and AIDS-related complex (ARC) to determine toxity and to establish appropriate doses. They found promising examples of patients who gained weight and patients with increases in CD4+ T-lymphocytes and in delayed hypersensitivity reactions. Fischl, Richman, Grieco, et al. (1987) promptly initiated a randomized trial comparing placebo treatment with AZT, given in 250 mg capsules every four hours (protocol BW02 in Table 11.1). One hundred sixty patients with AIDS and 122 with advanced ARC were enrolled between February and June of 1986. The study was terminated in September 1986 after a mean duration on study of 4 months and after 20 deaths. The study was stopped earlier than planned because 19 of the 20 deaths were from the placebo group. Thus, AZT had been shown to prolong life in patients with advanced HIV disease. On the basis of this study, the FDA approved the use of AZT for patients with AIDS or advanced AIDS-related complex and for patients with CD4+ T-cells below 200 cells/μl.

11.2.2 Less Advanced HIV Disease

The early success of AZT in patients with AIDS and advanced ARC led to studies to evaluate AZT in patients with less advanced HIV disease (Table 11.1). In a study of "mildly symptomatic" patients with initial CD4+ T-cell levels between 200 and 800 cells/μl, Fischl, Richman, Hansen, et al. (1990) found that AZT (200 mg every 4 hours) retarded the development of the earliest of AIDS, death or advancing AIDS-related complex compared to placebo. After a mean duration on study of 10 months on AZT and 9 months on placebo, there were 2 deaths, 5 cases of AIDS and 8 cases of AIDS-related complex among the 360 patients assigned to AZT, compared to 0 deaths, 21 AIDS cases and 15 cases of AIDS-related complex among the 351 patients on placebo (protocol ACTG016, Table 11.1). Similar results were found among 1338 asymptomatic patients with initial CD4+ T-lymphocyte levels below 500 cells/μl (Volberding, Lagakos, Koch, et al., 1990). That trial compared 428 patients on placebo with 453 patients who received 500 mg each day (100 mg every 4 hours while awake) and with 457 patients who received 1500 mg AZT each day (300 mg every 4 hours while awake). The rate of developing AIDS was about 2.4 times greater among patients on placebo than among patients on AZT treatment, and the rate of developing AIDS or advanced AIDS-related complex was about 1.9 times greater (protocol ACTG019, Table 11.1). Severe anemia developed in 6.3% of those on the 1500 mg/day AZT regimen, compared with 1.1% of those on 500 mg/day AZT and 0.2% of those on placebo. Moreover, AIDS and AIDS-related complex was retarded at least as much by the lower dose of AZT as by the larger dose. An independent study of low-dose AZT (600 mg/day) versus high-dose AZT (1500 mg/day) in patients with a history of *Pneumocystis carinii* pneumonia and with mean CD4+ T-cell level of 87 cells/μl confirmed that patients given the lower dose of AZT had less severe anemia, less neutropenia, and somewhat longer survival than the group treated with 1500 mg/day (Fischl, Parker, Pettinelli, et al., 1990).

On the basis of data from these trials, the Food and Drug Administration lowered the recommended daily dose of AZT to 500 mg/day, and on March 2, 1990, the FDA broadened indications for AZT to include patients with CD4+ T-cell counts of 500 cells/μl or less.

The decision to recommend that even asymptomatic patients with CD4+ T-cell levels of 500 cells/μl be given AZT was controversial because the clinical trials had been stopped before a survival benefit had been established. Indeed, among those with CD4+ T-cell levels between 200 and 500 cells/μl initially, only six deaths occurred during the study reported by Volberding, Lagakos, Koch, et al. (1990) (personal communication from Professor Lagakos), and only two deaths occurred during the study by Fischl, Richman, Hanson, et al., 1990.

The FDA Antiretroviral Advisory Committee had been persuaded that there were enough demonstrated benefits from early administration of AZT to justify its expanded use in those with less advanced HIV disease. Treatment improvements in CD4+ T-cell levels had been demonstrated and clinical benefits in retarding AIDS had been proven. It was at least plausible that these improvements would translate into improved survival. However, some physicians believed that more evidence of survival benefit was needed before endorsing the widespread use of AZT in early HIV disease (Ruedy, Schechter, and Montaner, 1990). They argued that known hematologic and other toxicities of AZT and possible unknown long-term toxicities might outweigh short-term benefits of AZT treatment. A recent analysis of adverse reactions to treatment with 1200 mg of AZT per day in

Table 11.1 Data from Selected Controlled Clinical Trials on HIV Disease

	Study Population	Treatments	Endpoints	AZT	Placebo	Risk Ratio[b]	Comment
Advanced Disease							
BW02[a]	Patients with AIDS or advanced AIDS-related complex (ARC)	1500 mg AZT daily vs. placebo	Death	1/137	19/145	.05	AZT prolongs life in patients with advanced disease
			Opportunistic infections	24	45	.56	
S.F. community prophylaxis trial[c]	AIDS or AIDS-related complex	Inhaled pentamidine 30 mg vs. 150 mg vs. 300 mg	PCP	*300 mg*	*150 mg*	*30 mg*	Higher doses of pentamidine prevent PCP, especially among those with a previous history of PCP
				28/139	32/134	41/135	
						.72	
Less Advanced Disease							
ACTG016[d]	No AIDS; early ARC with CD4+ T-cell levels between 200–800/μl	1200 mg AZT daily vs. placebo	*AIDS or advanced ARC	13/360	36/351	.35	AZT prolongs the time to AIDS or advanced ARC and to AIDS alone
			AIDS	5	21	.23	
			Death	2	0	—	

Table 11.1 (Continued)

Less Advanced Disease, cont'ed

			1500 mg	500 mg	Placebo	
ACTG019[f]	Asymptomatic without ARC or AIDS; CD4+ T-cells < 500/μl	1500 mg AZT daily vs. 500 mg daily vs. placebo				AZT prolongs the time to AIDS or ARC and to AIDS alone
		[a]AIDS or ARC	19/457	17/453	38/428	.52
		AIDS	14	11	33	.41
		Death	3	1	4	—
			Early AZT	*Later AZT*		
VA298[g]	No AIDS; signs or symptoms of ARC present; CD4+ T-cell between 200–500/μl	Early AZT (1500 mg daily) vs. later AZT after AIDS or CD4+ T-cells < 200/μl				AZT prolongs the time to AIDS, but no survival benefit is seen
		[a]AIDS or death	38/170	48/168		.78
		AIDS	28	48		.57
		Death	23	20		1.23

[a]Fischl, Richman, Grieco, et al. (1987).

[b]Risk ratio computed as the ratio of hazard rates if the data are given; otherwise as the ratio of proportions with events.

[c]Leoung, Feigal, Montgomery, et al. (1990); risk ratio compares 30 mg to the two higher doses.

[d]Fischl, Richman, Hansen, et al. (1990).

[e]Protocol-defined primary endpoint.

[f]Volberding, Lagakos, Koch, et al. (1990); risk ratio compares both AZT doses to placebo.

[g]Hamilton, Hartigan, Simberkoff, et al. (1992).

protocol ACTG016 (see Table 11.1) indicates that the benefits of delaying progression to AIDS are offset, in many cases, by severe symptomatic reactions (Gelber, Lenderking, Cotton, et al., 1992). Moreover, substantial HIV resistance to AZT had been demonstrated in vitro in viral isolates from 5 of 15 patients who had received AZT for 6 months or more (Larder, Darby, and Richman, 1989). In addition, although patients with advanced HIV disease obtained an impressive survival benefit from AZT initially (Fischl, Richman, Grieco, et al., 1987), the mortality rate increased rapidly after this initial respite (Fischl, Richman, Causey, et al., 1989). As of February 1, 1988, about 22 months after the initiation of AZT in patients with advanced HIV disease, 68 (47%) of those 144 patients initially assigned to AZT had died. Thus it was at least theoretically possible that asymptomatic patients whose CD4+ T-lymphocytes were stable at values somewhat below 500 cells/μl might be well advised to wait to initiate AZT therapy until CD4+ T-cell levels declined or symptoms developed. By waiting, they could avoid AZT toxicity and AZT resistance.

A recently published trial (Hamilton, Hartigan, Simberkoff, et al., 1992) compared early AZT treatment (1500 mg/day) with delayed AZT treatment in 338 patients at Veterans Administration Hospitals (Protocol VA298 in Table 11.1). These patients had initial CD4+ T-lymphocyte levels between 200 and 500 cells/μl. Those assigned to delayed AZT were given placebo pills initially but were monitored every four months for falling CD4+ T-cell levels and advancing clinical signs. Any patient whose CD4+ T-cell levels fell below 200 cells/μl or who developed AIDS was given AZT (1500 mg/day) at that time. This trial confirmed the results of previous studies that early use of AZT prolonged the time to AIDS, but, unfortunately, no survival benefit was demonstrated. There were 23 deaths among the 170 patients assigned to early AZT treatment and 20 deaths among the 168 patients assigned to delayed AZT treatment. Because there were only 43 deaths, it is possible that a modest survival benefit exists either for early AZT treatment or for delayed AZT treatment but was obscured by random error. The relative hazard for death comparing early to delayed AZT was 1.23, however, with 95% confidence interval (0.63, 2.27). An ongoing study in Europe, the Concorde 1 Trial, may provide additional data on the survival benefit from early use of AZT. Early treatment with AZT at the lower dose of 500 mg/day may produce a survival benefit compared to later treatment with AZT, but this hypothesis has not been studied.

In summary, while AZT has been shown to prolong survival in those with AIDS and advanced AIDS-related complex, and to retard the onset of AIDS in people with less advanced HIV disease, there is no consensus as to the best time to initiate AZT therapy in patients with less advanced disease. Some of these patients may benefit by waiting.

11.3 APPROACHES TO THERAPY BASED ON THE PATHOPHYSIOLOGY OF HIV DISEASE

The development of AZT was prompted by the knowledge that HIV was a retrovirus. AZT probably acts to inhibit reverse transcription (Figure 1.2) through its metabolites, some of which may be competitive inhibitors of the normal substrate for reverse transcription, thymidine 5'-triphosphate, and some of which are incorporated into the DNA chain, thereby terminating its further development. Mitsuya, Yarchoan, and Broder (1990) review the activities of a broad family of antiretroviral nucleosides like AZT and describe many potential points of attack on HIV based on an understanding of the viral life cycle (Figure 1.2).

Among the possible interventions they describe are: (1) blocking viral attachment to the cell by means of antibodies to the virus or to cellular CD4+ receptors or by genetically engineered soluble CD4 proteins; (2) blocking fusion of the virus with the target cell with specific drugs or antibodies; (3) using drugs to block entry of viral RNA into the target cell and to prevent uncoating of the RNA; (4) blocking reverse transcription of RNA into DNA with drugs like AZT; (5) blocking the normal degradation of viral RNA with RNase inhibitors; (6) blocking the viral DNA from entering the cell nucleus; (7) blocking the integration of viral DNA into the host DNA; (8) preventing the transcription of viral DNA back into viral RNA; (9) blocking the translation of viral messenger RNA into viral protein; (10) interfering with viral regulatory processes mediated through regulatory proteins such as *tat* and *rev*; (11) inhibiting a viral protease that is necessary to cleave viral proteins into mature products; (12) inhibiting chemical reactions such as glycosylation that are needed to produce mature viral components; (13) preventing efficient packaging of viral RNA into the developing virus; and (14) blocking the process of budding whereby mature viruses leave the infected cell.

In addition to therapies directed at HIV, there is a need to treat the many complications of HIV infection and immune deficiency, including opportunistic infections, malignancies, wasting syndrome, and neurologic disorders.

With so many possible interventions, there is some reason to hope that effective therapeutic strategies could be devised, especially if one considers the use of combinations of agents directed at different viral targets. To evaluate some of the many possible approaches, a large clinical trial program was established by the National Institutes for Allergy and Infectious Diseases. It was and is a major organizational, administrative and scientific challenge and accomplishment to coordinate hundreds of investigators, thousands of patients, and millions of data items in an effort to assess multiple promising therapeutic avenues simultaneously.

As of October 28, 1991, 202 trials were pending initiation or had been initiated by the AIDS Clinical Trials Group (National Institute of Allergy and Infectious Diseases, Division of AIDS, 1991). Of the 146 trials that had already been initiated, 19 were preliminary pharmacologic studies, 41 involved treatments of the primary HIV infection, 38 were directed at opportunistic infections, 13 at AIDS-related cancers, 3 at neurologic complications, 20 at pediatric HIV disease, and 12 at other issues.

A major effort has been made to study alternative antiretroviral therapies such as 2′,3′-dideoxyinosine (ddI) and 2′,3′-dideoxycytidine (ddC). In July 1991, FDA's Antiretroviral Advisory Committee recommended the use of ddI for individuals who were resistant or intolerant to AZT. This recommendation was based on improvements in CD4+ T-cell levels seen in phase I trials (Lambert, Seidlin, Reichman, et al. 1990; Cooley, Kunches, Saunders, et al., 1990) and in an ongoing randomized trial comparing ddI with AZT.

Recent news accounts (*The Wall Street Journal*, January 20, 1992) indicate that Hoffman-La Roche has halted comparative trials of ddC versus AZT because 59 of 320 people who took ddC died, compared to 33 of 315 who took AZT. Nonetheless, ddC is still being studied as an alternative for people who find AZT intolerable and for use in combination with AZT.

Substantial progress has been made in preventing and treating opportunistic infections that result from immunodeficiency. Observational data (Golden, Chernoff, Hollander, et al., 1989) suggested that inhaled pentamidine could reduce the rate of recurrence of *Pneumocystis carinii* pneumonia (PCP) by 50%, and a subsequent randomized trial comparing three doses of pentamidine (30 mg every 2 weeks, 150 mg every 2 weeks, or 300 mg every 4 weeks) demonstrated that the two higher doses reduced the incidence of PCP by 28%, compared to the 30 mg dose (Leoung, Feigal, Montgomery, et al., 1990). These data and data relating CD4+ T-cell levels to the risk of PCP were the basis of Public Health Service recommendations that prophylaxsis against PCP be instituted in patients with a previous episode of PCP as well as in patients whose CD4+ T-cell levels were below 200 cell/μl or constituted less than 20% of total lymphocytes (CDC, 1989c). Numerous controlled clinical trials have been published comparing the effectiveness and toxicities of various agents to prevent and treat PCP and the myriad other infectious complications of HIV disease.

11.4 OBSERVATIONAL STUDIES

Demonstrations of the efficacy of AZT, pentamidine, and other agents in controlled clinical trials have permitted the rapid licensing and introduction of these treatments into clinical practice. Clinical trials provide convincing evidence of efficacy because random allocation of treatments to patients reduces the possibility that an apparently favorable treatment effect is the result of assigning a preponderance of healthier patients to that treatment. In contrast, observational studies to determine treatment efficacy do not include a random treatment assignment. Such studies may be hard to interpret, not only because the quality of data on prognostic factors and follow-up is often less than in clinical trials, but principally because the healthier patients may preferentially be given one treatment or another (Byar, 1980). Thus, observational data are not usually relied on for proof of efficacy. Nonetheless, observational data may provide useful confirmation of clinical trial results and may give an indication of how well a therapy is performing in general medical practice.

11.4.1 Increased Survival

Several researchers have studied cohorts of patients diagnosed with AIDS in various years and investigated whether survival, measured from the date of AIDS diagnosis, is improving with calendar year of diagnosis. Such an improvement would be consistent with the introduction of AZT into general practice in March 1987 and with increasing use of agents to prevent and treat PCP and other opportunistic infections. Harris (1990b) studied 36,847 AIDS cases who were reported to CDC before September 1987 and who had been diagnosed between January 1984 and September 1987. Various procedures such as linkage of AIDS case reports with death certificates were used to ascertain vital status as of June 30, 1989. One-year survival improved from 45.1% for those diagnosed in 1984–5 to 50.9% for those diagnosed in 1986–7, but the improvements were mainly found among AIDS cases whose initial AIDS-defining condition was PCP. For such patients, the 1-year survival improved from 42.7% to 54.5%. Lemp,

Payne, Neal, et al. (1990) studied 4323 AIDS cases from San Francisco and found an improvement in median survival from about 10 months for AIDS patients diagnosed before 1986 to 12 and 16 months respectively for patients diagnosed in 1986 and 1987. They also noted that the improvement was largely confined to patients whose initial diagnosis was PCP. Moore, Hidalgo, Sugland, and Chaisson (1991) studied 1028 patients in the Maryland AIDS Registry and found improvements in median survival from about 10 months for patients diagnosed before 1986 to 13 and 15 months respectively for patients diagnosed in 1986 and in 1987–9.

These registry based studies demonstrate modest but consistent improvements in survival following AIDS diagnosis (Table 11.2). Some of this apparent improvement may be due to basic limitations in studies of this type. The follow-up information is obtained by linkage with death certificate reports and other passive surveillance methods. Increasing delays in reporting AIDS-related deaths or increasing proportions of AIDS-related deaths that are never reported as such (see Chapter 7) could explain a portion of the apparent improvement in survival rates. In addition, increasing awareness of treatments for PCP in 1986 and thereafter could have led some patients to seek diagnosis and treatment at an earlier stage of disease. Thus, earlier diagnosis of PCP could explain some portion of the survival improvements. To investigate this possibility, one would want to know CD4+ T-cell levels at the time of diagnosis, but registries usually do not provide this type of information.

It is difficult to obtain reliable, detailed treatment information from registry studies. Nonetheless, Lemp, Payne, Neal, et al. (1990) abstracted data on AZT use from medical records. For many patients, such information was not available. The median survival of 461 AIDS patients diagnosed in San Francisco in 1986–7 who never received AZT was 14 months, compared to 21 months for 172 patients who received AZT. Moore, Hidalgo, Sugland, and Chaisson (1991) determined AZT use from various sources, including insurance claims for 714 patients diagnosed with AIDS after April 1987. They found that the median survival was only 6 months for those who never received AZT, compared to 25 months for those who did receive AZT. In both these studies, part of the improvement in survival associated with AZT may be due to AIDS diagnosis at an earlier stage of disease among people who have good access to medical care.

A bias may account for much of the apparent benefit of AZT for prolonging life in these two studies. Both Lemp, Payne, Neal, et al., and Moore, Hidalgo, Sugland, and Chaisson compared AIDS patients who

Table 11.2 Estimates of Median Survival (in months) Following AIDS Onset Based on AIDS Registry Data

Type of AIDS-Defining Condition	1985 or Earlier	1986	1987	1988	1989	Location
			Year of Diagnosis			
All cases	10	12	16			U.S.[a]
	11	12	16			San Francisco[b]
	10	13	14	15	15	Maryland[c]
Pneumocystis carinii pneumonia (PCP)	9	12	16			U.S.[a]

[a]Data on PCP from figure 1 in Harris (1990b). Data for all cases in U.S. from Professor J.E. Harris (personal communication) as described in Gail, Pluda, Rabkin, et al. (1991).

[b]Lemp, Payne, Neal, et al. (1990).

[c]Moore, Hidalgo, Sugland, and Chaisson (1991).

received AZT at some point in their illness with patients who never received AZT. However, a patient who died shortly after AIDS diagnosis would have had little chance to receive AZT. Thus, this comparison group probably included a disproportionate number of patients with poor survival. In fact, the median survival of 6 months in the untreated group described by Moore, Hidalgo, Sugland, and Chaisson is only about half as long as the median survival of patients treated in 1986, before AZT was available (see Fätkenheuer, Stützer, Salzberger, and Schrappe, 1991, and Table 11.2). This bias does not affect the analyses of temporal trends in survival following AIDS diagnosis as shown in Table 11.2.

Despite their limitations, the studies in Table 11.2 provide evidence that survival following AIDS diagnosis increased over the 1980s. Registry studies of this type have the advantage that they are usually based on broad and representative populations.

11.4.2 Delay in Progression to AIDS

Clinical trial data provided strong evidence that AZT can delay the onset of AIDS in AIDS-free patients with advanced ARC (protocol BW02 in Table 11.1) and with less advanced HIV disease (protocols ACTG016, ACTG019, and VA298 in Table 11.1). Schechter, Craib, Le, et al. (1989b) reported a reduction in AIDS incidence coincident with the use of AZT in some members of a cohort of homosexual men in Vancouver. Nonetheless, it was hard to imagine how treatment of a few thousand patients with AZT beginning in 1987 might account for sudden improvements in national AIDS incidence trends seen among homosexual and bisexual men beginning in mid-1987 (Figure 7.4). Gail, Rosenberg, and Goedert (1990a) used "consistently" defined AIDS incidence data through June 30, 1987 (open squares in Figure 7.4) to project future consistently defined AIDS incidence (solid line) beyond mid-1987. Consistently defined AIDS refers to the surveillance definition in use before broadening the definition in the fall of 1987 (Section 7.5), but the consistently defined series includes cases diagnosed on the basis of presumptive clinical data and makes allowance for cases diagnosed under the broadened definition who would subsequently be diagnosed under the pre-1987 surveillance definition. Note that the consistently defined AIDS incidence curve suddenly flattens after mid-1987 (solid squares in Figure 7.4) and falls well below the lower 95% confidence bounds of AIDS projections. This sudden improvement is not fully explained by making back-calculated projections that allow for no infections after mid-1985 (dash-dot line in Figure 7.4).

Based on efficacy measurements from clinical trial data, Gail, Rosenberg, and Goedert (1990a) calculated that only about 5000–7000 gay men needed to have been treated with AZT or other agents beginning in mid-1987 to account for the sudden improvements in national AIDS incidence trends in the last half of 1987, even though hundreds of thousands of gay men were infected. If the AZT were used to treat only the sickest AIDS-free patients (e.g., those with CD4+ T-cell levels below 200 cells/μl), a small amount of drug could have a dramatic impact. Rosenberg, Gail, Schrager, et al. (1991) subsequently reported that 3204 AIDS-free homosexual and bisexual men with severe immunodeficiency received AZT in the initial period of controlled distribution between March 31, 1987, and September 18, 1987. Others received AZT after this period, and still others received AZT as the result of participation in clinical trials.

Data on AZT use in the San Francisco Men's Health Study indicated that the amounts of treatment in use in the last half of 1987 and first half of 1988 could explain the improvements in AIDS incidence seen in San Francisco, Los Angeles and New York City (see Figure 8.8; and table 1 in Gail, Rosenberg, and Goedert, 1990a).

Additional support for the hypothesis that AZT and other treatments are affecting national AIDS incidence trends comes from separate analyses in various risk groups. Groups such as intravenous drug users that are not expected to have good access to treatment show no improvement in AIDS incidence trends in the last half of 1987 (Figure 11.1). Rosenberg, Gail, Schrager, et al. (1991) found that the

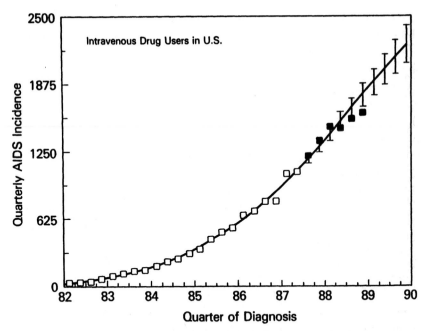

Figure 11.1 Projected and observed quarterly AIDS incidence among intravenous drug users in the United States. Projections were based on consistently defined AIDS incidence counts through June 30, 1987 (open squares), as described by Gail, Rosenberg, and Goedert (1990a). Vertical lines indicate 95% confidence limits, and solid squares depict quarterly AIDS incidence beginning in July 1987. (Source: Adaptation of figure 3 in Gail, Rosenberg, and Goedert, 1990a.)

risk groups that received substantial amounts of AZT initially were the groups that showed improvements in AIDS incidence trends beginning in mid-1987. Fife and Mode (1992) found improvements in AIDS incidence trends beginning in 1987 for residents of Philadelphia who resided in census tracts in the highest tercile of income, regardless of race. No such improvements were seen among those living in census tracts in the lowest tercile of income.

Data such as these strongly suggest that treatment had an impact on AIDS incidence trends, especially from mid-1987 to mid-1988, and that treatment should be taken into account in projecting AIDS incidence (Chapter 8). However, the longer term incidence of AIDS will be determined primarily by trends in the HIV infection curve. Moreover, surveillance data do not permit one to obtain precise estimates of the effects of AZT. Other agents, such as pentamidine, are probably playing a role. Some of the improvements in AIDS incidence trends may be due to increases in reporting delays or in underreporting, although recent evidence does not support this explanation (Buehler, Berkelman, and Stehr-Green, 1992). It has been argued that some of the improvements could be explained by antecedent decreases in the infection rate, provided it is also true that the hazard rate of the AIDS incubation distribution levels off after 6 or 7 years, even without treatment. Further discussion of these issues is found in Segal and Bacchetti (1990); Gail, Rosenberg, and Goedert (1990a, 1990b); Gail and Rosenberg (1992); and Bacchetti, Segal, and Jewell (1992, 1993).

Graham, Zeger, Park, et al. (1991) studied the effects of AZT and PCP prophylaxis in 2516 seropositive homosexual and bisexual male members of the Multicenter AIDS Cohort Study. Unlike registry studies, this cohort study provided data on the stage of disease (CD4 + T-cells > 500, 350–500, 200–349 without symptoms, 200–349 with symptoms, <200 without symptoms and <200 with symptoms), data on treatment use, and active follow-up data for AIDS incidence at 6-month intervals. AZT was consistently associated with slower rates of progression to AIDS in all patients whose initial CD4 + T-cell levels were below 350 cells/μl, and PCP prophylaxis was associated with a further reduction in the rates of AIDS incidence among patients already receiving AZT. The authors conclude that PCP prophylaxis is effective and that the efficacy of AZT demonstrated in clinical trials "can be translated to the population level."

Gardner, Brundage, McNeil, et al. (1992) found that the rate of progression from advanced immunodeficiency to AIDS decreased successively in cohorts of U.S. Army personnel first evaluated in 1986, 1987, and 1988. These data again suggest that improvements in treatment are having an impact in general medical practice.

11.5 SPECIAL PROBLEMS AND DESIGN ISSUES IN CLINICAL TRIALS FOR HIV DISEASE

11.5.1 Spectrum of Disease

HIV poses special challenges in clinical studies. The spectrum of HIV disease is extremely broad. A recently infected patient may well live more than 10 years without any treatment. A patient whose CD4 + T-cell level has fallen to 200 cells/μl needs treatment that can reconstitute immune competence and prevent opportunistic infections and other complications of immunodeficiency. A patient whose CD4 + T-cell level is 10 cells/μl needs agents that prevent and treat complications of immunodeficiency, such as PCP, cytomegalovirus, disseminated tuberculosis or non-Hodgkins lymphoma. Thus the needs for treatment are diverse, leading to competiton for resources and a necessary proliferation of studies. This problem is compounded by the fact that even among a single class of treatments, such as those directed at attacking HIV, there are many possible approaches (Section 11.3).

The fact that large numbers of young people have suddenly become seriously ill adds urgency to the search for treatments. The pace of conventional approaches to drug development, evaluation, and licensing is slow. The AIDS epidemic has forced a reexamination of many of the classical standards, including the need for and choice of a proper control arm, the need for randomization, and the reliance on death or other clinical evidence as endpoints, rather on less extreme indicators of progression (Green, Ellenberg, Finkelstein, et al., 1990; Byar, Schoenfeld, Green, et al., 1990; Ellenberg, Finkelstein, and Schoenfeld, 1992). We now discuss some of these difficulties and proposals to deal with them.

11.5.2 "Expanded Access" Versus the Need to Promote Participation in Controlled Trials

Many patients with advanced HIV disease, including many who could not tolerate AZT or for whom AZT appeared to be losing its effectiveness, were unwilling or unable to participate in comparative clinical trials and demanded access to alternative therapies, even unproven therapies. On September 28, 1989, the FDA approved the request of the Bristol-Myers Squibb company to begin clinical trials comparing ddI with AZT and, at the same time, FDA allowed certain patients who had failed on AZT or could not tolerate it to receive ddI. On May 20, 1990, the Public Health Service formalized these procedures and proposed in the *Federal Register* that promising investigational AIDS drugs be made available to patients with clinically significant HIV disease, provided the patient could not tolerate standard treatments or such treatments were no longer effective, and provided the patient could not participate in controlled clinical trials. This new mechanism for access to investigational drugs was termed the *parallel track*.

This proposal raised two principal concerns. First, it was possible that those given investigational drugs might suffer serious toxicities and complications and that the means to monitor toxicity would be inadequate. For example, it was reported in March 1990 that the death rate was 10 times higher among those patients given ddI by Bristol-Myers Squibb on a compassionate basis than among patients enrolled in clinical trials of ddI (Institute of Medicine, 1991, page 30). Although it was thought that the high death rate was due in part to the poor states of health of those given ddI outside the clinical trials program, it was not possible to rule out the possibility that some of the excess mortality was attributable to misuse or toxicities from ddI.

A second concern was that patients who received investigational drugs on the parallel track would not be available to participate in controlled clinical trials, thereby retarding studies to determine efficacy and toxicity. By January 1991, it was estimated that 14,000 patients were receiving ddI through expanded access, compared to 1600 patients who were participating in clinical trials (Institute of Medicine, 1991, page 32). Many scientists felt that the program of expanded access had slowed the clinical trials to some extent, but the impact was hard to quantify.

Statisticians have considered ways to promote participation in controlled clinical trials by communicating with AIDS advocates to help them understand essential features of design and by modifying the design, where possible, to make participation easier and more attractive (Byar, Schoenfeld, Green, et al., 1990; Green, Ellenberg, Finkelstein, et al., 1990; Ellenberg, Finkelstein, and Schoenfeld, 1992). Although these adaptations are potentially important in ensuring the success of these trials, clinical trials in AIDS research must adhere to sound principles of clinical trial practice (Friedman, Furberg, and DeMets, 1984; Pocock, 1983; Meinert, 1986) to produce scientifically convincing results.

Broadening eligibility criteria can enhance participation. Exclusions designed solely to assure a homogeneous study population could be eliminated. Losses in statistical precision that arise from studying heterogeneous populations can be reduced by the use of stratified analyses or regression models that adjust for important covariates. Exclusionary criteria designed to delineate which clinical trial is best for a given type of patient or to protect certain types of patients from harm would be retained. By broadening eligibility criteria, one would hope to provide an appropriate clinical study for most patients, and one would hope that conclusions derived from such studies would be broadly applicable.

A major factor in assuring good participation in trials of HIV disease is to make sure that the comparisons made are useful for managing HIV infected patients and that both the potential patients and their physicians are "substantially uncertain" as to which regimen being compared will turn out to produce the most favorable results (Byar, Schoenfeld, Green, et al., 1990). Placebo-controlled trials were certainly justifiable before AZT had been shown to be effective in patients with advanced disease; such trials may still be advisable in patients with early HIV disease. However, the use of placebo controls would no longer be medically relevant, ethical or feasible in studies of more advanced disease. Instead, patients and doctors would be interested in comparing new agents, or combinations of agents, with a standard regimen, such as AZT at 500 mg/day (Fleming, 1990; Cooper, 1990). Such studies may be able to demonstrate that a new regimen is as good as or better than standard therapy, but, if the new regimen is worse than standard therapy, it may still be better than no treatment at all. Deciding whether the new treatment is better than no treatment by comparing current results with "historical controls" who received no treatment is problematic (Byar, 1979). Time trends in the nature of the population studied, in the diagnostic methodology used to determine initial prognostic categories, and in ancillary supportive care may render the historical control population incomparable to the population under current study. Such time trends usually favor the treatments under current study, because patients treated previously often had more advanced disease and received less adequate ancillary care. Furthermore, adjustment procedures needed to correct for differences between the historical control population and the current population may be inadequate because of lack of knowledge about what factors are prognostic and what mathematical procedures should be used for adjustment, and because required covariate information may be missing for historical controls.

Sometimes it may be convincing to compare various doses of a drug in randomized trials. This strategy led to the useful result that lower doses of AZT were associated with lower toxicity and improved survival compared to higher doses (Fischl, Parker, Pettinelli, et al., 1990). Likewise, the randomized trial showing that higher doses of pentamidine prevented PCP more effectively than a low dose (Leoung, Feigal, Montgomery, et al., 1990) was instrumental in persuading experts of the usefulness of pentamidine for PCP prophylaxis (CDC, 1989c). Of course, dose comparisons may be hard to interpret, especially if no differences in responses are found. In that case, both doses may be ineffective or both may be effective.

Rarely there will be no attractive therapeutic option to a proposed new treatment, and an uncontrolled experiment may be convincing. Byar, Schoenfeld, Green, et al., (1990) refer to FDA's approval of ganciclovir for the treatment of retinitis caused by cytomegalovirus (CMV) and attempt to define those few circumstances where an uncontrolled trial may be justified. CMV retinitis was known to progress to blindness in most patients, and no effective treatment was available for comparison. Uncontrolled studies of ganciclovir demonstrated benefit in more than eighty percent of patients treated (Mills, Jacobson, O'Donnell, et al., 1988) and convinced FDA officials of efficacy.

A degree of flexibility on the part of clinical investigators and statisticians can help accommodate the needs of patients and improve trial participation and compliance. For example, the study by Hamilton, Hartigan, Simberkoff, et al. (1992) addressed whether immediate use of AZT was better than delayed use of AZT in AIDS-free patients with CD4+ T-cells in the range 200–500 cells/μl. Because patients knew they were being carefully monitored and would receive AZT as soon as the CD4+ T-cell level fell below 200 cells/μl or an AIDS-defining event occurred, they were willing to continue in the study in large numbers, even after public announcements and information provided by the trial's investigators that AZT could prolong the time to an AIDS-defining event. The question answered by this trial is not the same as whether AZT is better than no treatment, and patients' willingness to continue indicates that the trial was addressing a question of practical clinical importance.

When the Public Health Service announced new guidelines recommending that PCP prophylaxis be used in patients with CD4+ T-cell levels below 200 cells/μl, clinical investigators had to decide whether to modify their ongoing trials. Because PCP constitutes nearly half the initial AIDS-defining events in many risk groups (Table 1.1), the decision to administer pentamidine according to these guidelines required a prolongation of ongoing trials in order to retain original levels of statistical power, which depends mainly on the number of endpoint events. By adopting a flexible approach and changing protocols to conform with guidelines for PCP prophylaxis, investigators protected the interests of their patients and answered potentially useful questions about the efficacy of treatment in the presence of PCP prophylaxis.

Byar, Schoenfeld, Green, et al. (1990) and Ellenberg, Finkelstein, and Schoenfeld (1992) discuss some of the promise and some of the difficulties associated with enrolling the same patient in multiple studies to accommodate multiple needs for treatment, as well as more formal factorial designs.

Broadening eligibility requirements, making sure that comparisons are useful and meaningful to patients as well as to clinical investigators, and adopting a flexible stance that vigilantly protects patients' interests while preserving scientific validity are ways that organizers of clinical trials can encourage broad participation in such trials and decrease reliance on the parallel track. Communication with patient advocates is essential to promote participation because politically active advocacy groups, such as ACT UP, can encourage patients to participate. Perhaps more importantly, the dialogue between those who plan clinical trials and patient advocates can help define clinical questions that urgently require study and can identify aspects of a design that might discourage participation (Ellenberg, Finkelstein, and Schoenfeld, 1992).

11.5.3 Surrogate Endpoints

One of the most vexing problems in designing trials of HIV disease is selecting an appropriate endpoint. In patients with AIDS or advanced HIV disease, it is likely that information on survival will be forthcoming, and whatever endpoint is chosen for such studies, survival will be of interest. For patients with less advanced disease, such as AIDS-free patients with $200-500$ CD4$+$ T-cells/μl, it is still important to know whether a new treatment prolongs survival, but it is also clinically important to establish whether a new treatment can reduce morbidity by prolonging the time to AIDS, for example. Two clinical trials for such patients successfully demonstrated that AZT prolonged the time to AIDS, but these trials were stopped before information on survival was available (Section 11.2). In this setting, if the ultimate purpose of the trial had been to show that AZT prolonged survival, then the clinical endpoints that were used, development of AIDS or advanced AIDS-related complex (Volberding, Lagakos, Koch, et al., 1990; Fischl, Richman, Hansen, et al., 1990) would have been regarded as "surrogates." Often, the term *surrogate endpoint* refers to a change in laboratory measurements, such as CD4$+$ T-cell levels falling below 200 cells/μl. Jacobson, Bacchetti, Kolokathis, et al., (1991) and Moss (1990) discuss the possible use of a variety of laboratory measurements as surrogate endpoints or studying HIV disease.

Underlying the concept of surrogate endpoint is the supposition that there is a primary endpoint of dominant clinical importance, such as survival time. A surrogate endpoint is any other endpoint chosen for reasons of ease of study or practicality in the hope that one can learn about treatment effects on the primary endpoint indirectly through studies on the surrogate endpoint. Amato and Lagakos (1990) and Byar, Schoenfeld, Green, et al. (1990) discuss clinical relevance and the feasibility and reliability of a measurement as factors that should be taken into account when selecting an endpoint.

Sometimes changes in laboratory markers are used to modify

treatments, as in protocol VA298 in which AZT was given to patients whose CD4+ T-cell levels fell below 200 cells/μl (Section 11.2). This use of a marker can be considered to be an integral part of the treatment strategy, rather than a surrogate measure of treatment efficacy.

There are good reasons for wishing to rely on surrogate endpoints, particularly in patients with early HIV disease. A major motivation is the desire to accelerate the clinical trial process, thereby saving clinical trial resources and facilitating rapid approval of new treatments. In a cohort of patients with early HIV disease, it could take years before a sufficient number of deaths have occurred to investigate a treatment effect on survival, whereas surrogate responses, such as rates of change of CD4+ T-cell levels, could be detected in a much shorter time.

A second motivation for relying on surrogate endpoints concerns patient compliance and rapid changes in HIV therapeutics. A treatment of interest in 1990 might be irrelevant in 1995, and it is likely that many patients who were assigned to treatments in 1990 will desire to stop those treatments or try new ones if their HIV disease progresses, as indicated by declines in CD4+ T-cells or the onset of AIDS, for example. Thus standard "intention to treat" comparisons of those initially assigned to various treatment groups in 1990 may be hard to interpret when the trial ends in, say, 1997.

The problem with relying on surrogate endpoints is, of course, that treatment effects on such endpoints may not reflect treatment effects on the endpoint of primary interest. In order to interpret trials based on surrogate endpoints with confidence, one must understand the mechanism of treatment action, as illustrated in Figure 11.2. In this model, one can progress to the main endpoint either directly from the initial state of early HIV disease (path 3) or be successively experiencing a surrogate event (path 1) and then the main endpoint (path 2). We make the semi-Markov assumption that the hazards corresponding to paths 1, 2 and 3 depend only on the time spent in the antecedent state and not on when the patient arrived in the antecedent state.

If the *only* effect of treatment is to reduce the hazard in path 1, and if patients never travel path 3, then an effect of treatment on the surrogate will reliably anticipate a treatment effect in the same direction on the main endpoint. This is a special case of the stringent condition proposed by Prentice (1989) to define an adequate surrogate for hypothesis testing, namely that the hazard of developing the main endpoint, conditional on the surrogate history to that point in time, be independent of treatment. In symbols, this condition is $\lambda\{t|X(t), T\} = \lambda\{t|X(t)\}$, where $\lambda\{t|X(t), T\}$ is the instantaneous hazard of the

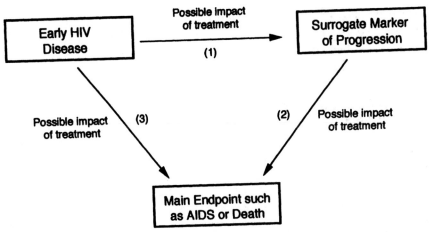

Figure 11.2 Relationships between treatment, the main endpoint, and a surrogate endpoint.

main endpoint at time t given treatment assignment T and given the entire history of the surrogate information, $X(t)$, up to time t. The quantity $\lambda\{t|X(t)\}$ is defined similarly but does not depend on treatment. In the present example, if a person still had early HIV disease at time t, his or her hazard of developing the main endpoint would be zero, regardless of treatment. Likewise if the patient had experienced the surrogate endpoint but not yet developed AIDS, his or her hazard would be the same, regardless of treatment.

Machado, Gail, and Ellenberg (1990) illustrated the effects of surrogate markers using the model in Figure 11.2 under assumptions that violate Prentice's condition. They chose parameters to model a clinical study in which patients were initially AIDS-free with CD4+ T-cell levels of 400 cells/μl. They defined the surrogate event as a CD4+ T-cell level falling below 200 cells/μl and the main endpoint as development of AIDS. In favorable cases, they found that reliance on the surrogate endpoint could reduce the required time of study from 6.5 years for the main endpoint to 3 years. However, reliance on the surrogate led to serious overestimates of treatment efficacy if treatment had serious delayed toxicity (an adverse impact on path 2 in Figure 11.2), or if treatment had only transient beneficial effects (treatment has a favorable impact on path 1 but no effect on paths 2 or 3).

Empirical studies by De Gruttola, Wulfsohn, Fischl, and Tsiatis (1992) and by Tsiatis, Dafni, De Gruttola, et al. (1992) indicate that CD4+ T-cell levels do not reflect the full benefit of AZT in prolonging the survival of patients with AIDS or AIDS-related complex. They found that at six months after randomization, patients on AZT with

CD4+ T-cell counts of 100 cells/μl has an annual hazard of death of .090/year compared to 0.620/year for patients with the same CD4+ T-cell level on placebo. AZT did boost the CD4+ T-cell levels initially in these studies, but the improvements in CD4+ T-cell levels were completely insufficient to explain the dramatic improvements in survival. Such data suggest that AZT is having favorable impacts on paths 2 and 3 in Figure 11.2, as well as on path 1. Perhaps this result is not surprising in view of the findings of Justice, Feinstein, and Wells (1989) that, among patients with AIDS, the number of major clinical signs and symptoms, such as dyspnea and weight loss, is of dominant prognostic value. Similar empirical studies are needed to determine the extent to which CD4+ T-cell levels reflect the benefits of preventing AIDS in patients with early HIV disease.

These examples demonstrate that it is not sufficient for a surrogate endpoint to be prognostic in order for that endpoint to give a clear indication of treatment efficacy on the main endpoint. In addition, the mechanism of action of the proposed treatment must be understood. If a new drug is a member of a class of drugs whose mechanism of action has been well defined, it may be plausible to assume a known mechanism of action. But even in cases where one has reason to believe that the mechanism of drug action is well understood, there may be surprises. For example, a recent study of the drugs encainide and flecainide to suppress life-threatening ventricular arrhythmias in patients recovering from myocardial infarctions demonstrated effective suppression of such arrhythmias. Based on a plausible mechanism of action, one would assume that suppression of arrythmias should lead to improved survival. Nonetheless, the trial was stopped early because it was found that the mortality rate was over twice as high among those patients given encainide or flecainide as among patients given placebo (Echt, Liebson, Mitchell, et al., 1991).

11.5.4 Monitoring AIDS Trials

Independent data monitoring boards (DMB) are usually appointed to determine when a trial should be terminated. The DMB has the important responsibilities of protecting the interests of patients who are participating in clinical trials and trying to assure that the trial will produce scientifically useful and convincing information. Adhering to these two objectives may become difficult as information on treatment efficacy and toxicity accumulates. The DMB must decide when to terminate a study, either because an important scientific goal has been reached, because continuation would adversely affect patients in the trial, or because no useful scientific purpose is served by continuing. Survey papers describe practical aspects of monitoring clinical trials (Armitage, 1991; DeMets, 1987) as well as statistical approaches to monitoring the principal endpoint (Gail, 1982, 1984).

Many of the challenges of studying HIV disease that we have previously described create difficulties in the monitoring process. In particular, if the main endpoint of the trial is not clearly identified or if there are multiple endpoints of importance, it is vital that the DMB work with the principal investigators to agree on the central purpose of the trial and on some hierarchy of importance for endpoints.

The rapid pace of scientific advance in HIV disease poses special challenges to the DMB. If the accepted standard of medical care changes during the course of the trial, as occurred in 1989 when the Public Health Service recommended prophylaxis against PCP for all patients with CD4+ T-cell levels below 200 cells/μl, the DMB may need to recommend protocol modifications or even termination of a trial if the required modification would destroy the scientific value of the trial.

The DMB may be forced to terminate a trial if the question under study is convincingly answered by another trial. For example, during the summer of 1989, the National Institutes of Allergy and Infectious Diseases announced that two studies of AZT versus placebo in AIDS-free patients had been terminated because they had shown that AZT could delay the time to AIDS or advancing AIDS-related complex. These studies were later published by Volberding, Lagakos, Koch, et al. (1990) and Fischl, Richman, Hanson, et al. (1990), as described previously. The DMB for the cooperative study of AIDS-free patients by the Veterans Administration (VA) seriously considered terminating protocol VA298 in view of these encouraging results. However, there were important differences between the VA study and the other studies that led to a continuation of the VA trial, later published by Hamilton, Hartigan, Simberkoff, et al. (1992). First, the therapeutic questions were different, because the VA trial compared early versus later use of AZT, whereas the other trials compared AZT versus placebo. Second, the VA population contained proportionately more black and Hispanic patients than the other trials. Third, the VA trial promised to provide valuable new information on whether AZT prolonged life. Finally, at the time the decision to continue the VA trial was taken, in late 1989, there was no internal evidence that AZT prolonged the time to death or to the combined endpoint of AIDS or death (Simberkoff, Hartigan, Hamilton, et al., 1993).

In this rapidly evolving scientific context, it is important that patients be kept informed regarding treatment options and that they be reminded of their right to withdraw from the study. In March 1990, the FDA approved broader indications for AZT, including treatment of all patients with CD4+ T-cell levels below 500 cells/μl. The DMB for the VA trial recommended that all patients on that study be advised in writing of the FDA recommendation and that they be asked to sign a new informed consent document informing them of their option either to continue on study medication or to withdraw from the study and receive treatment at no expense. Seventy-four percent chose to continue on blinded study treatment (Simberkoff, Hartigan, Hamilton, et al., 1992).

It is clear from these examples that a DMB may be forced to deal with many unanticipated contingencies, arising both from internal data and from external circumstances. It is therefore important that the DMB include members with a broad range of experience and knowledge in basic medical science, clinical medicine and statistics. It may be advisable to include members with formal training in medical ethics and advocates who understand the special needs of the patient population. It may be helpful in rare instances to invite outside experts to provide additional information and perspective before the DMB takes a particular decision.

11.6 VACCINE TRIALS

Since the discovery that AIDS was caused by a specific retrovirus, HIV, there has been an urgent desire and effort to develop vaccines to prevent further infections. The biology of HIV poses special problems, however (Berzofsky, 1991). First, the envelope protein of HIV is highly variable, not only among strains in different infected individuals but also among strains that evolve within a single infected individual. Thus, it may be difficult to develop a vaccine that will lead to the production of neutralizing antibody that is effective against the broad range of HIV strains. Second, HIV can spread from cell to cell as well as through the blood stream. To fight cell-to-cell spread requires a cytotoxic response, mediated by cells like CD8+ cytotoxic T-lymphocytes, as well as a humoral response (antibody production) mediated by B-lymphocytes. However, both B-lymphocytes and cytotoxic T-cells require the adequate functioning of CD4+ T-cells, known as helper T-lymphocytes (Section 1.2). Unfortunately, HIV destroys CD4+ T-cells, which limits the host's ability to mount either an effective humoral or cytotoxic immune response. Finally, once viral

DNA has been integrated into the DNA of cells of the host, it may remain latent and protected from immunologic defenses.

Effective vaccines have been made against simian immunodeficiency virus (SIV), which produces a disease in monkeys very similar to AIDS, as reviewed by Berzofsky (1991). Those vaccines provided some protection against infection for monkeys who were later challenged with SIV, and the protection against the development of fatal immunodeficiency was even better. However, some of this protection was based on antibody to antigens from human cells in which the SIV had been grown (Stott, 1991; Le Grand, Vaslin, Vogt, et al., 1992). Recent data demonstrate that SIV viral envelope antigens are sufficient to protect *Macaca fascicularis* monkeys against intravenous challenge with SIV (Hu, Abrams, Barber, et al., 1992), and human cellular antigens have been shown to inhibit infection of cultured cells by both HIV-1 and SIV (Arthur, Bess, Sowder, et al., 1992). Preliminary encouraging results have shown that vaccines can prevent HIV-1 infection in chimpanzees.

Although such animal studies are vital to vaccine research, there are important limitations on this type of study. Apart from humans, only great apes, such as the chimpanzee, and the monkey, *Macaca nemestrina*, are known to be susceptible to HIV infection (Agy, Frumkin, Corey, et al., 1992). Animals such as the chimpanzee are in short supply for medical research. More importantly, there are significant interspecies differences in the host response to HIV infection. For example, champanzees do not become ill following HIV infection. Thus, one cannot infer from a specific animal study that a particular vaccine will be effective either in preventing infection or in preventing the development of significant disease in humans. Inevitably, studies of safety and efficacy in humans are required. Stablein (1990) and Dixon and Rida (1991) discuss aspects of the design of such human studies.

11.6.1 Goals of Vaccine Trials in Humans

One potential application of vaccines is as immunotherapy to prevent or retard the progression of illness in patients who are already infected. For example, Redfield, Birx, Ketter, et al. (1991) have carried out preliminary studies showing that immunization with a molecularly cloned HIV envelope protein, gp160, was safe and elicited humoral (B cell) and cell-mediated (T cell) responses. They concluded that the therapeutic value of such immunization warrants further study. Such studies would likely be performed in patients with early HIV disease who still have the capacity to mount an immune response. Difficult design issues include selecting an appropriate endpoint and special monitoring for possible adverse effects of immunization in this comparatively healthy population. However, such clinical trials of immunotherapy pose very similar challenges to those described in Sections 11.2 and 11.5 for other therapeutic clinical trials in patients with early HIV disease.

The evaluation of vaccination to protect an uninfected population raises new issues. One goal might be to prevent HIV infection altogether. For example, one might monitor vaccinated and unvaccinated patients with serial Western blot assays to determine whether there were fewer new infections in the vaccinated group than in the unvaccinated group. We discuss design aspects of such a study later.

A second goal might be to reduce the incidence of clinically detectable immunodeficiency in an uninfected population. Many vaccines do not prevent infection but only bolster the host's response to infection so as to prevent clinical disease. If one relied on CD4+ T-cell levels as an endpoint, such a trial might take only a few more years than a study of incident HIV infection. However, if one defined the endpoint as the onset of AIDS or AIDS-related complex, such a trial would require many years and tens of thousands of patients. Therefore, we consider the design of a trial to measure the effectiveness of a vaccine to prevent infection. Similar considerations would apply to the designing of a trial to study vaccine effectiveness in preventing disease, but the effort required would be more daunting.

11.6.2 Design Considerations for a Vaccine Trial to Prevent Infection

Finding an appropriate study population will pose major problems. Even high-risk populations in the United States have annual infection incidence rates of the order of 1% per year (Table 3.8). Such infection rates necessitate a study involving many thousands of participants as described below. If the study were to be performed in an underdeveloped part of the world where infection rates were higher, one would need to resolve the ethical and political issues surrounding such experimentation, and one would need to make sure that the infrastructure was in place to follow patients carefully, to obtain samples for immunological analysis, and to carry out such analyses using sophisticated techniques, such as the Western blot procedure.

Once a suitable population is identified, it will be necessary to screen potential participants using a sensitive assay, such as the EIA (Chapter 6), to eliminate subjects who are already infected from the study. Counseling will be needed for those already infected, and potential study participants would need to be advised of the purpose and risks of the study and of precautions that everyone should take to avoid HIV infection. Such advice may reduce the HIV infection rate, necessitating a larger study. Patients who consent to participate are eligible for randomization.

Individual randomization is an important ingredient of a good vaccine trial. Each subject should have an independent chance of being assigned either to vaccine treatment or to placebo immunization. An alternative to individual randomization is cluster randomization (Cornfield, 1978). For example, one might locate several clinics for sexually transmitted diseases or several clinics for drug treatment and randomly assign each clinic to receive either vaccine or placebo immunization for all its uninfected patients. However, the chance of infection depends strongly on the local prevalence of infection in a community, and people with similar levels and types of risk behavior may tend to congregate. Therefore it is likely that there will be significant intraclinic correlation of infections, which reduces the statistical efficiency of the cluster randomization design (Cornfield, 1978). It is probably unnecessary to stratify the randomization and to use a balancing scheme to obtain balance within strata, because sufficient balance will usually be obtained by simple randomization in a trial involving thousands of subjects (Lachin, 1988). Nonetheless, baseline covariate information on important determinants of the risk of infection—such as baseline self-reports of the numbers and types of behaviors known to lead to infection, location, race, sex, and age—should be gathered to permit adjustments for these factors in the analysis.

A crucial issue is how to define the event of "new infection." A definition must be chosen that is equally applicable to the vaccinated and placebo groups. However, vaccination will produce changes in the Western blot assay, necessitating a change in the usual definitions of HIV infection. For example, one widely used definition is the presence of antibody to any two of the following protein sets: p24, gp41, and either gp120 or gp160. If a vaccine included no other HIV proteins but gp120, a new definition of infection might be: the presence of antibody to any two of p24, gp41, or gp160. Such a definition would reduce the sensitivity of the Western blot procedure because people who had p24 and gp120, for example, would no longer be defined as "infected." If more complicated vaccines were used, such as killed whole HIV, then immunologic assays like the Western blot might become useless for monitoring infection because all vaccinated subjects would develop multiple antibodies to proteins like p24, gp41, gp120, and gp160, even in the absence of infection. In this case, it might be necessary to rely on viral isolation techniques or a polymerase chain reaction assay (Section 6.5) to define infection. However, the technical and logistical demands of these approaches are substantial, and their specificity is not as high as EIA with Western blot confirmation (Chapter 6). Whatever laboratory definition of infection is adopted, it seems important to maintain very high levels of specificity (Chapter 6) to avoid serious dilution effects and the need for enormous sample sizes, as described below. Losses of sensitivity, though they necessitate somewhat larger sample sizes, are not as deleterious.

It is likely that some study participants will determine whether active vaccine or placebo has been administered. This "unblinding" of treatment assignment poses two problems. Some subjects who know they received active vaccine may feel protected and increase their levels of risky behavior. This phenomenon would reduce the apparent benefits of vaccination. Nonetheless, all such subjects should be included in the analysis of the vaccine trial, which is designed to evaluate the overall effectiveness of the strategy of vaccination.

Unblinding can also contribute to bias from "differential loss to follow-up." Loss to follow-up is said to be "nondifferential" if the expected difference in the proportions infected between the two study arms is the same among subjects who are lost to follow-up as among all subjects originally randomized. Otherwise, loss to follow-up is "differential." Differential loss to follow-up could arise, for example, if high-risk subjects who find out that they have received active vaccine tend to remain on the study, whereas high risk subjects who discover they received placebo tend to lose interest and be lost to follow-up. In this case, subjects who remain in follow-up on the placebo arm will have a lower infection rate than all those originally assigned to the placebo arm, whereas those who remain in follow-up on the active vaccine arm will have a higher infection rate than all those originally assigned to vaccine. A treatment comparison based on those who remain in follow-up will therefore tend to underestimate the effectiveness of vaccine, in this hypothetical example. This example illustrates the importance of minimizing loss to follow-up and of trying to ensure that subjects with particularly high or low risks are no more likely to be lost from one study arm than from the other. Effective blinding promotes this latter condition.

11.6.3 Definition of Vaccine Efficacy

Let p_1 be the probability that a member of a vaccinated cohort becomes infected during the course of the study, and let p_0 be the corresponding probability for unvaccinated controls. Although the following ideas hold for more general experimental designs, we assume for simplicity that the initially uninfected cohorts are fully enrolled at time $t = 0$ and that the study ends at time $t = \tau$, when all participants are tested to determine final infection status. The protective efficacy of a vaccine is defined as

$$E = 1 - R \equiv 1 - p_1/p_0, \tag{11.1}$$

which is estimable from the observed proportions infected, without any assumptions about the mechanism of action of the vaccine. When the vaccine prevents infection completely, the efficacy is unity. Note that the protective efficacy has the same mathematical form as Levin's (1953) "attributable risk" for a study of disease etiology and therefore can be estimated either by cohort or case-control methods (Walter, 1976).

Smith, Rodrigues, and Fine (1984) consider the mechanisms of action for a vaccine. Suppose $\lambda_0(t)$ is the hazard rate for infection of a member of the unvaccinated cohort. Then, under Model 1, the effect of vaccination is to reduce the hazard of infection to $\lambda_1(t) = \theta\lambda_0(t)$, where $0 \leqslant \theta \leqslant 1$. From Model 1, we calculate

$$E = 1 - \{1 - (1 - p_0)^\theta\}/p_0, \tag{11.2}$$

where

$$p_0 = 1 - \exp\left\{-\int_o^\tau \lambda_0(t)dt\right\}.$$

For experiments, such as we are considering, in which p_0 is small, we find that $E = 1 - R$ is nearly equal to $1 - \theta$.

Under Model 2 of Smith, Rodrigues, and Fine (1984), the effect of the vaccine is to render a proportion $1 - \alpha$ of the population completely immune and to have no effect on the remainder of the population. Under this model

$$E = 1 - \alpha p_0/p_0 = 1 - \alpha. \tag{11.3}$$

Understanding the mechanism of action is important if one wants to apply the results of a vaccine trial with rare events to another setting. For example, consider a setting in which the probability of infection for a member of an unvaccinated cohort, p_0^*, is large. If Model 1 is correct, the efficacy E^* computed by substituting p_0^* and θ into equation (11.2) will be smaller than the protective efficacy observed in the original experimental setting with small infection rates. This is because the right hand side of equation (11.2) decreases monotonically to zero as p_0 increases to unity, reflecting the fact that all vaccinees eventually get infected under Model 1.

By contrast, if Model 2 is correct, the same protective efficacy $E^* = 1 - \alpha$ will be found for a population with higher infection rates, p_0^*, as for the original population, because the right hand side of equation (11.3) does not depend on p_0.

The hazard $\lambda_0(t)$ can be related to quantities in epidemic models (Chapter 9). Let μ denote the number of new partners that a susceptible subject contacts per unit time. Let β_0 be the chance that an infected partner will transmit the disease to the susceptible subject during the partnership and let $y(t)$ be the proportion of people in the population who are infected at time t. Then, under the assumption that the susceptible subject has an equal chance of establishing contact with any member of the population, $\lambda_0(t) = \mu\beta_0 y(t)$, Haber, Longini, and Halloran (1991) define the efficacy of vaccination as $1 - \beta_1/\beta_0$, where β_1 is the chance that an infected individual will transmit disease to a vaccinated uninfected partner. This definition is equivalent to Model 1 above, because $\lambda_1(t)/\lambda_0(t) = \beta_1/\beta_0$; thus β_1/β_0 corresponds to θ in Model 1. Based on a simple epidemic model, Harber, Longini, and Halloran (1991) suggest that $1 - \beta_1/\beta_0$ be estimated from $1 - \{\log(1 - p_1)/\log(1 - p_0)\}$, which exceeds $E = 1 - R$ in equation (11.1).

Usually, the mechanism of action of a vaccine will be unknown at the time of initial studies. We therefore rely on the definition of protective efficacy in equation (11.1), which can be estimated without further assumptions.

11.6.4 Sample Size Considerations

We base our test for vaccine effect on the estimated proportions infected, $\hat{p}_0$ and $\hat{p}_1$, in the unvaccinated and vaccinated groups respectively. If infections are rare, as we assume, essentially the same sample size requirements would be obtained whether we were following the patients serially to establish the date at which infection occurred, or, as we assume, only at the end of the experiment to determine whether or not infection had occurred (Gail, 1985).

In the case of rare infections with equal numbers of subjects in the vaccinated and unvaccinated groups, the chi-square statistic for comparing the proportions infected in the two groups is very nearly equal to $(X_1 - X_0)^2/(X_1 + X_0)$, where X_i is the number of infections in group i ($i = 1$ for vaccinated and $i = 0$ for unvaccinated). We are assuming for now that the methods used to detect infection have perfect sensitivity and specificity. The total required sample size, $2N$, needed to assure power $1 - \beta = 0.9$ for a two-sided $\alpha = 0.05$ level test is given by

$$2N = 2(p_0 + p_1)(Z_{\alpha/2} + Z_\beta)^2/(p_0 - p_1)^2$$
$$= 2(1 + R)(Z_{\alpha/2} + Z_\beta)^2/p_0(1 - R)^2, \tag{11.4}$$

where $Z_{\alpha/2}$ is the $1 - \alpha/2$ quantile of the standard normal distribution and Z_β is the $1 - \beta$ quantile of the standard normal distribution.

From equation (11.4), it is clear that the required sample size varies nearly inversely as the square of the vaccine efficacy, $E = 1 - R$, and inversely with the probability of infection in the placebo group, p_0.

For simplicity, we imagine a 2-year study in which all subjects accrue at time zero and are examined for infection 2 years later. We assume that the hazard of infection is constant at 0.0101 per person year in the unvaccinated group, so that $p_0 = 1 - \exp(-2 \times 0.0101) = 0.02$. From equation (11.4) we calculate that the total number of subjects required to detect efficacy values $E = 1 - R$ of 0.75, 0.5, 0.25, and 0.10 are respectively 2336, 6306, 29,430, and 199,701. The required sample size increases rapidly with decreasing efficacy. Nonetheless, it may be useful to detect a vaccine efficacy of only 0.25, because such a vaccine might prevent a large number of infections.

Even these large required sample sizes do not reflect possible complications that require even larger samples. To illustrate these complications, we make comparisons to the previous case of $E = 1 - R = 0.5$ and $2N = 6306$. There are factors that can reduce p_0, necessitating a corresponding increase in sample size (equation (11.4)). If the advice given to study participants to limit risky behaviors reduces the chance of infection in the placebo group by 25% to $p_0 = 0.015$, the study size increases by the factor $1/0.75$ to 8408 (Table 11.3). Suppose the modified laboratory criteria for detecting infection are perfectly specific but have a sensitivity of only 80%. Then the observable rate of infection in placebo patients will be $p_0 = 0.80 \times 0.02 = 0.016$, and the required sample size increases by the factor $1/0.80$ to 7883.

Dilution factors that decrease apparent vaccine efficacy can have an important impact on sample size. Suppose for example that of the 1% of subjects who are infected in the year before recruitment, 10% of these were infected within the silent "window" before antibodies develop and just before recruitment (Section 6.4). Thus

Table 11.3 Sensitivity of Sample Size Calculations to Various Departures from Ideal Conditions

Conditions	Required Total Sample Size (2N)
Ideal conditions with $E = 1 - R = 0.5$ and $p_0 = 0.02$	6306
Factors that reduce p_0	
Advice given to study participants reduces the probability of infection in the placebo group to $p_0 = 0.015$	8408
Laboratory test has sensitivity 0.80 but perfect specificity	7883
Dilution effects	
Screening procedure allows infected subject to constitute 0.1% of the study population	6734
Vaccination requires 6 months to induce immunity	12,145
Laboratory criterion has perfect sensitivity but specificity only	
0.95	29,930
0.99	10,660

Note: Size was computed from equation 11.4 with $Z_{\alpha/2} = 1.96$ and $Z_\beta = 1.282$, corresponding to size 0.05 and power 0.9 for the two-sided test.

$0.1 \times 10\% = 0.1\%$ of the subjects entering the trial are already infected. The apparent infection rate in the placebo group at the end of the trial will then have expectation $p'_0 = 0.001 + 0.999 \times 0.02 = 0.021$ and the corresponding expectation for the vaccinated group is $p'_1 = 0.001 + 0.999 \times 0.02 \times 0.5 = 0.011$, assuming $R = 0.5$. Substituting p'_0 and p'_1 in equation (11.4), we obtain a total required sample of 6734, which is 6.7% more than 6306, the number needed with perfect screening. Note that the efficacy has been diluted from $E = 1 - R = 0.5$ to $1 - (0.011/0.021) = 0.476$.

Another type of dilution occurs if it takes a period of time, say 6 months, before the vaccine offers protection. Then, assuming $R = 0.5$, the rate of infection in the vaccinated group would be $p'_1 = (6/24) \times 0.02 + (18/24) \times 0.02 \times 0.5 = 0.0125$, instead of $p_1 = 0.01$, the rate of infection if the effect of vaccination is instantaneous. Applying equation (11.4), we obtain $2N = 12,145$, instead of 6734, an 80% increase. The efficacy is diluted to $1 - (0.0125/0.02) = 0.375$.

Lack of specificity of the laboratory criteria for infection can also cause serious dilution of the apparent vaccine efficacy. Suppose the new criterion has perfect sensitivity, but specificity 0.95. Then, assuming

$R = 0.5$, $p'_0 = 0.02 + 0.98 \times 0.05 = 0.0690$ and $p'_1 = 0.01 + 0.99 \times 0.05 = 0.0595$. The corresponding total sample size is $2N = 29,930$, almost five times the sample size required if the test has perfect specificity. The efficacy has been diluted to $1 - (0.0595/0.0690) = 0.138$. Even if the laboratory criterion has a specificity of 99%, the required sample size increases to 10,660 (Table 11.3).

Further adaptations are required to account for the fact that accrual takes place over time, that the final assessment of infection status may take place some time after accrual ends, and that some patients will be lost to follow-up (Rubinstein, Gail, and Santner, 1981). In particular, one can reduce the required number of subjects by extending the duration of follow-up, because the power of these studies depends on the total number of infections observed. Doubling the trial duration will roughly double p_0 in equation (11.4), thus halving the number of subjects required. Loss-to-follow-up is usually of minor importance under the assumption that those subjects who are lost are representative of their respective treatment groups. Lakatos (1986, 1988) gives very general methods to account for lag times before treatment effect, loss to follow-up and other factors.

The requirement to have very large trials, as indicated in Table 11.3, poses serious logistical problems and indicates the difficulty of carrying out such trials. Moreover, exposing large uninfected populations to the risks of vaccination, even in an experimental setting, requires a careful evaluation of potential risks and benefits. However, data from such trials would certainly be needed before one would risk exposing the general population or even special exposure groups to the risks of vaccination. Meier (1957) and Schonberger, Bregman, Sullivan-Bolyai, et al. (1979) discuss such risks for the polio and Swine flu vaccination programs, respectively.

References

Agresti, A., Mehta, C. R., and Patel, N. R. (1990). Exact inference for contingency tables with ordered categories. *Journal of the American Statistical Association* **85**: 453–58.

Agy, M. B., Frumkin, L. R., Corey, L., et al. (1992). Infection of *Macaca nemestrina* by human immunodeficiency virus type-1. *Science* **257**: 103–6.

Aitkin, M., and Clayton, D. (1980). The fitting of exponential, Weibull and extreme value distributions to complex censored survival data using GLIM. *Applied Statistics* **29**: 156–63.

Alter, H. J., Epstein, J. S., Swenson, S. G., et al. (1990). Prevalence of human immunodeficiency virus type 1 p24 antigen in U.S. blood donors—an assessment of the efficacy of testing in donor screening. *New England Journal of Medicine* **323**: 1312–17.

Amato, D. A., and Lagakos, S. W. (1990). Considerations in the selection of endpoints for AIDS clinical trials. *Journal of Acquired Immune Deficiency Syndromes* **3** (Suppl. 2): S62–S68.

Anderson, R. M. (1988a). The role of mathematical models in the study of HIV transmission and the epidemiology of AIDS. *Journal of Acquired Immune Deficiency Syndromes* **1**: 241–56.

Anderson, R. M. (1988b). The epidemiology of HIV infection: Variable incubation plus infectious periods and heterogeneity in sexual activity. *Journal of the Royal Statistical Society A* **151**: 66–93.

Anderson, R. M. (1989). Mathematical and statistical studies of the epidemiology of HIV. *AIDS* **3**: 333–46.

Anderson, R. M., Blythe, S. P., Gupta, S., and Konings, E. (1989). The transmission dynamics of the human immunodeficiency virus type 1 in the male homosexual community in the United Kingdom: The influence of changes in sexual behavior. *Philosophical Transactions of the Royal Society of London B* **325**: 45–98.

Anderson, R. E., Lang, W., Shiboski, S., et al. (1990). Use of β_2-microglobulin level and CD4 lymphocyte count to predict development of acquired immunodeficiency syndrome in persons with human immunodeficiency virus infection. *Archives of Internal Medicine* **150**: 73–77.

Anderson, R. M., and May, R. M. (1988). Epidemiological parameters of HIV transmission. *Nature* **333**: 514–19.

Anderson, R. M., May, R. M., Boily, M. C., et al. (1991). The spread of HIV-1 in Africa: Sexual contact patterns and the predicted demographic impact of AIDS. *Nature* **352**: 581–89.

Anderson, R. M., Medley, G. F., May, R. M., and Johnson, A. M. (1986). A preliminary study of the transmission dynamics of the human immunodeficiency virus (HIV), the causative agent of AIDS. *IMA Journal of Mathematics Applied in Medicine and Biology* **3**: 229–63.

Armitage, P. (1955). Tests for linear trends in proportions and frequencies. *Biometrics* **11**: 375–86.

Armitage, P. (1991). Interim analysis in clinical trials. *Statistics in Medicine* **10**: 925–37.

Arthur, L. O., Bess, J. W., Sowder II, R. C., et al. (1992). Cellular proteins bound to immunodeficiency viruses: Implications for pathogenesis and vaccines. *Science* **258**: 1935–38.

Association of State and Territorial Public Health Laboratory Directors (1987). *Second Consensus Conference on HIV Testing: Report and Recommendations.* March 16–18, Atlanta, Georgia.

Auerbach, D. M., Darrow, W. W., Jaffe, H. W., and Curran, J. W. (1984). Cluster of cases of the acquired immune deficiency syndrome: Patients linked by sexual contact. *The American Journal of Medicine* **76**: 487–92.

Auger, I., Thomas, P., De Gruttola, V. (1988). Incubation Period for Pediatric AIDS Patients. *Nature* **336**: 575–77.

Ayer, M., Brunk, H. D., Ewing, G. M., et al. (1955). An empirical distribution function for sampling with incomplete information. *Annals of Mathematical Statistics* **26**: 641–47.

Bacchetti, P. (1990). Estimating the incubation period of AIDS by comparing population infection and diagnosis patterns. *Journal of the American Statistical Association* **85**: 1002–08.

Bacchetti, P., and Jewell, N. P. (1991). Nonparametric estimation of the incubation period of AIDS based on a prevalent cohort with unknown infection times. *Biometrics* **47**: 947–60.

Bacchetti, P., and Moss, A. R. (1989). Incubation period of AIDS in San Francisco. *Nature* **338**: 251–53.

Bacchetti, P., Segal, M., and Jewell, N. P. (1992). Uncertainty about the incubation period of AIDS and its impact on backcalculation. In Jewell, N., Dietz, K., and Farewell, V. (eds.), *AIDS Epidemiology: Methodological Issues*, pp. 61–80. Boston: Birkhäuser.

Bacchetti, P., Segal, M., and Jewell, N. P. (1993). Back-calculation of HIV infection rates (with discussion). *Statistical Science* (in press).

Baecker, U., Weinauer, F., Cathof, A. G., et al. (1988). HIV antigen screening in blood donors. In *Program and Abstracts of the Fourth International Conference on AIDS*, vol. 2, p. 364, Abstract 7757. June 12–16, Stockholm, Swedish Ministry of Health and Social Affairs.

Bailey, N. T. J. (1975). *The Mathematical Theory of Infectious Diseases and Its Applications*. London: Griffen.

Baltimore, D. (1970). RNA-dependent DNA polymerase in virions of RNA tumor viruses. *Nature* **226**: 1209–11.

Barré-Sinoussi, F., Chermann, J. C., Rey, F., et al. (1983). Isolation of a T-lymphotropic retrovirus from a patient at risk for acquired immune deficiency syndrome (AIDS). *Science* **220**: 868–71.

Becker, N. G. (1989). *Analysis of Infectious Disease Data.* London: Chapman and Hall.

Becker, N. G., Watson, L. F., and Carlin, J. B. (1991). A method of non-parametric back-projection and its application to AIDS data. *Statistics in Medicine* **10**: 1527–42.

Begg, C. B. (1987). Biases in the assessment of diagnostic tests. *Statistics in Medicine* **6**: 411–23.

Berkley, S., Naamara, W., Okware, S., et al. (1990). AIDS and HIV infection in Uganda—are more women infected than men? AIDS **4**: 1237–42.

Berman, S. M. (1990). A stochastic model for the distribution of HIV latency time based on T4 counts. *Biometrika* **77**: 733–41.

Berzofsky, J. A. (1991). Approaches and issues in the development of vaccines against HIV. *Journal of Acquired Immune Deficiency Syndromes* **4**: 451–59.

Biggar, R. J., and the International Registry of Seroconverters (1990). AIDS incubation distribution in 1891 HIV seroconverters from different exposure groups. *AIDS* **4**: 1059–66.

Bishop, Y. M. M., Fienberg, S. E., and Holland, P. W. (1975). *Discrete Multivariate Analysis: Theory and Practice.* Cambridge, Mass.: MIT Press.

Blanche, S., Rouzioux, C., Moscato, M.-L. G., et al. (1989). A prospective study of infants born to women seropositive for human immunodeficiency virus type 1. *New England Journal of Medicine* **320**: 1643–48.

Bloom, D. E., and Carliner, G. (1988). The economic impact of AIDS in the United States. *Science* **239**: 604–10.

Blower, S. M., Hartel, D., Dowlatabadi, H., et al. (1991). Drugs, sex and HIV: A mathematical model for New York City. *Philosophical Transactions of the Royal Society of London. B* **321**: 171–87.

Bowen, P. A., Lobel, S. A., Caruana, R. J., et al. (1988). Transmission of human immunodeficiency virus (HIV) by transplantation: Clinical aspects and time course analysis of viral antigenemia and antibody production. *Annals of Internal Medicine* **108**: 46–48.

Bregman, D. J., and Langmuir, A. D. (1990). Farr's law applied to AIDS projections. *Journal of the American Medical Association* **263**: 1522–25.

Bremermann, H. J., and Anderson, R. W. (1990). Mathematical models of HIV infection. I. Threshold conditions for transmission and host survival. *Journal of Acquired Immune Deficiency Syndromes* **3**: 1129–34.

Breslow, N. E., and Day, N. E. (1990). *Statistical Methods in Cancer Research*, Vol. 1, *The Analysis of Case-Control Studies*. Lyon France: International Agency for Research on Cancer.

Breslow, N. E., and Day, N. E. (1987). *Statistical Methods in Cancer Research*. Vol. 2, *The Design and Analysis of Cohort Studies*. Lyon, France: International Agency for Research on Cancer.

Broder, S. (1988). The life cycle of human immunodeficiency virus as a guide to the design of new therapies for AIDS. In DeVita, V. T., Jr., Hellman, S., and Rosenberg, S. A. (eds.), *AIDS Etiology, Diagnosis, Treatment and Prevention*, pp. 78–86. Philadelphia: Lippincott.

Brookmeyer, R. (1989). More on the relation between AIDS cases and HIV prevalence. *New England Journal of Medicine* **321**: 1547–48.

Brookmeyer, R. (1991). Reconstruction and future trends of the AIDS epidemic in the United States. *Science* **253**: 37–42.

Brookmeyer, R., and Damiano, A. (1989). Statistical methods for short-term projections of AIDS incidence. *Statistics in Medicine* **8**: 23–34.

Brookmeyer, R., Dondero, T., Farber, S., et al. (1989). *Report of the Expert Panel on HIV Seroprevalence Estimates and AIDS Case Projection Methodologies*, New York City Department of Health.

Brookmeyer, R., and Gail, M. H. (1986). Minimum size of the acquired immunodeficiency syndrome (AIDS) epidemic in the United States. *Lancet* **2**: 1320–22.

Brookmeyer, R., and Gail, M. H. (1987). Biases in prevalent cohorts. *Biometrics* **43**: 739–49.

Brookmeyer, R., and Gail, M. H. (1988). A method for obtaining short-term projections and lower bounds on the size of the AIDS epidemic. *Journal of the American Statistical Association* **83**: 301–08.

Brookmeyer, R., Gail, M. H., Polk, B. F. (1987). The prevalent cohort study and the acquired immunodeficiency syndrome. *American Journal of Epidemiology* **126**: 14–24.

Brookmeyer, R., and Goedert, J. J. (1989). Censoring in an epidemic with an application to hemophilia-associated AIDS. *Biometrics* **45**: 325–35.

Brookmeyer, R., and Liao, J. (1990a). Statistical modelling of the AIDS epidemic for forecasting health care needs. *Biometrics* **46**: 1151–63.

Brookmeyer, R., and Liao, J. (1990b). The analysis of delays in disease reporting: Methods and results for the acquired immunodeficiency syndrome. *American Journal of Epidemiology* **132**: 355–65.

Brookmeyer, R., and Liao, J. (1992). Statistical methods for reconstructing infection curves. In Jewell, N., Dietz, K., and Farewell, V. (eds.), *AIDS Epidemiology: Methodologie Issues*, pp. 39–60. Boston: Birkhäuser.

Brundage, J. F., Burke, D. S., Gardner, L. I., et al. (1990). Tracking the spread of the HIV infection epidemic among young adults in the United States: Results of the first four years of screening among civilian applicants for U.S. military service. *Journal of Acquired Immune Deficiency Syndromes* **3**: 1168–80.

Brundage, J. F., Gardner, L., McNeil, J., et al. (1990). Progression of HIV disease during the early stages: Estimating rates of decline of CD4+ T-lymphocytes. *Abstracts of the VIth International Conference on AIDS,* vol. 1, p. 282, Abstract Th.C. 628. June 20–24, San Francisco.

Brundage, J. F., McNeil, J. G., Miller, R. N., et al. (1990). The current distribution of CD4+ T-lymphocyte counts among adults in the United States with human immunodeficiency virus infections: Estimates based on the experience of the U.S. Army. *Journal of Acquired Immunodeficiency Syndromes* 3: 92–94.

Buehler, J. W., Berkelman, R. L., and Stehr-Green, J. K. (1992). The completeness of AIDS surveillance. *Journal of Acquired Immune Deficiency Syndromes* 5: 257–64.

Burke, D. S., Brundage, J. F., Herbold, J. R., et al. (1987). Human immunodeficiency virus infections among civilian applicants for United States military service, October 1985 to March 1986. Demographic factors associated with seropositivity. *New England Journal of Medicine* **317**: 131–36.

Burke, D. S., Brundage, J. F., Redfield, R. R., et al. (1988). Measurement of the false positive rate in a screening program for human immunodeficiency virus infections. *New England Journal of Medicine* **319**: 961–64.

Busch, M. P., Eble, B. E., Khayam-Bashi, H., et al. (1991). Evaluation of screened blood donations for human immunodeficiency virus type 1 infection by culture and DNA amplification of pooled cells. *New England Journal of Medicine* **325**: 1–5.

Byar, D. P. (1979). The necessity and justification of randomized clinical trials. In Tagnon, H. J., and Stagnet, M. J. (eds.), *Controversies in Cancer: Design of Trials and Treatment,* pp. 75–82. New York: Masson.

Byar, D. P. (1980). Why data bases should not replace randomized trials. *Biometrics* **36**: 337–42.

Byar, D. P., Schoenfeld, D. A., Green, S. B., et al. (1990). Design considerations for AIDS trials. *New England Journal of Medicine* **323**: 1343–48.

Cahoon-Young, B., Chandler, A., Livermore, T., et al. (1989). Sensitivity and specificity of pooled versus individual sera in a human immunodeficiency virus antibody prevalence study. *Journal of Clinical Microbiology* **27**: 1893–95.

Carroll, R. J., and Ruppert, D. (1988). *Transformation and Weighting in Regression.* London: Chapman and Hall.

Castillo-Chavez, C., ed. (1989). *Lecture Notes in Biomathematics 83: Mathematical and Statistical Approaches to AIDS Epidemiology.* Berlin: Springer-Verlag.

Castillo-Chavez, C., Cooke, K. L., Huang, W., and Levin, S. A. (1989a). On the role of long incubation periods in the dynamics of acquired immunodeficiency syndrome (AIDS), part 1: Single population models. *Journal of Mathematical Biology* **27**: 373–98.

Castillo-Chavez, C., Cooke, K. L., Huang, W., and Levin, S. A. (1989b). On the role of long incubation periods in the dynamics of acquired immunodeficiency syndrome (AIDS), part 2: Multiple group models. In Castillo-Chavez, C. (ed.), *Lecture Notes in Biomathematics 83: Mathematical and Statistical Approaches to AIDS Epidemiology,* pp. 200–15. Berlin: Springer-Verlag.

Centers for Disease Control (1981a). Pneumocystis pneumonia—Los Angeles. *Morbidity and Mortality Weekly Report* **30**: 250–52.

Centers for Disease Control (1981b). Kaposi's sarcoma and Pneumocystis pneumonia among homosexual men—New York City and California. *Morbidity and Mortality Weekly Report* **30**: 305–08.

Centers for Disease Control (1982a). Update on acquired immune deficiency syndrome (AIDS)—United States. *Morbidity and Mortality Weekly Report* **31**: 507–14.

Centers for Disease Control (1982b). Opportunistic infections and Kaposi's sarcoma among Haitians in the United States. *Morbidity and Mortality Weekly Report* **31**: 353–61.

Centers for Disease Control (1982c). Possible transfusion-associated acquired immune deficiency syndrome (AIDS)—California. *Morbidity and Mortality Weekly Report* **31**: 652–54.

Centers for Disease Control (1982d). *Pneumocystis carinii* pneumonia among persons with hemophilia A. *Morbidity and Mortality Weekly Report* 31: 365–67.

Centers for Disease Control (1982e). Unexplained immunodeficiency and opportunistic infections in infants—New York, New Jersey, California. *Morbidity and Mortality Weekly Report* 31: 665–67.

Centers for Disease Control (1982f). A cluster of Kaposi's sarcoma and *Pneumocystis carinii* pneumonia among homosexual male residents of Los Angeles and Orange Counties, California. *Morbidity and Mortality Weekly Report* 31: 305–07.

Centers for Disease Control (1983). Immunodeficiency among female sexual partners of males with acquired immune deficiency syndrome (AIDS). *Morbidity and Mortality Weekly Report* 31: 697–98.

Centers for Disease Control (1984). Update: acquired immunodeficiency syndrome (AIDS)—United States. *Morbidity and Mortality Weekly Report* 32: 688–91.

Centers for Disease Control (1985a). Provisional Public Health Service inter-agency recommendations for screening donated blood and plasma for antibody to the virus causing acquired immunodeficiency syndrome. *Morbidity and Mortality Weekly Report* 34: 1–5.

Centers for Disease Control (1985b). Revision of the case definition of acquired immunodeficiency syndrome for national reporting—United States. *Morbidity and Mortality Weekly Report* 34: 373–75.

Centers for Disease Control (1986). Classification system for T-lymphotropic virus type III/lymphadenopathy-associated virus infections. *Morbidity and Mortality Weekly Report* 35: 334–39.

Centers for Disease Control (1987a). Survey of non-U.S. hemophilia treatment centers for HIV seroconversions following therapy with heat-treated concentrates. *Morbidity and Mortality Weekly Report* 36: 121–24.

Centers for Disease Control (1987b). Human immunodeficiency virus infection in the United States: A review of current knowledge. *Morbidity and Mortality Weekly Report* 36 (Suppl. 6): 1–48.

Centers for Disease Control (1987c). Public Health Service guidelines for counseling and antibody testing to prevent HIV infection and AIDS. *Morbidity and Mortality Weekly Report* 36: 509–15.

Centers for Disease Control (1987d). Revision of the CDC surveillance case definition for acquired immunodeficiency syndrome. *Morbidity and Mortality Weekly Report* 36 (Suppl. 1): 1–15.

Centers for Disease Control (1988). Update: Serologic testing for antibody to human immunodeficiency virus. *Morbidity and Mortality Weekly Report* 36: 833–45.

Centers for Disease Control (1989a). AIDS and human immunodeficiency virus infection in the United States: 1988 update. *Morbidity and Mortality Weekly Report* 38 (Suppl. 4): 1–38.

Centers for Disease Control (1989b). Interpretation and use of the Western Blot assay for serodiagnosis of human immunodeficiency virus type 1 infections. *Morbidity and Mortality Weekly Report* 38 (Suppl. 7): 1–7.

Centers for Disease Control (1989c). Guidelines for prophylaxis against *Pneumocystis carinii* pneumonia for persons infected with human immunodeficiency virus. *Morbidity and Mortality Weekly Report* 38 (Suppl. 5): 1–9.

Centers for Disease Control (1990a). Estimates of HIV prevalence and projected AIDS cases: Summary of a workshop, October 31–November 1, 1989. *Morbidity and Mortality Weekly Report* 39: 110–19.

Centers for Disease Control (1990b). MMWR surveillance for HIV-2 infection in blood donors—United States, 1987–1989. *Morbidity and Mortality Weekly Report* 39: 829–31.

Centers for Disease Control (1990c). Update: Serologic testing for HIV-1 antibody—United States, 1988 and 1989. *Morbidity and Mortality Weekly Report* 39: 380–83.

Centers for Disease Control (1990d). *HIV/AIDS Surveillance Report*, December 1990.

Centers for Disease Control (1991a). Pilot study of a household survey to determine HIV seroprevalence. *Morbidity and Mortality Weekly Report* **40**: 1–5.

Centers for Disease Control (1991b). *National HIV Serosurveillance Summary: Results through 1990.* Atlanta, Georgia: U.S. Department of Health and Human Services, Publication No. HIV/NCID/11-91/011.

Centers for Disease Control (1992a). *HIV/AIDS Surveillance Report,* January 1, 1992, 1–22.

Centers for Disease Control (1992b). 1993 Revised classification system for HIV infection and expanded surveillance case definition for AIDS among adolescents and adults. *Morbidity and Mortality Weekly Report* 41 (No. RR-17): 1–18.

Centers for Disease Control (1992c). Projections of the number of persons discussed with AIDS and the number of immunosuppressed HIV infected persons—United States, 1992–1994. *Morbidity and Mortality Weekly Report* 44 (No. RR-18): 1–29.

Chaisson, M. A., Stoneburner, R. L., Lifson, A. R., et al. (1990). Risk factors for human immunodeficiency virus type 1 (HIV-1) infection in patients at a sexually transmitted disease clinic in New York City. *American Journal of Epidemiology* **131**: 208–20.

Chernoff, H. (1954). On the distribution of the likelihood ratio. *Annals of Mathematical Statistics* **25**: 573–78.

Chin, J. (1990). Current and future dimensions of the HIV/AIDS pandemic in women and children. *Lancet* **336**: 221–24.

Chin, J., and Lwanga, S. K. (1991). Estimation and projection of adult AIDS cases: A simple epidemiological model. *Bulletin of the World Health Organization* **69**: 399–406.

Chin, J., and Mann, J. (1989). Global surveillance and forecasting of AIDS. *Bulletin of the World Health Organization* **67**: 1–7.

Chin, J., Sato, P. A., and Mann, J. M. (1990). Projections of HIV infections and AIDS cases to the year 2000. *Bulletin of the World Health Organization* **68**: 1–11.

Chmiel, J. S., Detels, R., Kaslow, R. A., et al. (1987). Factors associated with prevalent human immunodeficiency virus (HIV) infection in the Multicenter AIDS Cohort Study. *American Journal of Epidemiology* **126**: 568–77.

Clark, S. J., Saag, M. S., Don Decker, W., et al. (1991). High titres of cytopathic virus in plasma of patients with symptomatic primary HIV-1 infection. *New England Journal of Medicine* **324**: 954–60.

Cleary, P. D., Barry, M. J., Mayer, K. H., et al. (1987). Compulsory premarital screening for the human immunodeficiency virus. Technical and public health considerations. *Journal of the American Medical Association* **258**: 1757–62.

Clumeck, N., Mascart-Lemone, F., De Maubeuge, J., et al. (1983). Acquired immune deficiency syndrome in Black Africans. *Lancet* **1**: 642.

Clumeck, N., Sonnet, J., Taelman, H., et al. (1984). Acquired immunodeficiency syndrome in African patients. *New England Journal of Medicine* **310**: 492–97.

Clumeck, N., Taelman, H., Hermans, P., et al. (1989). A cluster of HIV infection among heterosexual people without apparent risk factors. *New England Journal of Medicine* **321**: 1460–62.

Coates, R. A., Soskolne, C. L., Read, S. E., et al. (1986). A prospective study of male sexual contacts of men with AIDS related conditions (ARC) or AIDS. *Canadian Journal of Public Health* **77** (Suppl. 1): 26–32.

Cohen, N. D., Muñoz, A., Reitz, B. A., et al. (1989). Transmission of retroviruses by transfusion of screened blood in patients undergoing cardiac surgery. *New England Journal of Medicine* **320**: 1172–76.

Colgate, S. A., Stanley, E. A., Hyman, J. M., et al. (1988). *A Behavior Based Model of the Initial Growth of AIDS in the United States.* Technical Report LA-UR-88-2396 of the Theoretical Division of the Los Alamos National Laboratory.

Comeau, A. M., Harris, J.-A., McIntosh, K., et al. (1992). Polymerase chain reaction in detecting HIV infection among seropositive infants: Relation to clinical status and age and to results of other assays. *Journal of Acquired Immune Deficiency Syndromes* 5: 271–78.

Cooley, T. P., Kunches, L. M., Saunders, C. A., et al. (1990). Once-daily administration of 2',3'-dideoxyinosine (ddI) in patients with the acquired immunodeficiency syndrome or AIDS-related complex: Results of a phase I trial. *New England Journal of Medicine* 322: 1340–45.

Coombs, R. W., Collier, A. C., Allain, J.-P., et al. (1989). Plasma viremia in human immunodeficiency virus infection. *New England Journal of Medicine* 321: 1626–31.

Cooper, E. C. (1990). Active control equivalence trials. *Journal of Acquired Immune Deficiency Syndromes* 3 (Suppl. 2): S77–S81.

Cornfield, J. (1978). Randomization by group: A formal analysis. *American Journal of Epidemiology* 108: 100–102.

Cox, D. R. (1972). Regression models and life-tables (with discussion). *Journal of the Royal Statistical Society, B,* 34: 187–220.

Cox, D. R. and Oakes, D. (1984). *Analysis of Survival Data.* London: Chapman and Hall.

Cumming, P. D., Wallace, E. L., Schorr, J. B., and Dodd, R. Y. (1989). Exposure of patients to human immunodeficiency virus through the transfusion of blood components that test antibody-negative. *New England Journal of Medicine* 321: 941–46.

Curran, J. W., Jaffe, H. W., Hardy, A. M., et al. (1988). Epidemiology of HIV infection and AIDS in the United States. *Science* 239: 610–16.

Curran, J. W., Morgan, W. M., Hardy, A. M., et al. (1985). The epidemiology of AIDS: Current status and future prospects. *Science* 229: 1352–57.

Daar, E. S., Moudgil, T., Meyer, R. D., and Ho, D. D. (1991). Transient high levels of viremia in patients with primary human immunodeficiency virus type 1 infection. *New England Journal of Medicine* 324: 961–64.

Darby, S. C., Doll, R., Thakrar, B., et al. (1990). Time from infection with HIV to onset of AIDS in patients with hemophilia in the UK. *Statistics in Medicine* 9: 681–89.

Darby, S. C., Rizza, C. R., Doll, R., et al. (1989). Incidence of AIDS and excess of mortality associated with HIV in hemophiliacs in the United Kingdom: Report on behalf of the directors of haemophilia centres in the United Kingdom. *British Medical Journal* 298: 1064–68.

Darrow, W. W., Echenberg, D. F., Jaffe, H. W., et al. (1987). Risk factors for human immunodeficiency virus (HIV) infections in homosexual men. *American Journal of Public Health* 77: 479–83.

Day, N. E., and Gore, S. M. (1989). Prediction of the number of new AIDS cases and the number of new persons infected with HIV up to 1992: The results of "back projection" methods. In *Short-term Prediction of HIV Infections and AIDS in England and Wales,* appendix 12. London: Her Majesty's Stationary Office.

De Cook, K. M., and Brun-Vézinet, F. (1989): Epidemiology of HIV-2 infection. *AIDS* 3 (Suppl. 1): S89–95.

Deffner, A., and Haeusler, E. (1985). A characterization of order statistic point processes that are mixed Poisson processes and mixed sample processes simultaneously. *Journal of Applied Probability* 22: 314–23.

De Gruttola, V., and Lagakos, S. W. (1989a). Analysis of doubly-censored survival data with applications to AIDS. *Biometrics* 45: 1–11.

De Gruttola, V., and Lagakos, S. W. (1989b). The value of AIDS incidence data in assessing the spread of HIV infection. *Statistics in Medicine* 8: 35–43.

De Gruttola, V., Lange, N., and Dafni, U. (1991). Modeling the progression of HIV infection. *Journal of the American Statistical Association* 86: 569–77.

De Gruttola, V., and Mayer, K. H. (1988). Assessing and modeling heterosexual spread of the human immunodeficiency virus in the United States. *Review of Infectious Diseases* **10**: 138–50.

De Gruttola, V., Seage, G. R., Mayer, K. H., and Horsburgh, C. R., Jr. (1989). Infectiousness of HIV between male homosexual partners. *Journal of Clinical Epidemiology* **42**: 849–56.

De Gruttola, V., and Tu, X. (1992). Modeling the relationship between disease progression and survival time. In Jewell, N., Dietz, K., Farewell, V. (eds.). *AIDS Epidemiology: Methodological Issues*, pp. 275–96. Boston: Birkhäuser.

De Gruttola, V., Tu, X. M., and Pagano, M. (1992). Pediatric AIDS in New York City: Estimating the distributions of infection, latency, and reporting delay and projecting future incidence. *Journal of the American Statistical Association* **87**: 633–40.

De Gruttola, V., Wulfsohn, M., Fischl, M. A., and Tsiatis, A. (1992*)*. Modeling the relationship between survival and CD4—lymphocytes in patients with AIDS and AIDS-related complex. *Journal of Acquired Immune Deficiency Syndromes* **6**: 359–65.

DeMets, D. L. (1987). Practical aspects in data monitoring: A brief review. *Statistics in Medicine* **6**: 753–60.

Department of Defense (1992). Prevalence of HIV-1 antibody in civilian applicants for military service, October 1985–March 1992. Tables prepared by the Division of HIV/AIDS, Centers for Disease Control, Atlanta, Georgia.

Detels, R., English, P., Visscher, B. R., et al. (1989). Seroconversion, sexual activity, and condom use among 2915 HIV seronegative men followed for up to 2 years. *Journal of Acquired Immune Deficiency Syndromes* **2**: 77–83.

De Vincenzi, I. (1992). Heterosexual transmission of HIV (letter). *Journal of the American Medical Association* **267**: 1919.

DeVita, V. T., Jr., Hellman, S., and Rosenberg, S. A., eds. (1988). *AIDS: Etiology, Diagnosis, Treatment and Prevention*. Philadelphia: Lippincott.

DeWys, W. D., Curran, J., Henle, W., and Johnson, G. (1982). Workshop on Kaposi's Sarcoma: Meeting Report. *Cancer Treatment Reports* **66**: 1387–90.

Diekmann, O., Heesterbeek, J. A. P., and Metz, J. A. J. (1990). On the definition and the computation of the basic reproductive ratio R_0 in models for infectious diseases in heterogeneous populations. *Journal of Mathematical Biology* **28**: 365–82.

Dietz, K. (1988). On the transmission dynamics of HIV (1988). *Mathematical Biosciences* **90**: 397–414.

Dietz, K., and Hadeler, K. P. (1988). Epidemiological models for sexually transmitted diseases. *Journal of Mathematical Biology* **26**: 1–25.

Dietz, K., and Schenzle, D. (1985). Mathematical models for infectious disease statistics. In Atkinson, A. C., and Fienberg, S. E. (eds.), *A Celebration of Statistics, ISI Centenary Volume*. New York: Springer-Verlag.

Dixon, D. O., and Rida, W. N. (1991). HIV vaccine trials: Some design issues including sample size calculation. Presentation at the American Statistical Association, August 1991, Atlanta, Georgia.

Dodd, R. Y. (1986). Testing for HTLV-III/LAV. In Menitove, J. E. and Kolins, J. (eds.), *AIDS*, pp. 55–78. Arlington, Virginia: American Association of Blood Banks.

Dodd, R. Y., and Fang, C. T. (1990). The Western immunoblot procedure for HIV antibodies and its interpretation. *Archives of Pathology and Laboratory Medicine* **114**: 240–45.

Dondero, T. J., St. Louis, M., Petersen, L., et al. (1989). Evaluation of the estimated number of HIV infections using a spreadsheet model and empirical data. Presented at a Workshop at the Centers for Disease Control, October 31–November 1, 1989, Atlanta.

Echt, D. S., Liebson, P. R., Mitchell, L. B., et al. (1991). Mortality and morbidity in patients receiving encainide, flecainide, or placebo: The cardiac arrythmia suppression trial. *New England Journal of Medicine* **324**: 781–88.

Efron, B. (1992). *The Jackknife, the Bootstrap and Other Resampling Plans*. Philadelphia: Society for Industrial and Applied Mathematics.

Efron, B. (1988). Logistic regression, survival analysis and the Kaplan-Meier curve. *Journal of the American Statistical Association* **83**: 414–25.

Eisenberg, B. (1989). The numbers of partners and the probability of HIV infection. *Statistics in Medicine* **8**: 83–92.

Eisenberg, B. (1991). The effect of variable infectivity on the risk of HIV infection. *Statistics in Medicine* **10**: 131–39.

Ellenberg, S. S., Finkelstein, D. M., and Schoenfeld, D. A. (1992). Statistical issues arising in AIDS clinical trials. *Journal of the American Statistical Association* **87**: 562–68.

Esteban, J. I., Shih, J. W.-K., Tai, C.-C., et al. (1985). Importance of Western Blot analysis in predicting infectivity of anti-HTLV-III/LAV positive blood. *Lancet* **2**: 1083–86.

European Collaborative Study (1991). Children born to women with HIV-1 infection: Natural history and risk of transmission. *Lancet* **337**: 253–60.

European Study Group (1989). Risk factors for male to female transmission of HIV. *British Medical Journal* **298**: 411–15.

Eyster, M. E., Gail, M. H., Ballard, J. O., et al. (1987). Natural history of human immunodeficiency virus infections in hemophiliacs: Effect of T-cell subsets, platelet counts and age. *Annals of Internal Medicine* **107**: 1–6.

Fahey, J. L., Taylor, J. M. G., Detels, R., et al. (1990). The prognostic value of cellular and serological markers in infection with human immunodeficiency virus type 1. *New England Journal of Medicine* **322**: 166–72.

Farzadegan, H., Polis, M., Wolinsky, S. M., et al. (1988). Loss of human immunodeficiency virus type 1 (HIV-1) antibodies with evidence of viral infection in asymptomatic homosexual men. A report from the Multicenter AIDS Cohort Study. *Annals of Internal Medicine* **108**: 785–90.

Fätkenheuer, G., Stützer, H., Salzberger, B., and Schrappe, M. (1991). Zidovudine and the natural history of AIDS. *New England Journal of Medicine* **325**: 1311–12.

Fauci, A. S. (1988). The human immunodeficiency virus: Infectivity and mechanisms of pathogenesis. *Science* **239**: 617–22.

Fienberg, S. E. (1980). *The Analysis of Cross-Classified Categorical Data*, 2d ed. Cambridge, Mass.: MIT Press.

Fife, D., and Mode, C. (1992). AIDS incidence and income. *Journal of Acquired Immune Deficiency Syndromes* **5**: 1105–10.

Fineberg, H. V. (1988). Education to prevent AIDS: Prospects and obstacles. *Science* **239**: 592–96.

Fischl, M. A., Parker, C. B., Pettinelli, C., et al. (1990). A randomized controlled trial of a reduced daily dose of zidovudine in patients with the acquired immunodeficiency syndrome. *New England Journal of Medicine* **323**: 1009–14.

Fischl, M. A., Richman, D. D., Causey, D. M., et al. (1989). Prolonged zidovudine therapy in patients with AIDS and advanced AIDS-related complex. *Journal of the American Medical Association* **262**: 2405–10.

Fischl, M. A., Richman, D. D., Grieco, M. H., et al. (1987). The efficacy of azidothymidine (AZT) in the treatment of patients with AIDS and AIDS-related complex. A double-blind placebo-controlled trial. *New England Journal of Medicine* **317**: 185–91.

Fischl, M. A., Richman, D. D., Hansen, N., et al. (1990). The safety and efficacy of zidovudine (AZT) in the treatment of subjects with mildly symptomatic human immunodeficiency virus type 1 (HIV) infection. A double-blind placebo-controlled trial. *Annals of Internal Medicine* **112**: 727–37.

Fleming, T. R. (1990). Evaluation of active control trials in AIDS. *Journal of Acquired Immune Deficiency Syndromes* **3** (Suppl. 2): S82–S87.

Fletcher, R. H., Fletcher, S. W., and Wagner, E. H. (1988). *Clinical Epidemiology: The Essentials*, 2d ed. Baltimore, Md.: Williams & Wilkins.

Friedland, G. H., and Klein, R. S. (1987). Transmission of the human immunodeficiency virus. *New England Journal of Medicine* **317**: 1125–35.

Friedland, G. (1989). Parenteral drug users. In Kaslow, R. A. and Francis, D. P. (eds.), *The Epidemiology of AIDS*, pp. 153–78. New York: Oxford University Press.

Friedman, L. A., Furberg, C. D., and DeMets, D. L. (1984). *Fundamentals of Clinical Trials*, 2d ed. Boston: Wright.

Freund, H. P., and Book, D. L. (1990). Determination of the spread of HIV from the AIDS incidence history. *Mathematical Biosciences* **98**: 227–41.

Gail, M. H. (1979). Some statistical methods for evaluating immunodiagnostic tests. In Herberman, R., and McIntire, R. (eds.) *Immunodiagnosis of Cancer*, pp. 20–37. New York: Marcel Dekker.

Gail, M. H. (1981), Evaluating serial cancer marker studies in patients at risk of recurrent disease. *Biometrics* **37**: 67–78.

Gail, M. H. (1982). Monitoring and stopping clinical trials. In Miké, V., and Stanley, K. E. (eds.), *Statistics in Medical Research: Methods and Issues with Applications in Cancer Research*, pp. 455–84. New York: Wiley.

Gail, M. H. (1984). Nonparametric frequentist proposals for monitoring comparative survival studies. In Krishnaiah, P. R., and Sen, P. K. (eds.), *Handbook of Statistics*, Vol. 4, pp. 791–811. Amsterdam: Elsevier Science.

Gail, M. H. (1985). Applicability of sample size calculations based on a comparison of proportions for use with the logrank test. *Controlled Clinical Trials* **6**: 112–19.

Gail, M. H. (1991a). A bibliography and comments on the use of statistical models in epidemiology in the 1980's. *Statistics in Medicine* **10**: 1819–85.

Gail, M. H. (1991b). Some statistical methods for immunodiagnostic cancer tests. In Herberman, R. B., and Mercer, D. W. (eds.), *Immunodiagnosis of Cancer*, pp. 13–25. New York: Marcel Dekker.

Gail, M. H., and Brookmeyer, R. (1988). Methods for projecting course of acquired immunodeficiency syndrome epidemic. *Journal of the National Cancer Institute* **80**: 900–11.

Gail, M. H., and Brookmeyer, R. (1990a). Projecting the incidence of AIDS. *Journal of the American Medical Association* **263**: 1538–39.

Gail, M. H., and Brookmeyer, R. (1990b). Modeling the AIDS epidemic. *AIDS Updates* **3**: 1–8.

Gail, M. H., Pluda, J. M., Rabkin, C. S., et al. (1991). Projections of the incidence of non-Hodgkin's lymphoma related to acquired immunodeficiency syndrome. *Journal of the National Cancer Institute* **83**: 695–701.

Gail, M. H., Preston, D., and Piantadosi, S. (1989). Disease prevention models of voluntary confidential screening for human immunodeficiency virus (HIV). *Statistics in Medicine* **8**: 59–81.

Gail, M. H., and Rosenberg, P. S. (1992). Perspectives on using back-calculation to estimate HIV prevalence and project AIDS incidence. In Jewell, N., Dietz, K., and Farewell, V. (eds.), *AIDS Epidemiology: Methodological Issues*, pp. 1–38. Boston: Birkhäuser.

Gail, M. H., Rosenberg, P. S., and Goedert, J. J. (1990a). Therapy may explain recent deficits in AIDS incidence. *Journal of Acquired Immune Deficiency Syndromes* **3**: 296–306.

Gail, M. H., Rosenberg, P. S., and Goedert, J. J. (1990b). Deficits in AIDS incidence (authors' reply). *Journal of Acquired Immune Deficiency Syndromes* **3**: 833–35.

Gallo, R. C., Salahuddin, S. Z., Popovic, M., et al. (1984). Frequent detection and isolation of cytopathic retroviruses (HTLV-III) from patients with AIDS and at risk of AIDS. *Science* **224**: 500–03.

Gardner, L. I., Brundage, J. F., McNeil, J. G., et al. (1992). Predictors of HIV-1 disease progression in early- and late-stage patients: the U.S. Army natural history cohort. *Journal of Acquired Immune Deficiency Syndromes* **5**: 782–93.

Gastwirth, J. L. (1987). The statistical precision of medical screening procedures: Application to polygraph and AIDS antibodies test data. *Statistical Science* **2**: 213–38.

Gastwirth, J. L., and Hammick, P. A. (1989). Estimation of the prevalence of a rare disease, preserving the anonymity of the subjects by group testing: Application to estimating the prevalence of AIDS antibodies in blood donors. *Journal of Statistical Planning and Inference* **22**: 15–27.

Gastwirth, J. L., and Johnson, W. O. (1991). Applicability of group testing as a quality control check on the sensitivity of screening tests applied in very low prevalence populations. (Submitted).

Gastwirth, J. L., Johnson, W. O., and Reneau, D. M. (1991). Bayesian analysis of screening data: Application to AIDS in blood donors. *The Canadian Journal of Statistics* **9**: 135–50.

Gayle, H. D., Keeling, R. P., Garcia-Tunon, M., et al. (1990). Prevalence of the human immunodeficiency virus among university students. *New England Journal of Medicine* **323**: 1538–41.

Gelber, R. D., Lenderking, W. R., Cotton, D. J., et al. (1992). Quality-of-life evaluation in a clinical trial of zidovudine therapy in patients with mildly symptomatic HIV infection. *Annals of Internal Medicine* **116**: 961–66.

General Accounting Office (1989). *AIDS Forecasting: Undercount of Cases and Lack of Key Data Weaken Existing Estimates.* Program evaluation and methodology division, 89-13, Washington, D.C., U.S. General Accounting Office.

Gerig, J. M., and Galant, A. R. (1975). Computing methods for linear models subject to linear parametric constraints. *Journal of Statistical Computation and Simulation* **3**: 283–96.

Goedert, J. J. (1990). Prognostic markers for AIDS. *Annals of Epidemiology* **1**: 129–39.

Goedert, J. J., Biggar, R. J., Melbye, M., et al. (1987). Effect of T4 count and cofactors on the incidence of AIDS in homosexual men infected with human immunodeficiency virus. *Journal of the American Medical Association* **257**: 331–34.

Goedert, J. J., Biggar, R. J. Weiss, S. H., et al. (1986). Three year incidence of AIDS in five cohorts of HTLV-III-infected risk group members. *Science* **231**: 992–95.

Goedert, J. J., Biggar, R. J., Winn, D. M., et al. (1984). Determinants of retrovirus (HTLV-III) antibody and immunodeficiency conditions in homosexual men. *Lancet* **2**: 711–16.

Goedert, J. J., and Blattner, W. A. (1988). The epidemiology and natural history of human immunodeficiency virus. In DeVita, V. T. Jr., Hellman, S., and Rosenbert, S. A. (eds.), *AIDS: Etiology Diagnosis, Treatment and Prevention*, pp. 33–60. Philadelphia: Lippincott.

Goedert, J. J., Eyster, M. E., Biggar, R. J., and Blattner, W. A. (1987). Heterosexual transmission of human immunodeficiency virus: Association with severe depletion of T helper lymphocytes in men with hemophilia. *AIDS Research and Human Retroviruses* **3**: 355–61.

Goedert, J. J., Kessler, C. M., Aledort, L. M., et al. (1989). A prospective study of human immunodeficiency virus type 1 infection and the development of AIDS in subjects with hemophilia. *New England Journal of Medicine* **321**: 1141–48.

Goedert, J. J., Mendez, H., Drummond, J. E., et al. (1989). Mother-to-infant transmission of human immunodeficiency virus type 1: Association with prematurity or low anti-gp120. *Lancet* **2**: 1351–54.

Goedert, J. J., Sarngadharan, M. G., Biggar, R. J., et al. (1984). Determinants of retrovirus (HTLV-III) antibody and immunodeficiency conditions in homosexual men. *Lancet* **2**: 711–16.

Goedert, J. J., Sarngadharan, M. G., Eyster, M. E., et al. (1985). Antibodies reactive with human

T cell leukemia viruses in the serum of hemophiliacs receiving factor VIII concentrate. *Blood* **65**: 492–95.

Golden, J. A., Chernoff, D., Hollander, H., et al. (1989). Prevention of *Pneumocystis carinii* pneumonia by inhaled pentamidine. *Lancet* **1**: 654–57.

Golub, A., and Gorr, W. (1990). *The Effect of Spatial Aggregation on Reported Growth of AIDS Cases*. Working paper 90-5, School of Urban and Public Affairs, Carnegie Mellon University.

Gonzales, J. J., and Koch, M. G. (1987). On the role of "transients" (biasing transitional effects) for the prognostic analysis of the AIDS epidemic. *American Journal of Epidemiology* **126**: 985–1005.

Gottlieb, M. S., Schroff, R., Schanker, H. M., et al. (1981). *Pneumocystis carinii* pneumonia and mucosal candidiasis in previously healthy homosexual men. Evidence of a new acquired cellular immunodeficiency. *New England Journal of Medicine* **305**: 1425–31.

Gould, P. (1988). *Understanding and Predicting the AIDS Epidemic in Geographic Space*. Working paper by the Penn State-Carnegie Mellon-Ohio State Consortium.

Graham, N. M. H., Zeger, S. L., Kuo, V., et al. (1991). Zidovudine use in AIDS-free HIV seropositive homosexual men in the Multicenter AIDS Cohort Study (MACS), 1987–1989. *Journal of Acquired Immune Deficiency Syndromes* **4**: 267–76.

Graham, N. M. H., Zeger, S. L., Park, L. P., et al. (1991). Effect of zidovudine and *Pneumocystis carinii* pneumonia prophylaxis on progression of HIV-1 infection to AIDS. *Lancet* **338**: 265–69.

Grant, R. M., Wiley, J. A., and Winkelstein, W. (1987). Infectivity of the human immunodeficiency virus: Estimates from a prospective study of homosexual men. *Journal of Infectious Diseases* **156**: 189–93.

Green, S. B., Ellenberg, S. S., Finkelstein, D., et al. (1990). Issues in the design of drug trials for AIDS. *Controlled Clinical Trials* **11**: 80–87.

Green, T. A., Karon, J. M., and Nwanyanwu, O. C. (1992). Changes in AIDS incidence trends in the United States. *Journal of Acquired Immune Deficiency Syndromes* **5**: 547–55.

Greene, W. C. (1991). The molecular biology of human immunodeficiency virus type 1 infection. *New England Journal of Medicine* **324**: 308–17.

Gwinn, M., Pappaioanou, M., George, J. R., et al. (1991). Prevalence of HIV infection in childbearing women in the United States: Surveillance using newborn blood samples. *Journal of the American Medical Association* **265**: 1704–08.

Haber, M., Longini, I. M., and Halloran, M. E. (1991). Measures of the effects of vaccination in a randomly mixing population. *International Journal of Epidemiology* **20**: 300–10.

Hamilton, J. D., Hartigan, P. M., Simberkoff, M. S., et al. (1992). A controlled trial of early versus late treatment with zidovudine in human immunodeficiency virus infection. Results of the Veterans Affairs Cooperative Study. *New England Journal of Medicine* **326**: 437–43.

Hanley, J. A., and McNeil, B. J. (1983). A method of comparing the areas under receiver operating characteristic curves derived from the same cases. *Radiology* **148**: 839–43.

Hardy, A. M., Starcher, E. T., and Morgan, W. M. (1987). Review of death certificates to assess completeness of AIDS case reporting. *Public Health Reports* **102**: 386–91.

Harris, J. E. (1990a). Reporting delays and the incidence of AIDS. *Journal of the American Statistical Association* **85**: 915–24.

Harris, J. E. (1990b). Improved short-term survival of AIDS patients initially diagnosed with *Pneumocystis carinii* pneumonia, 1984 through 1987. *Journal of the American Medical Association* **263**: 397–401.

Haseltine, W. A. (1989). Silent HIV infections. *New England Journal of Medicine* **320**: 1487–89.

Haseltine, W. A. (1991). Regulation of HIV-1 replication by *tat* and *rev*. In Haseltine, W. A., and Wong-Stahl, F. (eds.), *Genetic Structure and Regulation of HIV*, pp. 1–42. New York: Raven Press.

Hastie, T. J., and Tibshirani, R. J. (1990). *Generalized Additive Models*. London: Chapman and Hall.

Haverkos, H. W., and Edelman, R. (1989). Heterosexuals. In Kaslow, R. A., and Francis, D. P. (eds.), *The Epidemiology of AIDS*, pp. 136–52. New York: Oxford University Press.

Hessol, N. A., Lifson, A. R., O'Malley, P. M., et al. (1989). Prevalence, incidence, and progression of human immunodeficiency virus infection in homosexual and bisexual men in hepatitis B vaccine trials, 1978–1988. *American Journal of Epidemiology* **130**: 1167–75.

Hethcote, H. W. (1987). Mathematical models for the projection of AIDS incidence. Presented at the Johns Hopkins conference on statistical and mathematical modelling of the AIDS epidemic, November 1987.

Hethcote, H. W., and Van Ark, J. W. (1992a). *Lecture Notes in Biomathematics 95: Modeling HIV Transmission and AIDS in the United States*. Berlin: Springer-Verlag.

Hethcote, H. W., and Van Ark, J. W. (1992b). Weak linkage between HIV epidemics in homosexual men and intravenous drug users. In Jewell, N., Dietz, K., and Farewell, V. (eds.), *AIDS Epidemiology: Methodological Issues*, pp. 174–208. Boston: Birkhäuser.

Hethcote, H. W., Van Ark, J. W., and Karon, J. M. (1991). A simulation model of AIDS in San Francisco: II. Simulations, therapy and sensitivity analysis. *Mathematical Biosciences* **106**: 223–47.

Hethcote, H. W., Van Ark, J. W., and Longini, I. M., Jr. (1991). A simulation model of AIDS in San Francisco: I. Model formulation and parameter estimation. *Mathematical Biosciences* **106**: 203–22.

Hethcote, H. W., and Yorke, J. S. (1984). *Lecture Notes in Biomathematics 56: Gonorrhea Transmission Dynamics and Control*, chapter 5. Berlin: Springer-Verlag.

Hoff, R., Berardi, V. P., Weiblen, B. J., et al. (1988). Seroprevalence of human immunodeficiency virus among childbearing women: Estimation by testing samples of blood from newborns. *New England Journal of Medicine* **318**: 525–30.

Horsburgh, C. R., Jr., Qu, C. Y., Jason, I. M., et al. (1989). Duration of human immunodeficiency virus infection before detection of antibody. *Lancet* **2**: 637–40.

Horvitz, D. G., Folsom, R. E., Ezzati, T. M., and Massey, J. T. (1992). Assessment of nonresponse bias in the Dallas County HIV survey. (in preparation).

Horwitz, J. P., Chua, J., and Noel, M. (1964). Nucleosides V. The monomesylates of 1-(2′-deoxy-beta-d-lyxofuranosyl) thymine. *Journal of Organic Chemistry* **29**: 2076–78.

Hu, S.-L., Abrams, K., Barber, G. N., et al. (1992). Protection of macaques against SIV infection by subunit vaccines of SIV envelope glycoprotein gpl60. *Science* **255**: 456–59.

Hudson, C. P., Hennis, A. J. M., Kataaha, P., et al. (1988). Risk factors for the spread of AIDS in rural Africa: Evidence from a comparative socioepidemiological survey of AIDS, hepatitis B, and symphillis in southwestern Uganda. *AIDS* **2**: 255–60.

Hull, H. F., Bettinger, C. J., Gallaher, M. M., et al. (1988). Comparison of HIV-antibody prevalence in patients consenting to and declining HIV-antibody testing in an STD clinic. *Journal of the American Medical Association* **260**: 935–38.

Hyman, J. M., and Stanley, E. A. (1988). Using mathematical models to understand the AIDS epidemic. *Mathematical Biosciences* **90**: 415–73.

Imagawa, D., and Detels, R. (1991). HIV-1 in seronegative homosexual men. *New England Journal of Medicine* **325**: 1250–51.

Imagawa, D. T., Lee, M. H., Wolinsky, S. M., et al. (1989). Human immunodeficiency virus type 1 infection in homosexual men who remain seronegative for prolonged periods. *New England Journal of Medicine* **320**: 1458–62.

Institute of Medicine (1986). *Confronting AIDS: Directions for Public Health, Health Care, and Research.* Washington, D.C.: National Academy Press.

Institute of Medicine (1988). *Confronting AIDS: Update 1988.* Washington, D.C.: National Academy Press.

Institute of Medicine (1991). Expanding access to investigate therapies for HIV infection and AIDS: Conference Summary, March 12–13, 1990. Washington, D.C.: National Academy Press.

Isham, V. (1988). Mathematical modelling of the transmission dynamics of HIV infection and AIDS: A review. *Journal of the Royal Statistical Society A,* **151**: 5–30.

Isham, V. (1989). Estimation of the incidence of HIV infection. *Philosophical Transactions of the Royal Society of London, Series B* **325**: 113–21.

Italian Multicentre Study (1988). Epidemiology, clinical features, and prognostic factors of paediatric HIV infection. *Lancet* **2**: 1043–46.

Italian Seroconversion Study (1992). Disease progression and early predictors of AIDS in HIV-seroconverted injecting drug users. *AIDS* **6**: 421–26.

Jacobson, M. A., Bacchetti, P., Kolokathis, A., et al. (1991). Surrogate markers for survival in patients with AIDS and AIDS-related complex treated with zidovudine. *British Medical Journal* **302**: 73–78.

Jacquez, J. A., Simon, C. P., Koopman, J., et al. (1988). Modeling and analyzing HIV transmission: The effect of contact patterns. *Mathematical Biosciences* **92**: 119–99.

Jacquez, J. A., Simon, C. P., and Koopman, J. (1989). Structured mixing: Heterogeneous mixing by definition of activity group. In Castillo-Chavez, C. (ed), *Mathematical and Statistical Approaches to AIDS Epidemiology,* pp. 301–15. Berlin: Springer-Verlag.

Jaffe, H. W., Choi, K., Thomas, P. A., et al. (1983). National case-control study of Kaposi's sarcoma and Pneumocystis carinii pneumonia in homosexual men: Part 1, epidemiologic results. *Annals of Internal Medicine* **99**: 145–51.

Jason, J., Holman, R. C., Dixon, G., et al. (1986). Effects of exposure to factor concentrates containing donations from identified AIDS patients. *Journal of the American Medical Association* **256**: 1758–62.

Jewell, N. P. (1990). Some statistical issues in studies of the epidemiology of AIDS. *Statistics in Medicine* **9**: 1387–1416.

Jewell, N. P., and Kalbfleisch, J. D. (1992). Marker processes in survival analysis. In Jewell, N., Dietz, K., and Farewell, V. (eds.), *AIDS Epidemiology: Methodological Issues,* pp. 211–30. Boston: Birkhäuser.

Jewell, N. P., and Nielsen, J. P. (1993). A framework for consistent prediction rules based on markers. *Biometrika* **80**: 153–64.

Jewell, N. P., and Shiboski, S. C. (1990). Statistical analysis of HIV infectivity based on partner studies. *Biometrics* **46**: 1133–50.

Jewell, N. P., and Shiboski, S. C. (1992). The design and analysis of partner studies of HIV transmission. In Ostrow, D., and Kessler, R. (eds.), *Methodological Issues of AIDS Behavioral Research.* New York: Plenum Publishing.

Johnson, W. O., and Gastwirth, J. L. (1991). Bayesian inference for medical screening tests: Approximations useful for the analysis of acquired immune deficiency syndrome. *Journal of the Royal Statistical Society, Series B* **53**: 427–39.

Justice, A. C., Feinstein, A. R., and Wells, C. K. (1989). A new prognostic staging system for the acquired immunodeficiency syndrome. *New England Journal of Medicine* **320**: 1388–93.

Kakaiya, R. M., Cable, R. G., and Keltonic, J. (1987). Look back: The status of recipients of blood from donors subsequently found to have antibody to HIV. *Journal of the American Medical Association* **257**: 1176–77.

Kalbfleisch, J. D., and Lawless, J. F. (1989). Inference based on retrospective ascertainment: An analysis of data on transfusion related AIDS. *Journal of the American Statistical Association* **84**: 360–72.

Kalbfleisch, J. D., and Prentice, R. L. (1980). *The Statistical Analysis of Failure Time Data*. New York: John Wiley & Sons.

Kaplan, E. H. (1989). Needles that kill: Modelling human immunodeficiency virus transmission via shared drug injection equipment in shooting galleries. *Review of Infectious Diseases* **11**: 289–98.

Kaplan, E. H. (1990). Modeling HIV infectivity: Must sex acts be counted? *Journal of Acquired Immune Deficiency Syndromes* **3**: 55–61.

Kaplan, E. L., and Meier, P. (1958). Nonparametric estimation from incomplete observations. *Journal of the American Statistical Association* **53**: 457–81.

Karon, J., Dondero, T., and Curran, J. (1988). The projected incidence of AIDS and estimated prevalence of HIV infection in the United States. *Journal of Acquired Immune Deficiency Syndromes* **1**: 542–50.

Kaslow, R. A., and Francis, D. P., eds. (1989). *The Epidemiology of AIDS: Expression, Occurrence and Control of Human Immunodeficiency Virus Type 1 Infection*. New York: Oxford University Press.

Kaslow, R. A., Ostrow, D. G., Detels, R., et al. (1987). The Multicenter AIDS Cohort Study: Rationale, organization and selected characteristics of the participants. *American Journal of Epidemiology* **126**: 310–18.

Kim, M. Y., and Lagakos, S. W. (1990). Estimating the infectivity of HIV from partner studies. *Annals of Epidemiology* **1**: 117–28.

Kingsley, L. A., Detels, R., Kaslow, R., et al. (1987). Risk factors for seroconversion to human immunodeficiency virus among male homosexuals. *Lancet* **1**: 345–49.

Kingsley, L. A., Zhou, S. Y. J., Bacellar, H., et al. (1991). Temporal trends in human immunodeficiency virus type 1 seroconversion 1984–1989. A report of the Multicenter AIDS Cohort Study (MACS). *American Journal of Epidemiology* **134**: 331–39.

Kinsey, A. C., Pomeroy, W. B., and Martin, C. E. (1948). *Sexual Behavior in the Human Male*. Philadelphia: Sanders.

Kline, R. L., Brothers, T. A., Brookmeyer, R., et al. (1989). Evaluation of human immunodeficiency virus seroprevalence in population surveys using pooled sera. *Journal of Clinical Microbiology* **27**: 1449–52.

Knolle, H. (1990). Age preference in sexual choice and the basic reproduction number of HIV/AIDS. *Biometrical Journal* **32**: 243–56.

Koopman, J. S., Longini, I. M., Jacquez, J. A., et al. (1991). Assessing risk factors for transmission of infection. *American Journal of Epidemiology* **133**: 1199–1209.

Koopman, J., Simon, C., Jacquez, J., et al. (1988). Sexual partner selectiveness effects on homosexual HIV transmission dynamics. *Journal of Acquired Immune Deficiency Syndromes* **1**: 486–504.

Koopman, J. S., Simon, C. P., Jacquez, J. A., and Park, T. S. (1989). Selective contact within structured mixing with an application to HIV transmission risk from oral and anal sex. In Castillo-Chavez, C. ed., *Mathematical and Statistical Approaches to AIDS Epidemiology*, pp. 316–48. Berlin: Springer-Verlag.

Krämer, A., Wiktor, S. Z., Fuchs, D., et al. (1989). Neopterin: A predictive marker of acquired immune deficiency syndrome in human immunodeficiency virus infection. *Journal of Acquired Immune Deficiency Syndromes* **2**: 291–96.

Lachin, J. M. (1988). Properties of simple randomization in clinical trials. *Controlled Clinical Trials* **9**: 312–26.

Lagakos, S. W., Barraj, L. M., and De Gruttola, V. (1988). Nonparametric analysis of truncated survival data with application to AIDS. *Biometrika* **75**: 515–23.

Laird, N. M., and Ware, J. H. (1982). Random effects models for longitudinal data. *Biometrics* **38**: 963–74.

Lakatos, E. (1986). Sample size determination in clinical trials with time-dependent rates of losses and non-compliance. *Controlled Clinical Trials* **7**: 189–99.

Lakatos, E. (1988). Sample sizes based on the log-rank statistic in complex clinical trials. *Biometrics* **44**: 229–41.

Lambert, J. S., Seidlin, M., Reichman, R. C., et al. (1990). 2′,3′-dideoxyinosine (ddI) in patients with the acquired immunodeficiency syndrome or AIDS related complex. *New England Journal of Medicine* **322**: 1333–40.

Lange, N., Carlin, B., and Gelfand, A. (1992). Hierarchical Bayes models for the progression of HIV infection using longitudinal CD4 T-cell numbers. *Journal of the American Statistical Association* **87**: 615–32.

Lang, W., Perkins, H., Anderson, R. E., et al. (1989). Patterns of T lymphocyte changes with human immunodeficiency virus infection: From seroconversion to the development of AIDS. *Journal of Acquired Immune Deficiency Syndromes* **2**: 63–69.

Larder, B. A., Darby, G., and Richman, D. D. (1989). HIV with reduced sensitivity to zidovudine (AZT) isolated during prolonged therapy. *Science* **243**: 1731–34.

Law, C. G., and Brookmeyer, R. (1992). Effects of mid-point imputation on the analysis of doubly censored data. *Statistics in Medicine* **11**: 1569–78.

Lawless, J., and Sun, J. (1992). A comprehensive back-calculation framework for the estimation and prediction of AIDS cases. In Jewell, N., Dietz, K., and Farewell, V. (eds.), *AIDS Epidemiology: Methodological Issues*, pp. 81–104. Boston: Birkhäuser.

Lazzarin, A., Saracco, A., Musicco, A., et al. (1991). Man-to-woman sexual transmission of the human immunodeficiency virus. Risk factors related to sexual behavior, man's infectiousness, and woman's susceptibility. *Archives of Internal Medicine* **151**: 2411–16.

Le Grand, R., Vaslin, B., Vogt, G., et al. (1992). AIDS vaccine developments. *Nature* **355**: 684.

Lehmann, E. L. (1975). *Nonparametrics: Statistical Methods Based on Ranks*, chapter 1. San Francisco: Holden-Day.

Lemp, G. F., Payne, S. F., Neal, D., et al. (1990). Survival trends for patients with AIDS. *Journal of the American Medical Association* **263**: 402–06.

Lemp, G. F., Payne, S. F., Rutherford, G. W., et al. (1990). Projections of AIDS morbidity and mortality in San Francisco. *Journal of the American Medical Association* **263**: 1497–1501.

Leoung, G. S., Feigal, D. W., Montgomery, A. B., et al. (1990). Aerosolized pentamidine for prophylaxis against *Pneumocystis carinii* pneumonia. The San Francisco Community Prophylaxis Trial. *New England Journal of Medicine* **323**: 769–75.

Le Pont, F., Costagliola, D., Massari, V., and Valleron, A.-J. (1989). Blood donation and HIV infection: Impact of seroconversion delay on the sensitivity of the testing procedure. *Revue d' Epidemiologie et de Santé Publique* **37**: 97–102.

Levin, M. L. (1953). The occurrence of lung cancer in man. *Acta Unio Internationalis Contra Cancrum* **9**: 531–41.

Levy, J. A., ed. (1989). *AIDS Pathogenesis and Treatment*. New York: Marcel Dekker.

Liddell, F. D. K., McDonald, J. C., and Thomas, D. C. (1977). Methods for cohort analysis: Appraisal by application to asbestos mining (with discussion). *Journal of the Royal Statistical Society, Series A* **140**: 469–90.

Lifson, A. R., Darrow, W. W., Hessol, N. A., et al. (1990). Kaposi's sarcoma in a cohort of homosexual and bisexual men. Epidemiology and analysis for cofactors. *American Journal of Epidemiology* **131**: 221–31.

Longini, I. M., Jr. (1990). Modeling the decline of CD4+ T-lymphocyte counts in HIV-infected individuals. *Journal of Acquired Immune Deficiency Syndromes* **3**: 930–31.

Longini, I. M., Jr., Byers, R. H., Hessol, N. A., and Tan, W. Y. (1992). Estimating the stage-specific numbers of HIV infection using a Markov model and back-calculation. *Statistics in Medicine* **11**: 831–43.

Longini, I. M., Jr., Clark, W. S., Byers, R. H., et al. (1989). Statistical analysis of the stages of HIV infection using a Markov model. *Statistics in Medicine* **8**: 831–43.

Longini, I. M., Jr., Clark, W. S., Gardner, L. I., and Brundage, J. (1991). The dynamics of CD4+ T-lymphocyte decline in HIV infected individuals: A Markov modeling approach. *Journal of Acquired Immunodeficiency Syndromes* **4**: 1141–47.

Longini, I. M., Jr., Clark, W. S., Haber, M., and Horsburgh, R. J., Jr. (1989). The stages of HIV infection: Waiting times and infection transmission probabilities. In Castillo-Chavez, C. (ed.), *Lecture Notes in Biomathematics 83: Mathematical and Statistical Approaches in AIDS Epidemiology*, pp. 11–137. Berlin: Springer-Verlag.

Lui, K.-J., Darrow, W. W., and Rutherford, G. W. (1988). A model-based estimate of the mean incubation period for AIDS in homosexual men. *Science* **240**: 1333–35.

Lui, K.-J., Lawrence, D. N., Morgan, W. M., et al. (1986). A model based approach for estimating the mean incubation period of transfusion-associated acquired immunodeficiency syndrome. *Proceedings of the National Academy of Sciences, USA* **83**: 3051–55.

MacDonald, K. L., Jackson, J. B., Bowman, R. J., et al. (1989). Performance characteristics of serologic tests for human immunodeficiency virus type 1 (HIV-1) antibody among Minnesota blood donors. *Annals of Internal Medicine* **110**: 617–21.

Machado, S. G., Gail, M. H., and Ellenberg, S. S. (1990). On the use of laboratory markers as surrogates for clinical endpoints in the evaluation of treatment for HIV infection. *Journal of Acquired Immune Deficiency Syndromes* **3**: 1065–73.

Magder, L., and Brookmeyer, R. (1993). Analysis of infectious disease data from partner studies with unknown source of infection. *Biometrics* (in press).

Malone, J. L., Simms, T. E., Gray, C. G., et al. (1990). Sources of variability in repeated T-helper lymphocyte counts from human immunodeficiency virus type 1-infected patients: Total lymphocyte count fluctuations and diurnal cycle are important. *Journal of Acquired Immune Deficiency Syndromes* **3**: 144–51.

Mantel, N. (1963). Chi-square tests with one degree of freedom: Extension of the Mantel-Haenszel procedure. *Journal of the American Statistical Association* **58**: 690–700.

Marcus, R., and CDC Cooperative Needlestick Surveillance Group (1988). Surveillance of health care workers exposed to blood from patients infected with the human immunodeficiency virus. *New England Journal of Medicine* **319**: 1118–23.

Marion, S., and Schechter, M. (1991). An estimation of the number of persons in Canada infected with human immunodeficiency virus. Department of Health Care and Epidemiology, University of British Columbia.

Mariotto, A. B., Mariotti, S., Pezzotti, P., et al. (1992). Estimation of the acquired immunodeficiency syndrome incubation period in intravenous drug users: A comparison with male homosexuals. *American Journal of Epidemiology* **135**: 428–37.

Marmor, M., Friedman-Kien, A. E., Laubenstein, L., et al. (1982). Risk factors for Kaposi's sarcoma in homosexual men. *Lancet* **1**: 1083–87.

Marmor, M., Friedman-Kien, A. E., Zolla-Pazner, S., et al. (1984). Kaposi's sarcoma in homosexual men. A seroepidemiologic case-control study. *Annals of Internal Medicine* **100**: 809–15.

Massey, J. T., Ezzati, T. M., and Folsom, R. (1989). *Survey Methodology Requirements to Determine the Feasibility of the National Household Seroprevalence Survey.* Quality Assessment Task Force Report, National Center for Health Statistics, January 1989.

Massey, J. T., Ezzati, T. M., and Folsom, R. (1990). Statistical issues in measuring the prevalence of HIV infection in a household survey. *Proceedings of the Section on Survey Research Methods of the American Statistical Association*, pp. 160–69.

Masur, H., Michelis, M. A., Greene, J. B., et al. (1981). An outbreak of community-acquired *Pneumocystis carinii* pneumonia: Initial manifestation of cellular immune dysfunction. *New England Journal of Medicine* **305**: 1431–8.

May, R. M., and Anderson, R. M. (1987). Transmission dynamics of HIV infection. *Nature* **326**: 137–42.

May, R. M., and Anderson, R. M. (1988). Transmission dynamics of human immunodeficiency virus (HIV). *Philosophical Transactions of the Royal Society of London, Series B* **321**: 565–607.

Mayer, K. H., Stoddard, A. M., McCusker, J., et al. (1986). Human T-lymphotropic virus type III in high-risk antibody-negative homosexual men. *Annals of Internal Medicine* **104**: 194–96.

McCullagh, P., and Nelder, J. A. (1989). *Generalized Linear Models*, 2d ed. London: Chapman and Hall.

McDonald, J. W., and Diamond, I. D. (1990). On the fitting of generalized linear models with nonnegativity parameter constraints. *Biometrics* **46**: 201–06.

McKusick, L., Horstman, W., and Coates, T. J. (1985). AIDS and sexual behavior reported by gay men in San Francisco. *American Journal of Public Health* **75**: 493–96.

McMahan, C. A., Maxwell, L. C., and Shepherd, A. P. (1986). Estimation of the distribution of blood vessel diameters from the arteriovenous passages of microspheres. *Biometrics* **42**: 371–80.

McNeil, J. G., Brundage, J. F., Wann, Z. F., et al. (1989). Direct measurement of human immunodeficiency virus seroconversions in a serially tested population of young adults in the United States Army, October 1985 to October 1987. *New England Journal of Medicine* **320**: 1581–85.

Medley, G. F., Anderson, R. M., Cox, D. R., and Billard, L. (1987). Incubation period of AIDS in patients infected via blood transfusion. *Nature* **328**: 719–21.

Meier, P. (1957). Safety testing of poliomyelitis vaccine. *Science* **125**: 1067–71.

Meinert, C. L. (1986). *Clinical Trials: Design, Conduct and Analysis*. New York: Oxford University Press.

Melbye, M., Biggar, R. J., Ebbesen, P., et al. (1984). Seroepidemiology of HTLV-III antibody in Danish homosexual men: Prevalence, transmission, and disease outcome. *British Medical Journal* **289**: 573–75.

Mendelsohn, J., and Rice, J. (1982). Deconvolution of microfluorometric histograms with B splines. *Journal of the American Statistical Association* **77**: 748–53.

Menitove, J. E. (1986). Status of recipients of blood from donors subsequently found to have antibody to HIV. *New England Journal of Medicine* **315**: 1095–96.

Meyer, K. B., and Pauker, S. G. (1987). Screening for HIV: Can we afford the false positive rate? *New England Journal of Medicine* **317**: 238–41.

Miller, H. G., Turner, C. F., and Moses, L. E., eds. (1990); AIDS: *The Second Decade*. Washington, D.C.: National Academy Press.

Mills, J., Jacobson, M. A., O'Donnell, J. J., et al. (1988). Treatment of cytomegalovirus retinitis in patients with AIDS. *Review of Infectious Diseases* **10** (Suppl. 3): S522–31.

Mitsuya, H., Weinhold, K. J., Furman, P. A., et al. (1985). 3′-azido-3′-deoxythmidine (BW A509U): An antiviral agent that inhibits the infectivity and cytopathic effect of human T-lymphotropic virus type III/lymphadenopathy-associated virus in vitro. *Proceedings of the National Academy of Science* (USA) **82**: 7096–7100.

Mitsuya, H., Yarchoan, R., and Broder, S. (1990). Molecular targets for AIDS therapy. *Science* **249**: 1533–44.

Moore, R. D., Hidalgo, J., Sugland, B. W., and Chaisson, R. E. (1991). Zidovudine and the natural history of the acquired immunodeficiency syndrome. *New England Journal of Medicine*

324: 1412–16.

Morgan, W. M., and Curran, J. W. (1986). Acquired immunodeficiency syndrome: Current and future trends. *Public Health Reports* **101**: 459–65.

Moss, A. R. (1990). Laboratory markers as potential surrogates for clinical outcomes in AIDS trials. *Journal of Acquired Immune Deficiency Syndromes* **3** (Suppl. 2): S69–71.

Moss, A. R., and Bacchetti, P. (1989). Natural history of HIV infection. *AIDS* **3**: 55–61.

Moss, A. R., Bacchetti, P., Osmond, D., et al. (1988). Seropositivity for HIV and the development of AIDS or AIDS-related condition: Three year follow-up of the San Francisco General Hospital Cohort. *British Medical Journal* **296**: 745–50.

Moss, A. R., Osmund, D., Bacchetti, P., et al. (1987). Risk factors for AIDS and HIV seropositivity in homosexual men. *American Journal of Epidemiology* **125**: 1035–47.

Mosteller, F., and Tukey, J. W. (1977). *Data Analysis and Regression.* Reading, Massachusetts: Addison-Wesley.

Muñoz, A., Wang, M.-C., Bass, S., et al. (1989). Acquired immunodeficiency syndrome (AIDS)-free time after human immunodeficiency virus type 1 seroconversion in homosexual men. *American Journal of Epidemiology* **130**: 530–39.

National Institute of Allergy and Infectious Diseases, Division of AIDS (1991). *Thirteenth AIDS Clinical Trials Group Meeting Report,* December 2–5, 1991, Washington, D.C.

Newman, M. E. (1990). *The Development of Zidovudine (AZT) for the Treatment of AIDS.* Report from the National Cancer Institute Office of Cancer Communications, May 1990.

Nicolosi, A., Leite, M. L. C., Molinari, S., et al. (1992). Incidence and prevalence trends of HIV infection in intravenous drug users attending treatment centers in Milan and Northern Italy. *Journal of Acquired Immune Deficiency Syndromes* **5**: 365–73.

Nicolosi, A., Leite, M. L. C., Musicco, M., et al. (1992). Parenteral and sexual transmission of human immunodeficiency virus in intravenous drug users: A study of seroconversion. *American Journal of Epidemiology* **135**: 225–33.

Nold, A. (1980). Heterogeneity in disease-transmission modeling. *Mathematical Biosciences* **52**: 227–40.

Novick, L. F., Berns, D., Stricof, R., et al. (1989). HIV seroprevalence in newborns in New York State. *Journal of the American Medical Association* **261**: 1745–50.

Novick, L. F., Glebatis, D. M., Stricof, R. L., et al. (1991). II. Newborn seroprevalence study: Methods and results. *American Journal of Public Health* **81** (Suppl.): 15–21.

Nychka, D. (1988). Bayesian confidence intervals for smoothing splines. *Journal of the American Statistical Association* **83**: 1134–43.

Oleske, J., Minnefor, A., Cooper, R., et al. (1983). Immune deficiency syndrome in children. *Journal of the American Medical Association* **249**: 2345–49.

Ostertag, W., Roesler, G., Krieg, C. J., et al. (1974). Induction of endogenous virs and of thymidine kinase by bromodeoxyuridine in cell cultures transformed by Friend virus. *Proceedings of the National Academy of Sciences, USA* **71**: 4980–85.

O'Sullivan, F. (1986). A statistical perspective on ill-posed inverse problems. *Statistical Science* **1**: 502–27.

O'Sullivan, F., Yandell, B. S., Raynor, W. J., Jr. (1986). Automatic smoothing of regression functions in generalized linear models. *Journal of the American Statistical Association* **81**: 96–103.

Padian, N. Marquis, L., Francis, D. P., et al. (1987). Male-to-female transmission of human immunodeficiency virus. *Journal of the American Medical Association* **258**: 788–90.

Padian, N. S., Shiboski, S., and Jewell, N. P. (1990). The effect of number of exposures on the risk of heterosexual HIV transmission. *Journal of Infectious Diseases* **161**: 883–87.

Padian, N. S., Shiboski, S. C., and Jewell, N. P. (1991). Female-to-male transmission of human immunodeficiency virus. *Journal of the American Medical Association* **266**: 1164–67.

Pappaioanou, M., Dondero, T. J., Petersen, L. R., et al. (1990). The family of HIV seroprevalence surveys: Objectives, methods and uses of sentinel surveillance for HIV in the United States. *Public Health Reports* **105**: 113–19.

Payne, C. D. (1986). *The GLIM Manual Release 3.77*. Oxford: Numerical Algorithms Group.

Pepe, M. S., Self, S. G., and Prentice, R. L. (1989). Further results on covariate measurement errors in cohort studies with time to response data. *Statistics in Medicine* **8**: 1167–78.

Peterman, T., and Allen, J. (1989). Recipients of blood and blood products. In Kaslow, R. A., and Francis, D. P. (eds.), *The Epidemiology of AIDS*, pp. 179–93. New York: Oxford University Press.

Peterman, T. A., Stoneburner, R. L., Allen, J. R., et al. (1988). Risk of human immunodeficiency virus transmission from heterosexual adults with transfusion associated infections. *Journal of the American Medical Association* **259**: 55–58.

Petersen, L., Satten, G., and Dodd, R. (1992). Time period from infectiousness as blood donor to development of detectable antibody and the risk of HIV transmission from transfusion of screened blood. *Abstract MoC0091*, VIII International Conference on AIDS, Amsterdam, July 19–24, 1992.

Peterson, D., Willard, K., Altmann, M., et al. (1990). Monte Carlo simulation of HIV infection in an intravenous drug user community. *Journal of Acquired Immune Deficiency Syndromes* **3**: 1086–95.

Phair, J., Muñoz, A., Detels, R., et al. (1990). The risk of *Pneumocystis carinii* pneumonia among men infected with human immunodeficiency virus type 1. *New England Journal of Medicine* **322**: 161–165.

Phillips, A. N., Lee, C. A., Elford, J., et al. (1991). Serial CD4 lymphocyte counts and the development of AIDS. *Lancet* **337**: 389–92.

Phillips, A. N., Lee, C. A., and Elford, J. (1992). The cumulative risk of AIDS as the CD4 lymphocyte count declines. *Journal of Acquired Immune Deficiency Syndromes* **5**: 148–52.

Philips, D. (1962). A technique for the numerical solution of certain integral equations of the first kind. *Association for Computing Machinery Journal* **9**: 84–97.

Pickering, J., Wiley, J. A., Padian, N. S., et al. (1986). Modelling the incidence of acquired immunodeficiency syndrome (AIDS) in San Francisco, Los Angeles and New York. *Mathematical Modelling* **7**: 661–88.

Piot, P., Plummer, F. A., Mhalu, F. S., et al. (1988). AIDS: An international perspective. *Science* **239**: 573–79.

Pizzo, P. A., and Butler, K. M. (1991). In the vertical transmission of HIV, timing may be everything. *New England Journal of Medicine* **325**: 652–54.

Pocock, S. J. (1983). *Clinical Trials: A Practical Approach*. Chichester, U.K.: John Wiley & Sons.

Polk, B. F., Fox, R., Brookmeyer, R., et al. (1987). Predictors of the acquired immunodeficiency syndrome developing in a cohort of seropositive homosexual men. *New England Journal of Medicine* **316**: 61–66.

Popovic, M., Sarngadharan, M. G., Read, E., and Gallo, R. C. (1984). Detection, isolation and continuous production of cytopathic retroviruses (HTLV-III) from patients with AIDS and pre-AIDS. *Science* **224**: 497–500.

Prentice, R. L. (1982). Covariate measurement errors and parameter estimation in a failure time regression model. *Biometrika* **69**: 331–42.

Prentice, R. L. (1989). Surrogate endpoints in clinical trials: Definition and operational criteria. *Statistics in Medicine* **8**: 431–40.

Prentice, R. L., and Breslow, N. E. (1978). Retrospective studies and failure time models. *Biometrika* **65**: 153–58.

Press, W. H., Teukolsky, S. A., Vetterling, W. T., and Flannery, B. P. (1992). *Numerical Recipes in FORTRAN, the ART of Scientific Computing*, 2d ed. Cambridge, Mass.: Cambridge University Press.

Public Health Service (1986). Coolfont report: A PHS plan for prevention and control of AIDS and the AIDS virus. *Public Health Reports* **101**: 341–48.

Quinn, T. C., Glasser, D., Cannon, R. O., et al. (1988). Human immunodeficiency virus infection among patients attending clinics for sexually transmitted diseases. *New England Journal of Medicine* **318**: 197–203.

Quinn, T. C., Piot, P., McCormick, J. B., et al. (1987). Serologic and immunologic studies in patients with AIDS in North America and Africa. The potential role of infectious agents as cofactors in human immunodeficiency virus infection. *Journal of the American Medical Association* **257**: 2617–21.

Quinn, T. P., and Mann, J. (1989). HIV-1 infection and AIDS in Africa. In Kaslow, R. A., and Francis, D. P. (eds.), *The Epidemiology of AIDS*, pp. 194–220. New York: Oxford University Press.

Raboud, J., Reid, N., Coates, R. A., and Farewell, V. T. (1993). Estimating risks of progressing to AIDS when covariates are measured with error. *Applied Statistics* (in press).

Ragni, M. V., Kingsley, L. A., Nimorwicz, P., et al. (1989). HIV heterosexual transmission in hemophilia couples: Lack of relation to T4 number, clinical diagnosis, or duration of HIV infection. *Journal of Acquired Immune Deficiency Syndromes* **2**: 557–63.

Ranki, A., Valle, S. L., Krohn, M., et al. (1987). Long latency precedes overt seroconversion in sexually transmitted human immunodeficiency virus infection. *Lancet* **2**: 589–93.

Ransohoff, D. F., and Feinstein, A. R. (1978). Problems of spectrum and bias in evaluating the efficacy of diagnostic tests. *New England Journal of Medicine* **299**: 926–30.

Redfield, R. R., Birx, D. L., Ketter, N., et al. (1991). A phase I evaluation of the safety and immunogenicity of vaccination with recombinant gp160 in patients with early human immunodeficiency virus infection. *New England Journal of Medicine* **324**: 1677–84.

Redfield, R. R., Markham, P. D., Salahuddin, S. Z., et al. (1985). Heterosexually acquired HTLV-III/LAV disease (AIDS-related complex and AIDS). Epidemiologic evidence for female-to-male transmission. *Journal of the American Medical Association* **254**: 2094–96.

Redfield, R. R., Wright, D. C., and Tramont, E. C. (1986). The Walter Reed staging classification for HTLV-III/LAV infection. *New England Journal of Medicine* **314**: 131–32.

Reesink, H. W., Lelie, P. N., Huisman, J. G., et al. (1986). Evaluation of six enzyme immunoassays for antibody against human immunodeficiency virus. *Lancet* **2**: 483–86.

Remis, R. S., and Palmer, R. (1991). Modelling AIDS mortality from survival analysis to evaluate completeness of reporting. In *Abstracts from the VII International Conference on AIDS*, vol. 2, p. 48, Abstract W.C. 97. June 16–21, Florence.

Research Triangle Institute (1990). *National Household Seroprevalence Survey Feasibility Study Final Report*, Vol. 1. Research Triangle Institute, Research Triangle Park, N.C.

Rezza, G., Lazzarin, A., Angarano, G., et al. (1989). The natural history of HIV infection in intravenous drug users: Risk of disease progression in a cohort of seroconverters. *AIDS* **3**: 87–90.

Rogers, M. F., Qu, C.-Y., Rayfield, M., et al. (1989). Use of the polymerase chain reaction for early detection of the proviral sequences of human immunodeficiency virus in infants born to seropositive mothers. *New England Journal of Medicine* **320**: 1649–54.

Rosenberg, P. S. (1990). A simple correction of AIDS surveillance data for reporting delays. *Journal of Acquired Immune Deficiency Syndromes* **3**: 49–54.

Rosenberg, P. S., Biggar, R. J., Goedert, J. J., and Gail, M. H. (1991). Backcalculation of the number with human immunodeficiency virus infection in the United States. *American Journal of Epidemiology* **133**: 276–85.

Rosenberg, P. S., and Gail, M. H. (1990). Uncertainty in estimates of HIV prevalence derived by backcalculation. *Annals of Epidemiology* **1**: 105–15.

Rosenberg, P. S., and Gail, M. H. (1991). Back-calculation of flexible linear models of the human immunodeficiency virus infection curve. *Applied Statistics* **40**: 269–82.

Rosenberg, P. S., Gail, M. H., and Carroll, R. J. (1992). Estimating HIV prevalence and projecting AIDS incidence in the United States: A model that accounts for therapy and changes in the surveillance definition of AIDS. *Statistics in Medicine* **11**: 1633–55.

Rosenberg, P. S., Gail, M. H., and Massey, J. T. (1992). A comparison of HIV prevalence estimates from the Dallas County household HIV survey with estimates derived by backcalculation. (in preparation).

Rosenberg, P. S., Gail, M. H., and Pee, D. (1991). Mean square error of estimates of HIV prevalence and short-term AIDS projections derived by backcalculation. *Statistics in Medicine* **10**: 1167–80.

Rosenberg, P. S., Gail, M. H., Schrager, L. K., et al. (1991). National AIDS incidence trends and the extent of zidovudine therapy in selected demographic and transmission groups. *Journal of Acquired Immune Deficiency Syndromes* **4**: 392–401.

Rosenberg, P. S., Levy, M. E., Brundage, J. F., et al. (1992). Population-based monitoring of an urban HIV/AIDS epidemic: Magnitude and trends in the District of Columbia. *Journal of the American Medical Association* **268**: 495–503.

Royce, R. A., Luckman, R. S., Fusaro, F. E., and Winkelstein, W. (1991). The natural history of HIV-1: Staging classifications of disease. *AIDS* **5**: 355–64.

Rubinstein, L. V., Gail, M. H., and Santner, T. J. (1981). Planning the duration of a comparative clinical trial with loss to follow-up and a period of continued observation. *Journal of Chronic Diseases* **34**: 469–79.

Rubinstein, A., Sicklick, M., Gupta, A., et al. (1983). Acquired immunodeficiency with reversed T4/T8 ratios in infants born to promiscuous and drug-addicted mothers. *Journal of the American Medical Association* **249**: 2350–56.

Ruedy, J., Schechter, M., and Montaner, J. S. G. (1990). Zidovudine for early human immunodeficiency virus (HIV) infection: Who, when and how? *Annals of Internal Medicine* **112**: 721–23.

Ryder, R. W., Nsa, W., Hassig, S. E., et al. (1989). Perinatal transmission of the human immunodeficiency virus type 1 to infants of seropositive women in Zaire. *New England Journal of Medicine* **320**: 1637–42.

Sandler, S. G., Dodd, R. Y., and Fang, C. T. (1988): Diagnostic tests for HIV infection: Serology. In DeVita, V. T., Jr., Hellman, S., and Rosenberg, S. A. (eds.), *AIDS Etiology, Diagnosis, Treatment and Prevention*, pp. 121–36. Philadelphia: Lippincott.

San Francisco Department of Public Health (1991). Young men's survey, San Francisco, 1991. HIV seroprevalence among young gay and bisexual men. *San Francisco Epidemiological Bulletin* **7**: 31–33.

Sanathanan, L. (1972). Estimating the size of a multinomial population. *Annals of Mathematical Statistics* **43**: 142–52.

Sarngadharan, M. G., Popovic, M., Bruch, L., et al. (1984). Antibodies reactive with human T-lymphotropic retroviruses (HTLV-III) in the serum of patients with AIDS. *Science* **224**: 506–08.

Sattenspiel, L. (1987). Population structure and the spread of disease. *Human Biology* **59**: 411–38.

Schechter, M. T., Craib, K., Le, T., et al. (1989a). Progression to AIDS and predictors of AIDS in seroprevalent and seroincident cohorts of homosexual men. *AIDS* **3**: 347–53.

Schechter, M. T., Craib, K. J. P., Le, T. N., et al. (1989b). Influence of zidovudine on progression to AIDS in cohort studies. *Lancet* **1**: 1026–27.

Schonberger, L. B., Bregman, D. J., Sullivan-Bolyai, J. Z., et al. (1979). Guillain-Barré syndrome following vaccination in the national influenza immunization program, United States, 1976–1977. *American Journal of Epidemiology* **110**: 105–23.

Schwartz, J. S., Dans, P. E., and Kinosian, B. P. (1988). Human immunodeficiency virus test evaluation, performance and use: Proposals to make good tests better. *Journal of the American Medical Association* **259**: 2574–79.

Scott, G. B., Hutto, C., Makuch, R. W., et al. (1989). Survival in children with perinatally acquired human immunodeficiency virus type 1 infection. *New England Journal of Medicine* **321**: 1791–96.

Segal, M., and Bacchetti, P. (1990). Deficits in AIDS incidence (letter). *Journal of Acquired Immune Deficiency Syndromes* **3**: 832–33.

Self, S., and Pawitan, Y. (1992). Modeling a marker of disease progression and onset of disease. In Jewell, N., Dietz, K. Farewell, V. (eds.), *AIDS Epidemiology: Methodological Issues*, pp. 231–55. Boston: Birkhäuser.

Selik, R. M., Buehler, J. W., Karon, J. M., et al. (1990). Impact of the 1987 revision of the case definition of AIDS in the United States. *Journal of Acquired Immune Deficiency Syndromes* **3**: 73–82.

Sharples, K., Carlson, R., Skegg, D., and Paul, C. (1991). Short term projections of AIDS incidence in New Zealand. Department of Preventice and Social Medicine, University of Otago Medical School, Dunedin, New Zealand.

Shaw, G. M., Wong-Staal, F., and Gallo, R. C. (1988). Etiology of AIDS: Virology, molecular biology, and evolution of human immunodeficiency virus. In DeVita, V. T., Jr., Hellman, S., and Rosenberg, S. A. (eds.), *AIDS: Etiology, Diagnosis, Treatment and Prevention*, pp. 11–31. Philadelphia: Lippincott.

Sheppard, H. W., Ascher, M. S., Busch, M. P., et al. (1991). A multicenter proficiency trial of gene amplification (PCR) for detection of HIV-1. *Journal of Acquired Immune Deficiency Syndromes* **4**: 277–83.

Shiboski, S. C., and Jewell, N. P. (1992) Statistical analysis of the time dependence of HIV infectivity based on partner study data. *Journal of the American Statistical Association* **87**: 360–72.

Silverman, B. W. (1985). Some aspects of the spline smoothing approach to non-parametric regression curve fitting. *Journal of the Royal Statistical Society B* **47**: 1–52.

Simberkoff, M. S., Hartigan, P. M., Hamilton, J. D., et al. (1993). Ethical dilemmas in continuing a zidovudine trial after early termination of similar tests. *Controlled Clinical Trials* **14**: 6–18.

Sloand, E. M., Pitt, E., Chiarello, R. J., and Nemo, G. J. (1991). HIV testing: State of the art. *Journal of the American Medical Association* **266**: 2861–66.

Smith, P. G., Rodrigues, L. C., and Fine, P. E. M. (1984). Assessment of the protective efficacy of vaccines against common diseases using case-control and cohort studies. *International Journal of Epidemiology* **13**: 87–93.

Solomon, P. J., Fazekas de St. Groth, and Wilson, S. R. (1990). *Projections of the Acquired Immune Deficiency Syndrome in Australia Using Data to the End of September 1989*. National Center for Epidemiology and Population Health Working Paper, Australian National University.

Solomon, P. J., and Wilson, S. R. (1990). Accommodating change due to treatment in the method of back projection for estimating HIV infection incidence. *Biometrics* **46**: 1165–70.

Stablein, D. M. (1990). Challenges of HIV vaccine development. *Statistics in Medicine* **9**: 1425–31.

Stein, J. H., editor-in-chief (1990). *Internal Medicine*. Boston: Little Brown and Company.

Stevens, C. E., Taylor, P. E., Zang, E. A., et al. (1986). Human T-cell lymphotropic virus type III infection in a cohort of homosexual men in New York City. *Journal of the American Medical Association* **255**: 2167–72.

Stoneburner, R. L., Des Jarlais, D. C., and Benezra, D. (1988). A larger spectrum of severe HIV-1 related disease in intravenuous drug users in New York City. *Science* **242**: 916–19.

Stott, E. J. (1991). Anti-cell antibody in macaques. *Nature* **353**: 393.

St. Louis, M. E., Conway, G. A., Hayman, C. R., et al. (1991). Human immunodeficiency virus infection in disadvantaged adolescents: Findings from the U.S. Job Corps. *Journal of the American Medical Association* **266**: 2387–91.

St. Louis, M. E., Rauch, K. J., Petersen, L. R., et al. (1990). Seroprevalence rates of human immunodeficiency virus infection at sentinel hospitals in the United States. *New England Journal of Medicine* **323**: 213–18.

Tan, W. Y. (1992). *Stochastic Models of AIDS Epidemiology.* (in preparation).

Tan, W. Y., and Hsu, H. (1989). Some stochastic models of AIDS spread. *Statistics in Medicine* **8**: 121–36.

Tango, T. (1989). Estimation of haemophilia-associated AIDS incidence in Japan using individual dates of diagnosis. *Statistics in Medicine* **8**: 1509–14.

Taylor, J. M. G. (1989). Models for the HIV infection and AIDS epidemic in the United States. *Statistics in Medicine* **8**: 45–58.

Taylor, J. M. G., Cumberland, W. G., and Sy, J. P. (1992). *A Stochastic Model for Analysis of Longitudinal AIDS Data.* Technical Report, Division of Biostatistics, University of California, Los Angeles.

Taylor, J. M. G., Fahey, J. L., Detels, R., and Giorgi, J. V. (1989). CD4 percentage, CD4 number and CD4:CD8 ratio in HIV infection: Which to choose and how to use. *Journal of Acquired Immune Deficiency Syndromes* **2**: 114–24.

Taylor, J. M. G., Kuo, J.-M., and Detels, R. (1991). Is the incubation period of AIDS lengthening? *Journal of Acquired Immune Deficiency Syndromes* **4**: 69–75.

Taylor, J. M. G., Muñoz, A., Bass, S. M., et al. (1990). Estimating the distribution of times from HIV seroconversion to AIDS using multiple imputation. *Statistics in Medicine* **9**: 505–14.

Temin, H. M., Mitzutani, S. (1970). RNA-dependent DNA polymerase in virions of Rous sarcoma virus. *Nature* **226**: 1211–13.

Tikhonov, A. (1963). Solution of incorrectly formulated problems and the regulation method. *Soviet Mathematics* **5**: 1035–38.

Tindall, B., Swanson, E., and Cooper, D. A. (1990). Development of AIDS in a cohort of HIV seropositive homosexual men in Australia. *Medical Journal of Australia* **153**: 260–65.

Tsai, W.-Y., Goedert, J. J., Orazem, J., et al. (1993). A nonparametric analysis of the transmission rate of human immunodeficiency virus from mother to infant. *Biometrics* (in press).

Tsiatis, A. A., Dafni, U., De Gruttola, V., et al. (1992). The relationship of CD4 counts over time to survival of patients with AIDS: Is CD4 a good surrogate marker? In Jewell, N., Dietz, K., and Farewell, V. (eds.), *AIDS Epidemiology: Methodological Issues*, pp. 256–74. Boston: Birkhäuser.

Turnbull, B. W. (1974). Nonparametric estimation of a survivorship function with doubly censored data. *Journal of the American Statistical Association* **69**: 169–73.

U.S. Bureau of the Census (1991). *Statistical Abstract of the United States*, 111th ed. Washington, D.C.: U.S. Government Printing Office.

Van de Perre, P., Simonon, A., Msellati, P., et al. (1991). Postnatal transmission of human immunodeficiency virus type 1 from mother to infant. A prospective cohort study in Kigali, Rwanda. *New England Journal of Medicine* **325**: 593–98.

Van Druten, J. A. M., Reintjes, A. G. M., Jager, J. C., et al. (1990). HIV infection dynamics and intervention experiments in linked risk groups. *Statistics in Medicine* **9**: 721–36.

Vaupel, J. W., and Yashin, A. I. (1985). Heterogeneity's ruses: Some surprising effects of selection on population dynamics. *American Statistician* **39**: 176–85.

Vecchio, T. J. (1966). Predictive value of a single diagnostic test in unselected populations. *New England Journal of Medicine* **274**: 1171–73.

Volberding, P. (1989). HIV infection as a disease: The medical indications for early diagnosis. *Journal of Acquired Immune Deficiency Syndromes* **2**: 421–25.

Volberding, P. A., Lagakos, S. W., Koch, M. A., et al. (1990). Zidovudine in asymptomatic human immunodeficiency virus infection. A controlled trial in persons with fewer than 500 CD4-positive cells per cubic millimeter. *New England Journal of Medicine* **322**: 941–49.

von Sydow, M., Gaines, H., Sönnerborg, A., et al. (1988). Antigen detection in primary HIV infection. *British Medical Journal* **296**: 238–40.

Wahba, G. (1983). *A Comparison of GCV and GML for Choosing the Smoothing Parameter in the Generalized Spline Smoothing Problem.* Technical Report 712, Department of Statistics, University of Wisconsin.

Wahba, G. (1990). *Spline Models for Observational Data.* Philadelphia: Society for Industrial and Applied Mathematics.

Walter, S. D. (1976). The estimation and interpretation of attributable risk in health research. *Biometrics* **32**: 829–49.

Ward, J. W., Bush, T. J., Perkins, H. A., et al. (1989). The natural history of transfusion-associated infection with human immunodeficiency virus. Factors influencing the rate of progression to disease. *New England Journal of Medicine* **321**: 947–52.

Ward, J. W., Deppe, D. A., and Samson, S. (1987). Risk of human immunodeficiency virus infection from blood donors who later developed the acquired immunodeficiency syndrome. *Annals of Internal Medicine* **106**: 61–62.

Ward, J. W., Holmberg, S. D., Allen, J. R., et al. (1988). Transmission of human immunodeficiency virus (HIV) by blood transfusions screened as negative for HIV antibody. *New England Journal of Medicine* **318**: 473–78.

Ware, J. H. (1985). Linear models for the analysis of longitudinal studies. *The American Statistician* **41**: 95–101.

Warner, S. L. (1965). Randomized response: A survey technique for eliminating evasive answer bias. *Journal of the American Statistical Association* **60**: 63–69.

Waterman, M. (1974). A restricted least squares problem. *Technometrics* **16**: 135–36.

Weisberg, S. (1985). *Applied Linear Regression,* 2d ed. New York: John Wiley & Sons.

Weiss, S. H., Goedert, J. J., Gartner, S., et al. (1988). Risk of human immunodeficiency virus (HIV-1) infection among laboratory workers. *Science* **239**: 68–71.

Weiss, S. H., Goedert, J. J., Sarngadharan, M. G., et al. (1985). Screening test for HTLV-III (AIDS agent) antibodies: Specificity, sensitivity and applications. *Journal of the American Medical Association* **253**: 221–25.

Weiss, R., and Thier, S. O. (1988). HIV testing is the answer—what's the question? *New England Journal of Medicine* **319**: 1010–12.

Wieand, S., Gail, M. H., James, B. R., and James, K. L. (1989). A family of nonparametric statistics for comparing diagnostic markers with paired or unpaired data. *Biometrika* **76**: 585–92.

Wiley, J. A., and Herschkorn, S. J. (1988). Perils of promiscuity. *Journal of Infectious Disease* **158**: 500–501.

Wiley, J., A., Herschkorn, S. J., and Padian, N. S. (1989). Heterogeneity in the probability of HIV transmission per sexual contact: The case of male-to-female transmission in penile-vaginal intercourse. *Statistics in Medicine* **8**: 93–102.

Winkelstein, W., Jr., Lyman, D. M., Padian, N., et al. (1987). Sexual practices and risk of infection by the human immunodeficiency virus. The San Francisco Men's Health Study. *Journal of the American Medical Association* **257**: 321–25.

Winkelstein, W., Jr., Padian, N. S., Rutherford, G., and Jaffe, H. W. (1989). Homosexual men. In Kaslow, R. A., and Francis, D. P. (eds.), *The Epidemiology of AIDS*, pp. 117–35. New York: Oxford University Press.

Winkelstein, J. W., Royce, R. A., and Sheppard, H. W. (1990). Median incubation time for human immunodeficiency virus (HIV) [Letter]. *Annals of Internal Medicine* **112**: 797.

Winkelstein, W., Jr., Samuel, M., Padian, N. S., et al. (1987). The San Francisco Men's Health Study. III. Reduction in human immunodeficiency virus transmission among homosexual/bisexual men, 1982–1986. *American Journal of Public Health* **77**: 685–89.

Winkelstein, W., Jr., Wiley, J. A., Padian, N. S., et al. (1988). The San Francisco Men's Health Study: Continued decline in HIV seroconversion among homosexual/bisexual men. *Amerian Journal of Public Health* **78**: 1472–74.

Wolinsky, S. M., Rinaldo, C. R., Kwok, S., et al. (1989). Human immunodeficiency virus type 1 (HIV-1) infection a median of 18 months before a diagnostic Western Blot. *Annals of Internal Medicine* **111**: 961–72.

Wolinsky, S. M., Rinaldo, C., and Phair, J. (1990). Response to letter. *Annals of Internal Medicine* **112**: 797–98.

Woodward, J. A., Bonett, D. G., and Brecht, M. L. (1985). Estimating the size of a heroin abusing population using multiple-recapture census. In (eds.), Rouse, B., Kozel, N., and Richards, L., *Self-Report Methods of Estimating Drug Use: Meeting Current Challenges to Validity*, pp. 158–71. Washington, D.C.: National Institute of Drug Abuse, Monograph 57, DHHS Publication (ADM) 85-1402, U.S. Government Printing Office.

World Health Organization (1991). *1990 World Health Statistics Annual*, pages 31–35, Genève.

World Health Organization (1992). *1991 World Health Statistics Annual*, pages 30–32, Genève.

Yarchoan, R., Klecker, R. W., Weinhold, K. J., et al. (1986). Administration of 3′-azido-3′-deoxythimidine, an inhibitor of HTLV-III/LAV replication, to patients with AIDS or AIDS-related complex. *Lancet* **1**: 575–80.

Zeger, S. L., Liang, K.-Y., and Albert, P. S. (1988). Models for longitudinal data: A generalized estimating equation approach. *Biometrics* **44**: 1049–60.

Zeger, S. L., See, L.-C., and Diggle, P. J. (1989). Statistical methods for monitoring the AIDS epidemic. *Statistics in Medicine* **8**: 3–21.

Index

Printed in the United States
39888LVS00001B/174

9 780195 076417